CW00919726

SCARCE TITLE
w/ 33

Physicians, Colonial Racism, and Diaspora in West Africa

Physicians, Colonial Racism, and Diaspora in West Africa

Adell Patton, Jr.

University Press of Florida

GAINESVILLE • TALLAHASSEE • TAMPA • BOCA RATON
PENSACOLA • ORLANDO • MIAMI • JACKSONVILLE

01 00 99 98 97 96 6 5 4 3 2 1

Library of Congress Cataloging-in-Publication Data
Patton, Adell, 1936–
    Physicians, colonial racism, and diaspora in West
Africa/Adell Patton.
        p.   cm.
    Includes bibliographical references and index.
    ISBN 0-8130-1432-8 (alk. paper)
    1. Physicians—Africa, West—History.   2. Medi-
cine—Africa, West—History.   3. Physicians—
Africa, West—Political activity.   4. Africa, West—
Race relations.   I. Title.
R652.p38   1996
610'.966—dc20   95-45070

The University Press of Florida is the scholarly publishing agency for the State University System
of Florida, comprised of Florida A & M University,
Florida Atlantic University, Florida International
University, Florida State University, University
of Central Florida, University of Florida, University
of North Florida, University of South Florida, and
University of West Florida.

University Press of Florida
15 Northwest 15th Street
Gainesville, FL 32611

For my wife, Christine Zimmerman Patton,
my mother, Willie Wilson Patton;
and to the memories of
Adell Patton, Sr. (1912–1989), my father;
Rosie Lee Patton Moore (1917–1986), my aunt;
Clinton Lee Patton (1909–1960), my uncle; and
Henry Louis Baldwin (1936–1993), my cousin

Contents

Contents

Figures, Maps, and Tables

FIGURES

Preface

*I*magine that you are a physician born in British West Africa and cannot practice in your country. Or imagine that you are an African contemplating the study of medicine in Great Britain or an African with the medical degree in hand from a school in the United States. You hear about a British administrative action that will place you on a roster segregating you from your European, middle-class medical peers when you return to your country from Great Britain. Or, in another example from the United States, you learn that your medical training and degree are unacceptable to colonial authorities in your country of origin. This prohibitive policy will prevent you from making a living as a medical practitioner. The year is 1901 and colonialism is in full force; it marks the start of an era of restrictions and reduced opportunities for African medical professionals, a break from the previous century when African and West Indian physicians worked freely to protect the health of Africans and Europeans alike in West Africa.

But did this scenario actually occur? One day in July 1980 an archival clerk in the Public Record Office, London, England, handed over a document marked "CO [for Colonial Office] 879 102," dated

December 17, 1909, and, in disbelief, I read of these very charges
against the British colonial government by Mayfield Boyle, Sr. (MD,
1902, Howard University, Washington, D.C.), of Freetown, Sierra
Leone, West Africa. Over time, I came across a litany of these charges
of racial discrimination by other African physicians and, in a collective show of support, by a group of African and West Indian medical
students in Edinburgh, Scotland. Even a few colonial officials dis-
sented against the segregated policy and joined the African chorus.
Colonial officials even raised the issue of sexuality and whether
African and West Indian doctors should be allowed to have European
women as patients.

In spite of these conditions, however, African physicians reacted
and developed strategies for training and employment in their respective territories. They scrambled to the United States, Canada,
Great Britain, and Europe, and then back to the African continent
and, closer to the era of independence, to the former Soviet Union
and Eastern bloc countries. Still, all did not go well upon their return.
Under colonialism, African doctors dealt with pseudoscientific
racism and the dynamics of the changing power relations of white
over black. Under independence—and obviously under different circumstances—the doctors went through a process of conflict resolution that was resolved by indigenous procedures and policies for
training and certifying medical professionals.

The purpose of this book is to chronicle and analyze the social history of African doctors and their professional struggles in the African
diaspora and in West Africa during the period 1800 to 1985. This work
is intended for the use of the general public who wish to learn something about African history, especially African medical history. My
hope is that it will be useful to world health officials, African health
policymakers, African medical students, and academicians worldwide engaged in teaching general African history, comparative colonial history and law, comparative studies, the politics of health, medical history, the African diaspora, and the history of West Africa.

Although the precolonial history of Africa had been the subject of
my earlier research and graduate training, I approached this study

without any background in the politics of health, in medical history, or in the social history of medicine. I am indebted, therefore, to a number of people for their aid, and while I will not attempt to mention every person by name, I am appreciative of their assistance nevertheless.

First, I would like to express special appreciation to Professor Steven Feierman, who introduced me to the social history of medicine at the November 1978 African Studies Association (ASA) annual meeting in Baltimore. He asked me to chair his panel on Diseases and Social Change in Colonial Africa, and in the rushed reading of the panel papers I came upon a discussion of residential segregation in Professor K. David Patterson's paper, "Health in Urban Ghana: The Case of Accra, 1900–1940." This paper reported as follows: "Early in the century there were attempts to protect Europeans from malaria and yellow fever by making them live apart from Africans. Ironically, this policy was first suggested by an African physician, Dr. John Farrell Easmon, in 1893. His recommendation led to the construction of European bungalows in Victoriaborg. Segregation was official policy by 1901. An uninhabited 400-yard 'neutral zone' was established to protect Victoriaborg and the European area on the ridge."

For me, "segregation" is a provocative word based on experience, and educated Africans protested its implementation on a number of occasions in Anglophone West Africa. How could an African doctor, such as Easmon, advocate a policy to improve the health conditions of only Europeans and at the same time not consider the alternative health policy of improving the health conditions of any and every group of human beings in the town? I mulled over the question in my hotel from late in the night until dawn the next morning, when the scheduled ASA panel was to meet. Notwithstanding my intellectual naïveté about the use of the cordon sanitaire, Patterson's passage on the sensitive matter of segregation, and Easmon's role in its development, ignited my interest to pursue the Easmon family records. In time this book came to cover seven generations of African physicians and to expand well beyond the noted Easmon family. The social history of medicine became the natural specialty for self-training and analysis. Professors Feierman, Patterson, and Sandra T. Barnes have remained my scholarly companions in this endeavor since 1978, advising me at various stages in the development of the manuscript. Barnes next introduced me to Professor Magali Sarfatti Larson, whose sociological study of the professions served as an indispensable guide, and Larson further acquainted me with other authors specializing in the professions, such as Terence Johnson and Andrew Abbott. I owe limitless gratitude to Dr. Modupe Broderick for introducing me to African medical families in Sierra Leone long before my research reached the pilot project stage. The published works of Christopher Fyfe on Sierra Leone and David Kimble on Ghana (Gold Coast) served as continuous models for this study.

Howard University provided the initial funding for my research. I am grateful to Dr. Lorraine A. Williams, who, as vice president for academic affairs, provided the first grant for research on this book at the London Public Record Office through a Howard University faculty research grant in 1980. The Department of History supported the project thereafter for summer archival travels to London and to Freetown, Sierra Leone, in the summer of 1983, as did the African Studies and Research Program (Dr. Robert Cummings, director). In the fall of 1993 the Department of History again provided generous funding. Howard University supported me further with two research sabbaticals over a sixteen-year period. I am most grateful to this outstanding institution for its support; indeed, some of its medical graduates are featured in this study. Thanks also go to the undergraduate and graduate students who offered me endless encouragement to complete the project.

The Council for International Exchange of Scholars (CIES) of the U.S. Information Agency provided me with a Senior Fulbright Researcher grant to Sierra Leone in 1984 and 1985. I would like to express my gratitude especially to Linda Rhodes of CIES for her indispensable assistance with regard to the grant, which allowed for related archival study both in England and other areas of West Africa. Professor Magbailey Fyle, of the Institute of African Studies at Fourah Bay College, University of Sierra Leone, provided invaluable cooperation and assistance. Dr. Walter Awooner-Renner was a continuous consultant and critic of this book on both sides of the Atlantic, and he facilitated liaisons with doctors in Sierra Leone. Similarly, the famed Dr. Davidson Nicol (1924–94) was a constant source of inspiration and help in West Africa, the United States, and at Cambridge, England, in May 1992, and he was the first to recommend that I include a chapter on Africans who pursued medical training in the former USSR and Eastern bloc countries. I am grateful to the Ghana National Archives and to the late Charles Tettey, medical historian and librarian at the Ghana Teaching Hospital at Korle Bu. The archivist in charge of the Nigerian National Archives in Ibadan, B. L. Evborokhai, provided important assistance also. U.S. Ambassador Howard Jeter and his wife, Donice Jeter, sponsored my invaluable trip from London to Tanzania and Zanzibar to review the medical system in East Africa. Back in the United States, Bruce Martin, Library of Congress research facilities officer, assisted me in gaining access to that great institution over an extended period of time for my research, for which I am most grateful.

The Carter G. Woodson Institute of the University of Virginia at Charlottesville provided support through a senior fellow award. The institute also made available the computer programming staff for the production of the manuscript and gave me time away from teaching and sundry university obligations to write this book. The institute further supported me with a travel research grant in May 1992 to the Public Record Office to review materials declassified since my previous visit. I also wish to express my special gratitude to Professor Armstead Robinson (1947–95), director of the institute, Professor William Jackson, associate director for research, Gail Shirley, administrator, and Mary Rose, computer program manager, without whose assistance this book could have not been produced. Mary Farrer, computer assistant, Anthony Wilburn, and Lorice Washington were particularly helpful, especially with the tables. Joseph Miller and Jeanne Maddox Toungara were indispensable in the arrangement that enabled me to teach African history in the Corcoran Department of History at the University of Virginia. I owe my thanks to David Throup for assistance with computer software applicable to my research interest. And while I wish to acknowledge the Carter G. Woodson Institute for making me computer literate, I must also express thanks to the makers of the number two pencils with which the entire first draft of this book was written!

The following editors granted permission to incorporate portions of previously published articles in my name into the book: Professors Norman Bennett, and Margaret Jean Hay of the *International Journal of African Historical Studies* for the article on John Farrell Easmon; and Professor Alton Hornsby, Jr., of the *Journal of Negro History,* for the article on Mayfield Boyle. I am exceedingly grateful to these editors.

The manuscript focus benefited from the help of a number of persons. Since 1979 Calvin Sinnette, MD (Howard University School of Medicine), has contributed immensely to the study's classification of medical training and to ongoing discussions with regard to the design of the study. Professor Arthur Burt (Department of History, Howard University) read the entire manuscript and made numerous thematic and conceptual suggestions on how the imperial system worked in England, Africa, and the West Indies. His ideas made a great difference in the way the book came to be focused. Professor Georges Nzongola Ntalaja (African Studies Department, Howard University) allowed me to exploit his magnificent intellect and he encouraged me to consult with him continuously on comparative analysis. Dr. Gary King (coordinator of the Urban Health Research Program, Department of Community Medicine and Health Care, University of Connecticut Health Center) offered valuable, informative assistance on the professions.

Naomi Roslyn Patton, our daughter, also read the manuscript in its entirety and lent her gifted editorial hand with emendations. Christine Zimmerman Patton, my wife, commented on several chapters, and typed some of the manuscript. In honor of Christine's devotion and sacrifice to my scholarly interest, I dedicate this book to her. She agreed to share the dedication with my mother and in memory of my late father and some close relatives.

Almost every student and scholar can boast of persons who played an indelible role in their development. The following persons (in chronological order) played such a role in my life: Professor Henry Cheaney, distinguished professor emeritus, Kentucky State University, my mentor, who first encouraged me to study history; Professor Emma Lou Thornbrough (1913–94), distinguished professor emerita, Butler University, mentor and friend; Professor William Brown, University of Wisconsin-Madison; Dr. John Belknap, University of Wisconsin-Madison; Professor Crawford Young, distinguished professor, University of Wisconsin-Madison; Professor Jan Vansina, distinguished professor, University of Wisconsin-Madison; Professor Philip Curtin, distinguished professor, Johns Hopkins University; Professor Harold Lewis, emeritus (1908–93), Howard University; and Dr. Bennie Robinson, Kentucky State University.

Finally, the graphics and printing services of the University of Missouri-St. Louis should be thanked for the production of maps, figures, and final design of the study before going to press. Lasting gratitude is expressed to Murray Velasco, David Gellman, and Herman Nebel.

The views and interpretation of the data expressed in this book are solely my own.

Abbreviations

APC	All People's Congress
ASAPS	Anti-Slavery and Aborigines' Protection Society
BMA	British Medical Association
BMC	British Medical Council
ChB	Bachelor of Surgery
ChM	Master of Surgery
CMO	Chief Medical Officer
CMS	Church Missionary Society
CNA	Colonial Nursing Association
CPSU	Communist Party of the Soviet Union
DCH	Diploma of Child Health
DIH	Diploma International Health
DIL	Doctor International Law
DL	Diploma Licentiate
DMS	Director of Medical Services
DPH	Diploma of Public Health, London
DRCOG	Diploma of the Royal College of Obstetrics and Gynecology
DTMH	Diploma of Tropical Medicine and Hygiene
DTMP	Diploma of Tropical Medicine and Parasitology (Germany, Holland, Switzerland)

EBIM	Elections Before Independence Movement
FRCP	Fellow of the Royal College of Physicians (England)
FRCSE	Fellow of the Royal College of Surgeons of Edinburgh
FWACP	Fellow of the West African College of Physicians
GCC	Gold Coast Chronicle
GCI	Gold Coast Independent
HMOCS	Her (His) Majesty's Overseas Civil Service
LAH	Licentiate of Apothecaries Hall
LFPS	Licentiate of the Faculty of Physicians and Surgeons of Glasgow
Lic.	Licentiate (diploma to practice medicine)
LKQCP	Licentiate of the King's and Queen's College of Physicians of Ireland
LM	Licentiate of Midwifery, Royal College of Surgeons of Edinburgh; Licentiate of Midwifery, Ireland
LRCP	Licentiate of the Royal College of Physicians (England)
LRCP AND SLRCS	Licentiate of the Royal College of Surgeons of Ireland
LSA	Licentiate of the Society of Apothecaries, London
MBCH	Bachelor of Medicine; Master of Surgery
MD	Doctor of Medicine
MRCP	Member of the Royal College of Physicians (England)
MRC Path	Member of the Royal College of Pathologists
MRCS	Member of the Royal College of Surgeons (England)
NMO	Native Medical Officer
NMS	Native Medical Staff
PMO	Principal Medical Officer
RCP	Royal College of Physicians (England)
SLMDA	Sierra Leone Medical and Dental Association
SMO	Senior Medical Officer
USAID	U.S. Agency for International Development
WAFF	West Africa Frontier Force
WAMS	West Africa Medical Staff
WAYL	West Africa Youth League
WHO	World Health Organization

Introduction

*T*his book is about African physicians in West Africa from 1800 to 1985, a period when major issues revolved around the inequality of blacks in their own countries. How did Africans, -indigenous to their respective communities, come to be interested in Western medicine and where were they trained—in Africa or abroad? If it is assumed that these trained physicians had the right to practice the medical art in their countries of origin—and we learn that this was not so under colonialism—what circumstances gave rise to their becoming marginalized? How did African doctors respond to their plight of inequality and what form did their professional struggles take? Obviously medical autonomy was long in coming and only partially achieved during the political changes of the independence era—the 1960s. This book attempts to address these questions through in-depth analysis.

The objectives of this work are fourfold: to uncover the history of the development of the indigenous West African frontier medical community; to examine how some African physicians used their

medical training to introduce principles of Western scientific medicine into the lay community of West Africa; to determine the extent of
resistance by colonial officials to the efforts of African physicians to
achieve professional mobility in the colonial health services; and to
describe the response of African physicians to colonial resistance.

With regard to the first objective, it appears that many Africans
who later became medical doctors worked first in dispensaries established by the missionaries; their development will be traced beyond
these early origins. To fulfill the second objective, it must be borne in
mind that Western medicine was not well advanced in the United
States or Europe until the 1940s, when penicillin and a number of
other drugs first became available. Colonial officials could do little
about the treatment of diseases in Africa until the late 1930s, when
sulfa drugs were first introduced. In 1945 antibiotics made their first
appearance in Africa. Pathogenic agents could not be successfully
dealt with without proper hygienic measures, such as the provision of
clean water and other sanitary improvements. In northern Ghana, for
example, river blindness (onchocerciasis) had a long history, but
colonial officials did little to eradicate it until 1950. On the other
hand, there is adequate information available to achieve the third objective: to document colonial resistance to the professional development of African doctors and their ensuing struggles after 1901. The
documentation to support colonial resistance is closely related to the
information required in the fourth objective: the African physicians'
response.[1] It is appropriate, however, to explain how I went about
gathering data in order to answer these objectives.

Methodology figures prominently in the development of this
book. Collective biography is the investigation of common traits of a
group in history through a combined study of their lives. In the early
nineteenth century and until the last quarter of the twentieth century,
African medical students formed groups with common goals in West
Africa. First, they received training abroad in the Western world
under colonialism and then in socialist countries through the independence era. Indeed, medical schools were founded in twentieth-
century West Africa, but not in large enough numbers to comply with

the needs of medical services. Doctors, however, became medical practitioners as well as policymakers in West Africa. Collective biography permits the exploration of additional questions about social origins, inherited political and economic position, education, occupation, and comparative levels of competence. The method further allows us to examine the rise of political actions and their origins among African doctors, and how changing racism and imperial power impacted on colonialism and contributed to the way that African doctors were treated under the system.

The study next moves to social structure and social mobility to explain why some privileged groups were more successful in attaining medical training and becoming medical practitioners. Collective biography or prosopography (as described by ancient historians), therefore, provides us with the mechanism to examine group dynamics of the African medical profession in Anglophone West Africa.[2]

Primary archival data in England and West Africa cover the years from the early 1800s to around 1970, for declassified data in the various classes and groups available ended in the 1960s at the time of my last search in the Public Record Office, London, in May 1992. The concluding era of my study—the years from 1960 to 1985—was explored through actual fieldwork in West Africa in 1984–85. I recorded numerous oral interviews on the subject of medical history with African doctors, and I was a participant-observer of patient care in hospitals and clinics. These opportunities were indispensable to my fieldwork. The process of interviewing continued in meetings with African doctors from 1984 to 1992. These meetings served as variants to what doctors had to say about themselves and about each other, and they were a corrective to official policy data, data that roughly covered the years from 1918 through the 1970s.

Beginning in 1980, for example, I conducted interviews of British doctors who served in the Colonial Medical Service. The Rhodes House Archives at Oxford recently made available documents that corroborated their accounts. Subsequently, I interviewed African doctors residing in England. I even visited Tanzania and its island of

Zanzibar briefly in September 1984 before going on to Sierra Leone in October. Sierra Leone became my research base for the collection of archival data and recorded interviews for Anglophone West Africa. Jan Vansina's *Oral Tradition as History* (1985) guided my analysis and contributed to cross-cultural understanding. In January 1985 I visited Dr. Adelola Adeloye, neurosurgeon and medical historian, at the Ibadan Teaching Hospital, Nigeria, and conducted interviews during my stay. With Charles Tettey, the late medical historian and librarian, I observed the excellent multistory pediatric hospital facility at Korle Bu in Ghana, but with sadness recalled that the hospital had only two doctors for women to consult. Pregnant women were not getting adequate prenatal care. On the positive side, the private Link Road Clinic, owned by Dr. M. A. Barnor with the assistance of Dr. Charles Odamten Easmon, is an excellent facility and properly staffed.

I spent nearly a year in Freetown, Sierra Leone, and became aware of chronic shortages that sometimes impeded good patient care. Dr. Walter Awooner-Renner, who maintained a private practice, lent insulin to a doctor in the government hospital for a patient who had been in need of the drug for five days. This collaboration is frequent among doctors. I also witnessed a woman, who had apparently just left the operating table, washing her own clinical gown at the famous Connaught Hospital. In the same hospital the wards generally lacked uniform bed sheets and the patients were without uniform clothing. In spite of these poor conditions, there are numerous stories about heroic efforts made by doctors to save the lives of their patients.

Physicians and Generations

The historical study of African doctors and their residencies in the diaspora extends over several generations. This dimension is reflected in the organization of chapters in the book. The generations fall into the following periods: (1) 1790s1845; (2) 1853–1880s; (3) 1880s–1900; (4) 1900–1912; (5) 1912–World War II; (6) World War II–1950s; and (7) 1957–85. Chapter 1 explores the colonial medical systems in Africa (both Francophone and Anglophone). The consequences of differing certification requirements for African physicians trained in the

United States, England, and in Europe are also explained. African women doctors, the role of medical history, and a number of other important issues are also reviewed. Chapter 2 focuses on the African doctor from ancient times to 1800 and ends with the role of imperial power after 1800 and the introduction of Western medicine.

In part 2 the chapters rank the physicians into generations. Normally, the term "generation" refers to the human life span. In this study, generation means the time that African medical students were trained as a group and appeared on the Medical Register but in different decades of the nineteenth and twentieth centuries. This explains why the lengths in our divisions vary from twelve years to fifty-five. Chapters 3 and 4 take us to the end of the nineteenth century and examine generations 1, 2, and 3 with ethnography and collective biography. Chapter 5 explores generation 4 and the twentieth-century changes under formal colonial rule, such as the segregated roster for African doctors, and African reaction abroad and in West Africa. Chapters 6 and 7 are biographical in nature; these chapters first explore medical practice in the protectorate of Sierra Leone, and then the Canadian and British certification process in order to qualify for the Medical Register in Sierra Leone. Chapter 8 brings the book to the end of the colonial era and introduces the new problems faced by African students in the era of Cold War competition. Many sought medical training in the USSR and Eastern bloc countries. On their return to West Africa they brought with them a new medical culture and ideology to compete with established Western-influenced medical practices.

Alma-Ata and the Year 2000

A study of the African medical profession cannot be adequate without due regard for health conditions in the present and future. The World Health Organization (WHO) presented a guiding principle for African leaders, physicians, and health planners. On September 12, 1978, the body met at Alma-Ata (now Almaty), in the Kazakhstan Republic of the former Soviet Union, and issued the following declaration:

Table 1. *Number of physicians and population per physician in the United States, Canada, and Anglophone West Africa, late 1980s*

COUNTRY	TOTAL POP. (IN MILLIONS)	NO. OF PHYSICANS	POP. PER PHYSICIAN
United States	246.0	414,916	593
Canada	26.1	43,192	604
Nigeria	111.9	8,037	13,924
Ghana	14.4	1,665	8,625
Sierra Leone	4.0	190	20,858
Gambia	0.779	49	15,898

Source: PC Globe, Inc., Tempe, Arizona, 1987–89.

Governments have a responsibility for the health of their people which can be fulfilled only by the provision of adequate health and social measures. A main social target of governments, international organizations and the whole world community in the coming decades should be the attainment by all peoples of the world by the year 2000 of a level of health that will permit them to lead a socially and economically productive life. Primary health care is the key to attaining this target as part of development in the spirit of social justice.[3]

The urgent declaration at Alma-Ata is supported by the following comparative statistics on African doctors in Anglophone West Africa drawn from *PC Globe* (1987–89), and based on UN Reports 1990 (see tables 1 and 2). Health statistics are constantly changing in Africa and will continue to account for some of the statistical variances.

Table 2. *Crude birth rates, crude death rates, and infant-mortality rates for the ten nations with the highest infant-mortality rates and the United States, late 1980s*

COUNTRY	CRUDE BIRTHRATE (PER 1,000 POP.)	CRUDE DEATH RATE (PER 1,000 POP.)	INFANT-MORTALITY RATE (PER 1,000 POP.)
Afghanistan	47.5	23.9	183.0
Sierra Leone	47.2	29.0	175.0
Mali	50.4	21.7	175.0
North Yemen	55.0	22.0	175.0
Gambia	48.5	28.0	169.0
Malawi	53.2	20.8	157.0
Guinea	46.7	22.7	153.0
Central African Republic	43.9	19.1	148.0
Somalia	47.8	17.0	147.0
Mozambique	45.2	19.1	147.0
United States	15.7	8.7	10.0

Source: PC Globe, Inc., Tempe, Arizona, 1987–89.

PART ONE

Historical Background

African Physicians in Time Perspective

Introduction

This book is a history of African physicians who pioneered the constantly changing frontiers in the modern medical profession. Anglophone West Africa, with a combined population totaling over 138 million in 1990, is the focal geographical region of this study (see map 1), and includes the national states of Gambia, Ghana, Nigeria, and Sierra Leone. However, while the practice of medicine in Africa is over four thousand years old, the doctors in our study during the mid-nineteenth century were generally from Sierra Leone and thereafter from other countries in the region. Yet, because West Africa lacked medical schools to train them, Africans traveled through voluntary dispersal or diaspora to obtain medical training, first to areas under British control and then later to the United States and to non-Western areas of the world, before their return to Africa to practice their professions.

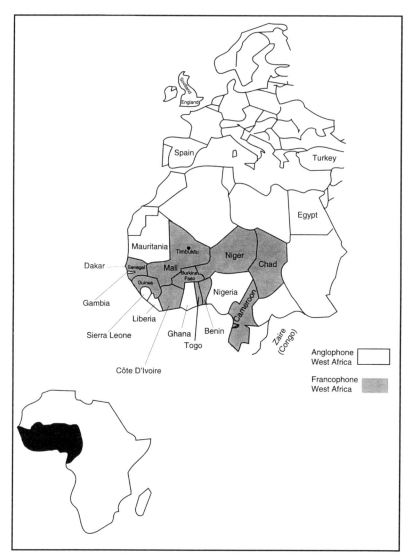

Map 1. Contemporary West Africa

In terms of their training and certification, the African physicians in this study fall into four categories of the cognitive elite: (1) the doctor trained in Western Europe, primarily in Great Britain and on the Continent, prior to and after World War II; (2) the doctor trained in the United States through the post-1900s, mostly at Howard

University and Meharry medical schools, and in Canada and the Caribbean for whom no chronology known to the author exists; (3) the doctor trained in the former USSR and in the socialist nations of Eastern Europe in the Cold War era; and (4) the most recent development in medical education—the African doctor trained wholly or partially in Africa.[1] The data in our study go beyond these confining catagories to encompass all medical training during the period examined.

Doctors trained in the West, the Soviet Union, and the Eastern bloc were recipients of two different medical cultures. Here, the term medical culture refers to the applied curriculum structure and general procedures followed toward specialization and transmitted to succeeding generations. This paradigm for the British was enunciated in 1858 and features long periods of training in general medicine and general surgery. Moreover, the British Medical Council condemned specialization at the initial stage; in the intricacies of the modern world the physician would find inestimable value in the study of chemistry, physics, biology, and mathematics, along with other professional subjects.[2] This system endowed doctors with broad expertise to handle diverse problems in health care and delivery systems in both central and isolated posts. Although American-trained African doctors were not allowed to go directly from the United States onto the Medical Register in West Africa until the independence era, the U.S. model was similar to the British medical system with regard to the broad nature of its training. Medical tensions arose after the 1960s with the introduction of the communist medical culture based on shorter periods of training and early specialization. Cold War competition between East and West complicated the introduction of this second medical culture in Anglophone West Africa.

Researchers Robert Melson and Howard Wolpe show how the concept of communalism functions as a unique feature in organizational behavior and as a mechanism for solidarity, a bond we find among African doctors working abroad as well as among those practicing in Africa. Communalism allowed Africans in medical training in Great Britain, Western Europe, the United States, Canada, the USSR, and the Eastern bloc to form close links with others sharing a common culture, purpose, and identity. These social ties served as the basis for networks back in the homeland: bonds that perpetuated group feeling or complementarity.[3] Upon completion of medical training, African doctors returned to their respective countries with their communal ties intact, only to encounter plural medical systems with divisions between them. Often a group within the divided systems sought mobility in the hierarchy in order to advance itself or to protect its rank and power; this encounter is called competitive communalism. Thus, complementarity or group interest formed the basis for defense in both *intraprofessional conflicts* (such as those between African doctors and European doctors) and in *interprofessional relations* (struggles against a competing profession, such as between Western medicine versus African herbalists). Africans doctors, however, had a difficult time making a living outside the government in the nineteenth century because there were few patients who trusted Western medicine. Hence, African doctors could do better in the British Colonial Medical Service, but this was at the expense of sacrificing their medical autonomy. Trained and certified physicians could put up their name plates and were allowed to practice, such as Herbert Christian Bankole-Bright, Albert Whiggs Easmon, Sir Kofo Abayomi, Dr. Curtis Adeniji-Jones, and Dr. Raymond Sarif Easmon. Easmon wrote numerous political articles in the *African Standard* (published in Sierra Leone) following World War II.

Throughout the nineteenth century and beyond, therefore, African doctors employed by the government were forced to deal with the British doctors sent to Africa by the colonial authorities. In a recent essay describing these medical men, Virginia Berridge observes: "They were the sons of 'men of the secondary professional classes or tradesmen,' of 'intelligent artisans' and sometimes tradesmen and domestic servants' families. Only 3 percent of Fellows of the Royal College of Surgeons in the period 1800–1889 could be classified as 'gentlemen' against 45 percent of navy officers in the period 1814–49."[4] In a profession that became increasingly overcrowded in the nineteenth century—as evidenced by the annual number of graduates in medicine from the medical teaching centers at Cambridge, Edinburgh, Oxford, and Glasgow—numerous doctors had to take on less desirable positions, such as the poor medical officer, in order to make ends meet. Employment in Africa constituted an attractive opportunity for some of these doctors from middle-class backgrounds. There, as representatives of British imperial power, they were unquestionably among the elite. With the beginning of the twentieth century and the triumph of colonialism, African doctors suffered through differential rates in salaries in the changing dynamics of power relations and had to contend with a lower status in the professional ranks. Imperial power, racist ideology, notions about black sexuality, and social stratification within the medical ranks intensified intraprofessional conflict and competition. African doctors felt betrayed. The changing imperial system reduced their rewards of promotion and status in ways remarkably different from those in the nineteenth century. Herein lies the common thread in each chapter of this book: intraprofessional conflict, altered by expanding colonialism, which fostered the protest behavior of the African doctors over several generations in the struggle for professionalism.

Certification in the medical profession implied equity of professional status. African doctors had trained alongside their European classmates and realized their full potential. Some of the Africans surpassed the Europeans in academic ability, and most returned to Africa with confidence, feeling themselves equal to the English middle-class civil servants who held power. Thus direct confrontations were unavoidable. Competitive communal responses ensued, and African medical networks in Anglophone West Africa acted as the catalyst for political action expressed in petitions, supportive attacks in the West African press, and outright withdrawal by some African doctors from the Colonial Medical Service, entering private practice instead. This kind of group activity is consistent with institutional communalism.

Intraprofessional conflict of a different sort occurred in the independence era. African doctors steeped in the medical culture of the West themselves now lodged complaints against the first generation of communist-trained African doctors. These Western-trained doctors charged that the new practitioners, with their specialized training, lacked appropriate clinical preparation for the more general needs of the African medical practice. Accusations soon surfaced between the two cultures. It appears that tensions accelerated more rapidly in countries lacking medical schools with teaching hospitals—such as Gambia and Sierra Leone—than in countries like Ghana and Nigeria possessing such infrastructures. Gambia and Nigeria had the smallest number of socialist-trained doctors within the region and thus there were fewer intraprofessional conflicts.

Even though they were constrained by political conditions in the colonial and independence eras, African medical elites manifested the general traits identified in Magali Sarfatti Larson's 1977 sociological study of general professionalism: (1) highly specialized skills based on lengthy training and esoteric or abstract knowledge; (2) legitimation of competence by certification; (3) organization through association; (4) a group code of ethics and concomitant exclusivity; and (5) commitment to public service. In a broad sense the components represent the ideal type, and the assimilation of these standards describes the process of professionalization.[5] We know today, as Andrew Abbott reminds us in his recent study, that many other occupational groups and organizations that may not have incorporated all of these components are no less professional than those of law and medicine. In this context abstract knowledge of systems by exclusive occupational groups and their control of certification still constitute the key element of a profession, and British colonial policy and power strongly influenced this process in Anglophone West Africa. African doctors conducted themselves in accordance with and in response to the government's exclusive monopoly of medical regulation. Hence, what history can tell us about this development forms a viable approach to the social history of the African medical doctor.

Jurisdiction or the authority of administration and control remains the most important component of the various elements characterizing the professions. Abbott reports that "models in which particular individuals occupy particular places at given times—called the vacancy model" and the vacancies themselves are spaces opened to mobility and available to individual aspirations and challenges to an existing system.[6] External forces, such as the expansive French and British medical systems, can either create or extinguish vacancies; this leads to interprofessional competition over who stays and who goes. For example, the traditional healer had been present in Africa from time immemorial; however, the practice of secrecy protected the healer's knowledge, and while some families became more powerful than others, families that did not have exclusive access to important knowledge could not drive out their rivals completely and occupy their spaces or vacancies.[7]

Western versus Traditional Medicine

This brings us to a brief assessment of the conflict between Western and traditional medicine. We must not forget that "professions are carnivorous competitors that grow in strength as they engulf jurisdictions."[8] The Western-trained doctor, upon his return to Africa, had to combat the traditional practitioners as well as his British and European peers. Confidence in the traditional healer was rooted in African tradition and custom. The Western doctor sought to superimpose medical practices and experiences learned outside of Africa on communities that had little or no respect for Western values. And this was only part of the dilemma. African healers would often direct their patients to the hospital when their treatments failed, and it did not take long for the efficaciousness of Western inoculations to be recognized among the communities, especially following the development of sulfa drugs in the mid-1930s and antibiotics in World War II, when physicians were able to attack most pathogenic bacteria effectively. One example is river blindness, or onchocerciasis, which decimated whole populations in the districts of Wa, Lawra (Lorha), Tumu, Navrongo (Navarra), Zuarungu, and Bawku (now the upper region of Ghana) in the northern territories of the Gold Coast, until the late B. B. Waddy, a British colonial doctor, finally convinced the British medical establishment of the serious nature of this disease in 1948 or 1949. Waddy's efforts forced the medical department to investigate the disease, and ophthalmological and entomological teams toured the region. By the 1950s measures to treat river blindness were in operation.[9] Hence, under the colonial medical systems of the French and British, traditional healers suffered diminishing status in the eyes of African patients, and only since the 1960s has Western pharmacology begun to recognize the efficacy of some traditional remedies.[10]

Doctors and Political Leadership

Since physicians historically have provided the prescription for patient well-being, they had educational and social advantages that enabled them to be accepted in elite circles and to be taken seriously as political candidates. Their professional credentials lent them prestige and also freed them from suspicions of corruption and self-interest that conventional politicians have always been subject to. Because of these factors, African physicians have long memories pertaining to their role in African development. While the health care needs of the African people remained in the forefront of their concerns, twentieth-century doctors often left their medical practice, sometimes permanently, in order to respond to the new dynamics of social change in politics, in nationalism, and in the liberation struggle. For example, John Randall (1855–1928) and Orisadipe Obasa (1863–1940) of Lagos went into politics and in 1908 founded the People's Union, the first political organization in Nigeria.[11] In 1920 Dr. Herbert Christian Bankole-Bright (1883–1958) of Freetown, Sierra Leone, used the Accra Conference of the National Congress of British West Africa to call for gradual self-government within the British Empire and promote resolutions on topics of medical and sanitary problems in the British territories of West Africa. Similarly, in Francophone West Africa, Dr. Félix Houphouët-Boigny (1905–93; *médecin Africain,* or African medical assistant, in 1925)[12] advised the Brazzaville Conference of 1944 on the need in each territory for an autonomous, mobile public health service to combat endemic diseases such as trypanosomiasis, malaria, leprosy, and treponematosis—all before becoming president for life of Côte d'Ivoire. Another physician, Milton Margai, became the first prime minister of the Sierra Leone republic in 1961. In the 1960s Dr. Hastings Kamuzu Banda, a Meharry Medical School graduate and former life president of the republic of Malawi, led his nation to independence from British rule. In the 1970s the late president Samora Moïsés Machel, a nurse, won independence for Mozambique in a national liberation struggle against the Portuguese; and his Portuguese compatriot Dr. Agostinho Neto led Angola to independence in the same era. More recently Dr. Ishaya Audu, a pediatrician from northern Nigeria, served as foreign secretary in the republic of Nigeria. These are only the most prominent examples of physicians turned politicians.

Traditionally, doctors became political leaders because medicine was one of the few professions that provided Africans with independence. After law and medicine, employment in the colonial government was the only other route for African elites to seek work; and colonial regulations, while allowing administrative action sanctioned by the government, prohibited all partisan political action. One observer noted that this had the effect of shackling 90 percent of the intelligentsia.

The Easmons were politically active because they were one of the few remaining families of Nova Scotian settler stock still to have an independent and rebellious character. With a deep sense of injury by the British—for they had fought in the War of Independence against the American colonies—they felt shortchanged for a variety of reasons to be explored later. They believed themselves to be equal to any European with their family history of one hundred years of education or more. The Easmons, however, were always downgraded, as were most Africans when the time came for promotions and various other forms of professional advancement. As a result, many doctors sought employment in the Colonial Medical Service for one or two years, then went into private practice, and joined the colonial Legislative Council at the turn of the twentieth century, there debating mostly against the government. This behavior of the doctors occurred throughout West Africa. In order to understand how this pattern unfolded, we must ascertain why African doctors had to confront imperial authority in the struggle for medical professionalism.

The Colonial Medical Service

Until colonial times African doctors had mobility within the British medical service of West Africa. This was possible because, unlike

France and Germany where the state created the institutions that trained professionals in order to assure a supply of civil servants and structured their operations accordingly, England and America lacked a real civil service infrastructure until the mid-1850s. And even the American system was based on political patronage until the Pendleton Act of 1883 reformed the system; it established a list of civil service jobs to be filled through set examination scores administered by the Civil Service Commission. English and American universities were in need of reform and showed little concern for the certification of knowledge.[13] This created personnel and staffing problems for England and its imperial system, especially in West Africa, at that time commonly known as the "white man's grave." Since the British had been occupying the West Indies for over two hundred years, they had a trained cadre there to help. Hence West Indians and newly trained Africans filled some of the staffing void with reasonable mobility. This all changed after the 1850s. With improvements in preventive health in the colonial era, more Europeans went to West Africa to staff positions. They became almost the only medical personnel of the colonial corporate system of the Colonial Office in London, which functioned mainly to protect the health of the European population. One historical turning point was the British Colonial Office's creation of an extremely conservative body, the West African Medical Staff (WAMS) in 1901.[14] This institution excluded African doctors from membership and placed them on a separate roster with lower salaries than the British doctors. This is explored fully in chapter 5. Medical sociologists, most notably Terence Johnson, have labeled similar structural changes as the "corporate patronage model."[15]

My working hypothesis for this book is that corporate patronage delayed the rise of African medical professionalism and most of the organizational features associated within this form of collegial authority. In addition, it contributed to the delay in medical autonomy discernable even today in African nations. This means that neither Western cultural transmission patterns nor the stages of development that a profession follows (often called professionalization) can explain the traits of the professions in the new African states. Johnson argues that the professions in the Third World share a collective experience that varies markedly from occupations in the industrialized world. The binary system of professions in colonial administrations and their legacy in the postcolonial states explain in large part this turn of development in diverse structures in the British Commonwealth. While a number of institutional relationships developed under colonialism, Johnson argues that corporate patronage was the most significant variable and the "reverse of professionalism in the sense that it is the client—a powerful, corporate client—which regulates the profession rather than the members of the occupation itself through associationism. Where corporate patronage prevailed, professionalism, with all the cultural and organizational attributes we have come to associate with this form of colleague authority, never developed."[16]

African doctors decried this system and acrimoniously accused the Europeans of racial discrimination.[17] Scientific expertise in the hands of European physicians gave them political leverage, since they could argue that their knowledge transcended national boundaries and hence their dictates had the status of universal truth. However, this factor did not reduce the role of nonmedical men, such as political officials, in the formulation of medical policy.[18] The point here is that European medical officers could use scientific expertise to support political decisions with total disregard of African interests, and they often did so, sometimes under the rubric of medical science. For example, T. S. Gale shows how attempts were made to protect Europeans from malaria and yellow fever by forcing them to live apart from Africans. In 1893, paradoxically, John Farrell Easmon, an African physician and the subject of chapter 4, first recommended this policy in the Gold Coast. If Easmon was intent upon becoming the consummate politician, his recommendation may well have endeared him to the European medical establishment and might explain his later promotion to chief medical officer of the Gold Coast medical establishment, notwithstanding the fact that the African community deplored the cordon sanitaire.

Even more disconcerting to the African physicians, however, was a medical policy that proscribed them from treating white patients, especially white women, except perhaps in mining areas with few or no

European doctors, or in situations where African doctors held re-
tainers with European firms. Here it must be remembered that the
European mind was already generally conditioned to a negative
image of Africans long before informal and formal rule—an image
formed through accepted notions and inextricably linked to pseudoscientific ideas about comparative mental ability and racial dominance.[19] So the dilemma of the African doctor trained in Western
medicine does have several dimensions. Sometimes these dimensions
may appear as unrelated, but considered together they suggest themes
that clarify the complexities of ethnic myths and suspicions, and explain the fear of whites dealing with the African doctor trained in a
European medical system.

African Physicians "In Their Place"

This leads to the final theme of this book: to chronicle and analyze the
African physicians' struggle for equality in the medical profession established under colonial rule in Anglophone West Africa. The nineteenth century witnessed the transfer of medical skills that were once
the monopoly of whites to blacks, whose skills were comparable to
those of the whites. Despite their qualifications, the colonial bureaucracy enforced distinctions that favored middle-class British medical
officers while denying opportunities to comparably trained Africans
in the same medical service. So the Africans became increasingly
marginalized in the medical profession. By 1900 colonialism was on
its way to complete establishment in Africa, and its effect could be
seen in changes in the Colonial Medical Service in West Africa. This
issue is detailed in chapter 4.

   The time frame of this book covers a span of approximately 185
years—from about 1800 to 1985—and the nineteenth century is crucial because that was when Africans were first trained in the tradition
of Western medicine under incipient colonialism. In 1900 colonialism triumphed with the inception of the Colonial Medical Service. But it was through political aspirations, along with the demand
for medical autonomy through African medical associations, that
changes occurred, including independence in most of Africa by 1960.

However, African doctors and their role in the advancement of medical knowledge will be addressed before the issue of how they came to be organized.

The French Colonial Medical System

Researcher M. A. Vaucel shows that the French colonial medical system in West Africa had little in common with the corporate patronage system of its British neighbor. The first overseas practitioners of French colonial medicine began in the seventeenth century, and by the eighteenth century the French Naval School of Medicine was established at Rochefort (1722), at Brest (1731), and Toulon (1732). Through these establishments official French medical practice was established overseas in the last years of the century.

Similar to the British situation, the majority of the French health services overseas were military, with doctors in large numbers due to the needs of the troops. These physicians were also available for the civilian population, and so the French medical service began.[20] In 1751 the military organized the first nationalized health services, and in 1763 the first inspectors and director generals of medicine, of pharmacy, and of botany were named, with authority over the navy and colonies. The organization of a new corps began in 1890, independent of the navy, and charged with the health services of the colonies and protectorates and under the direction of the minister of colonies.

The corps existed for ten years. In 1900 the Colonial Army was created as an arm of the War Department, and its health services were uniformly made up of doctors from the previous corps, to which were added the naval doctors who came as volunteers. Afterward, the school of Bordeaux, which was called the Health Service of the Navy and of the Colonies, became the common source of recruitment of doctors for the navy and of doctors for the colonial troops. The physicians of the Colonial Corps—called overseas troops in 1958 and naval troops in 1960—have always been more numerous than the actual needs of the military required.

Of the total number of doctors designated each month for overseas duty, 80 percent were placed outside the strict military command and assigned to work in Public Health Services of the overseas territories. The more senior general officer was the Director of Health Services under the Minister of the Colonies for France Overseas. Nevertheless, these military doctors represented more than 90 percent of the French medical personnel overseas in 1965. Further, the civilian cadre of medical assistants were organized by the French in Madagascar, Indochina, West Africa, and New Caledonia in the recent twentieth century.

Moreover, an efficacious development was the founding of local medical schools for the indigenous people at Pondicherry (India) in 1863; at Tananarive (Madagascar) in 1896, a year after occupation; at Hanoi (Vietnam) in 1902; at Dakar (Senegal) in 1918; and at Ayos (Cameroon) in 1928. After an average of four years at these institutions the doctors revealed themselves to be excellent clinicians. The British at first refused to consider African demands for local medical schools like those the French established until the late 1920s, but then they used the Dakar model in their fact-finding mission.

Unlike British West Africa, where African doctors trained in the West returned in larger numbers to practice medicine in their respective countries and where British policy sought to preserve African institutions under indirect rule, the French policy was direct rule through assimilation. Here, African societies were to be leveled, with French culture on top and with the perspective that Africans in Francophone territories be allowed to become citizens of France. French citizenship, however, was preserved initially to the Four Communes, or older cities of Senegal, long subject to the policy of assimilation. French education and language were requirements, and in the case of medicine one could attend medical school in France. Vaucel tries to prove that premature assimilation constituted a brain drain and caused a reduction in the number of Francophone African doctors available to the general population in the villages. As one might recall, the French and the British embarked upon developments during World War II to enhance self-sufficiency in the colonies, developments that proved to be important in preparing for decolonization. The state-guided initiative of the British was the Colonial Development and Welfare (CD and W) Acts. The French equivalent was FIDES (Fonds pour l'Investissement pour le Développement Economique et Social). While FIDES was a direct consequence of the war and gained support through gratitude for French Africa's help to free France under General de Gaulle's leadership, the impact of FIDES on increasing the numbers of African doctors in the region remains to be assessed.[21]

The French policy of assimilation was a costly proposition. It reduced the African to an inferior status in the same way the British policy did. In the area designated under the *indigénat* where Africans could be handed sentences of imprisonment by French authorities without trial or appeal, the French used the whip (*fouet* and *chicote*) to discipline the African, and the move toward assimilation made Francophone Africa an auxiliary of France.[22] French-speaking Africans, therefore, still preferred to go to France to begin their studies, either with a government scholarship or family support, and then, even more problematically, to stay for many years after obtaining the required MD in order to pursue specialized training. African economies could not support many physicians, and so the best use of the few was in broad, generalized practice, treating as many people as possible for the basic kinds of health and sanitation problems. The people with more unusual maladies, who might benefit from specialist attention in more affluent economies, were simply out of luck. The young African doctors, with their medical studies completed, were attracted to specializations that oriented them to work in large urban hospitals or in private practice; epidemiology did not seem to interest them, nor did laboratory research. The foundation established by the French, which tended to ignore rural areas, later caused problems under independence. The physicians' lengthy studies in France heightened social differences upon their return between themselves and the villagers. This state of affairs reduced the number of African doctors both in France and in Africa, which was manifested by the lower number of physicians willing to go back to their country of origin to work for their own government. Where there was a British exodus in Anglophone West Africa in the years before and after independence, the French medical assistance teams were able to prolong their stays in Africa from five to twenty years, depending upon the training success rates to recruit and train African doctors willing to serve in Africa.

French colonial policy, therefore, was one of integration, or incorporation of overseas territories into the metropolis. Consequently, there was no intention on the part of France to train a cadre of doctors in French colonial Africa, since there was no expectation of separation from France. For the British, however, colonial status was expected to be temporary.

Comparative Medical Certification

Some clarification of medical terminology is required because of the differences in certification procedures among the various national systems (see abbreviations).[23] In the European framework the term MD is a postgraduate medical degree; in order to practice medicine as a fully qualified professional one must obtain a bachelor of medicine (MB) degree and the bachelor of surgery (ChB) or bachelor of science (BS) degree. Only those individuals interested in accelerated research and further training work toward the doctorate of medicine (MD), a degree equivalent in the sciences and liberal arts to the Ph.D. but awarded in the clinical sciences.

In the United Kingdom the MRCS is the basic degree equivalent to the European MB or BS, and the FRCS is a professional postgraduate degree. Hence, membership or completion of a course of training in the Royal College of Surgeons of England (FRCS, Lic.) and in the Royal College of Physicians of London (FRCP, MRCP—basic degrees, LRCP, Extra-Lic., RCP) is another route to qualification as well as at Edinburgh, Glasgow, or Dublin. The LRCP is also a basic degree. In Dublin, the LRCP and S—Licentiate Apothecary Hall—is now banned and was in Ireland only; it was an outside licensing body. In England, the MRCS and LRCP represent qualifications obtained outside the university following five to six years of training and without the university exam; one may be licensed as a doctor after finishing the course of the outside licensing bodies (MRCS, LRCP, LAH, LRCP and S). In the Royal College of Surgeons, the MRCS is an honorary degree given by them.

Traditionally, many Africans en route to Western Europe matriculated at Edinburgh or Dublin, and because of the training connection
Fourah Bay College in Sierra Leone had with the Durham medical institution, an increasing number went there or to Newcastle-on-Tyne,
due to its Durham linkage (see map 2). This practice began in the
1850s and has continued over the last 130 years. James Africanus Beale
Horton (MRCS, LM, MD) and William Broughton Davies (MD),
both students at Fourah Bay College, were the first Africans to follow
this road to medical professionalism in 1859 and 1858 respectively,
through the auspices of the colonial government.

The certification requirement on the European Continent is more
comparable to that of the United States. Prior to World War II,

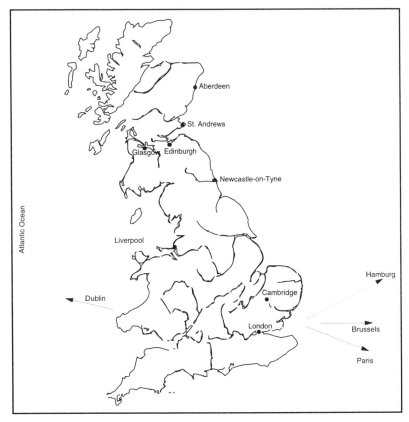

Map 2. Western European medical centers, nineteenth and twentieth centuries

France, Germany, Austria, Sweden, and Poland had generally the same system except that a distinction in terms of degrees did not exist. The German doctor, for example, was an *Arzt* or physician, with a level of training time comparable to the bachelor of medicine in Great Britain. In order to meet continental standards for the MD degree, a stage further was required: this involved academic research that had to be completed and defended. However, the bachelor of medicine (MB) from England and the doctorate of medicine (MD) from the Continent are generally treated equally by regulatory entities in some of the countries under review, although the degrees are absolutely different.

The doctorate of medicine (MD) in the United States generally first requires a bachelor's degree in a four-year undergraduate program, followed by an additional four years in a medical school. This MD, which is equivalent to the Ph.D., is a requirement for being licensed to practice.

The former Soviet Union certified with the MD degree, as did the socialist countries of Eastern Europe where Africans received training in the late 1950s through the 1970s. Both regions tended to encourage specialization very early.[24] By 1985 the former USSR had trained some 52,000 doctors from the Third World as specialists and revamped its medical requirements to be comparable to those degrees in most of the other countries affected by perestroika. This change will be explored in chapter 8.

African Women Physicians

In English-speaking West Africa women did not become medical doctors until after the first quarter of the twentieth century, some seventy years after their first male counterparts. Dr. Agnes Yewande Savage (MB, ChB), the daughter of Dr. Richard Akiwande Savage of Nigeria, graduated from Edinburgh in 1929, the first Nigerian woman to complete medical training. She finished her professional service in Ghana before retiring to England, where she died in 1965 at the age of fifty-eight.[25] The next Nigerian female to qualify was Dr. Abimbola

Awoliyi (née Akerele), who received her medical degree from the University of Dublin in 1938.

The rising interest in medical professionalism then reached Sierra Leone. Dr. Irene Cole Ihgodaro (MB, BS) graduated from Dunelm in July 1944; marriage, apparently, carried her on to Nigeria for medical practice. Dr. Sophie Elisabeth Jenner Wright (MRCS, LRCP) received her outside licensing body confirmation after completing a course of study in November 1944, and she went on to complete her basic university undergraduate degrees (MB, BS) in London in 1946. She is, of course, the daughter of the famed late Dr. Ernest J. Wright. Dr. Ola Elsie Palmira During (MD, BS), affectionately dubbed in the Krio language as the "pickin' doctor" (the children's doctor) in Sierra Leone, was next to qualify from Dunelm in 1950. Dr. Priscilla Rosamund Kasope Nicol (LRCP and S) followed in Ireland in 1953. Then came Dr. Marcella Gwynnie Ekua Davies (LRCP and S; LAH, LM, 1954, Coombe; DTMH, Liverpool; DPH, Liverpool; FWACP). In addition to serving as chief medical officer of Sierra Leone, Davies served as the WHO National program coordinator for Sierra Leone (see figure 1). Dr. June Spain Holst-Ronnes (MB, ChB) received her medical degree from St. Andrew's in 1955 and also became the mayor of Freetown. By the late 1950s a number of other Sierra Leone women had qualified as doctors.[26]

In colonial Ghana, Dr. Susan Gyankorama De-Graft Johnson (née Ofori-Atta; MB, ChB, 1947, Edinburgh; DRCOG, 1949; DCH, 1958) was the first woman to qualify as a physician; she pioneered in pediatrics. In 1950 she returned to Ghana and in time became medical officer in charge at Kumasi Hospital; later she assumed charge of the Princess Marie Louise Hospital for Women in Korle Bu and became affectionately known as "mmofra doctor" (children's doctor). Dr. Matilda Clerk (MB, ChB, 1949, Edinburgh; DTMH, 1952, England) was the second pioneer woman doctor to qualify as a medical officer; and she also served at the Princess Marie Louise Hospital for Women (now Accra Children's Hospital). Clerk and De-Graft Johnson both died in 1985.[27] Both Ghana and Nigeria obviously have a longer list of female doctors than is possible to mention here, but an additional

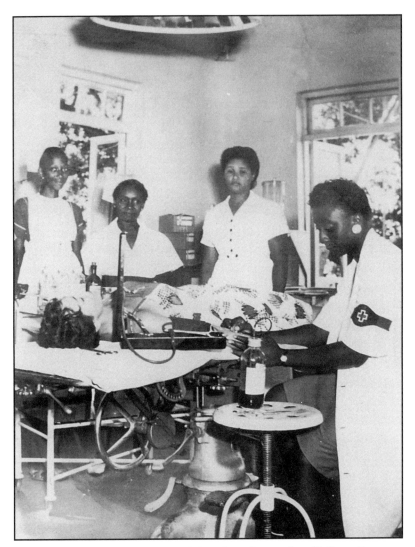

Figure 1. *Dr. Marcella Davies (right) with patient and staff, Sierra Leone, c. 1960. Courtesy of Marcella Davies.*

comment must be made. Unless they received their early secondary training in the science curriculum in England, some of these earlier pioneer women doctors encountered numerous obstacles on the road to professionalism. In a number of African countries colonial policy proscribed the teaching of science courses to Africans until the 1950s.

British Medical Culture and Reform

In 1858 the British established a General Medical Council (GMC) for the purpose of protecting the public from incompetent and uneducated practitioners. Prior to 1858, nineteen licensing agencies existed in Great Britain; the archbishop of Canterbury was among these. According to Spencer Brown, medicine was in a state of anarchy.[28] But with branches in England and Wales, Scotland, and Ireland, the GMC set new guidelines. Before physicians were allowed to practice medicine, their names had to appear on a list of what became known as the Medical Register. In addition, the GMC introduced the Medical Act as a reform effort to rid the profession of unqualified doctors and began to enforce the provisions of this legislation. One provision stated the eligibility requirements needed for the physician's name to be listed along with types of certification on its Medical Register before authorization was given to practice medicine.[29] The GMC mandated that students must pass certain types of examinations in designated subjects and must study in institutions that it recognized in order to become registered medical practitioners. Further, the council had the authority to control the licensing bodies to bring about a regularization of standards. This reform effort was a hallmark in the development of medical education; now removed from the politics of the modern state and health ministries, an autonomous national body regulated medical education. And the introduction of a strong British medical culture into Anglophone West Africa was a logical outcome of training African doctors in Britain and of the colonial policy mandated by the council. A general education in the natural sciences was urged for premed students, to be followed by graduate training for medical professionals. Even now, British medicine still adheres to this old and venerated principle.

In 1948 the National Health Service Act ended one of the nightmares of British medical education; aspiring physicians no longer had to pass the final qualifying exam that licensed them simultaneously to practice medicine, surgery, and midwifery. Hypothetically, the newly certified doctor was qualified to treat rare diseases, perform the most intricate operations, and deliver babies. Under the new act the qualifying doctor had only to complete a residency under supervision in a hospital and to complete two resident posts satisfactorily—one in medicine and one in surgery—before admission to the Medical Register. Further specialization in medicine, surgery, and obstetrics and gynecology required at least five more years of training after qualification; only then could the doctor practice unsupervised. It was within this medical culture, steeped in colonialism, that most African doctors were trained alongside their European counterparts. This meant that a medical culture that did not fit the Western model would be poorly tolerated. The U.S. medical system began to be accepted with reservations in the 1950s, and in Sierra Leone, at least, the German medical system (East and West) found acceptance because the German professors made periodic visits in the 1960s and 1970s to assess the progress of their past students. These professors often gave seminars with Sierra Leone doctors from other training backgrounds in attendance. The conflicts created by the convergence of various foreign medical cultures in Africa are explored further in chapter 8.

African Medical Schools

Francophone West Africa founded the first local medical schools for training, and independence created few difficulties for this region. The public health services continued to include the same number of French medical doctors with the same percentage of French military doctors as had practiced under colonialism, except for two African republics—Mali and Guinea—where, out of a total of fourteen doctors, twelve were foreigners and only two were of the French public health services. Hence, beyond Mali and Guinea, the unity of method and the homogeneity of teams, with some 230 French doctors, were maintained in Francophone West Africa.

In each republic the minister of health was African and assisted by a French adviser. Progress came slowly, however, for at first the local school of medicine—such as that in Dakar—just trained medical assistants, and only gradually was such an institution transformed into a full medical school with its own faculty, nurses' training, and a teaching hospital. In the cities of Dakar and Abidjan the transition was apparently made in the 1960s. The countries of Cameroon and the Congo followed. African governments wanted to invest in these schools because they brought national prestige, but the great demand made it difficult for the French to furnish teaching personnel for each African country.

Medical schools in Anglophone West Africa were a long time in coming. Sessional Paper 22 of 1928, which British colonial authorities placed on the table of the Legislative Council of Nigeria, contains the first reference ever to the establishment of a medical school in West Africa. This reference had the backing of the Colonial Office for a medical school to serve all of the colonies. And after an intensive study of the Dakar Training School for the medical assistant and pharmacy assistant, officials from the involved territories—Nigeria, Sierra Leone, Gold Coast—met in a series of conferences in 1927. The conferees, however, were unable to develop a common policy, and Nigeria decided to go its own way.

The Yaba Medical Training College, located some six miles from Lagos on the mainland, was the outcome, and in October 1930 officials opened the doors of the new teaching hospital. Its purpose until 1948 was to train medical assistants, not physicians, and to award them a diploma. After more extensive instruction the institution conferred the Diploma of Licentiate of the School of Medicine of Nigeria—the same Yaba school—which gave equivalency to forms of European degrees. In 1946 the Royal College of Surgeons, England, gave recognition to diploma holders retroactive to 1941–42.

The Yaba graduates were outstanding, and out of sixty-two, twenty-nine went on to achieve the MRCS and LRCP, after further study and clinical experience.[30] In 1948 the Yaba school began a transfer and merger with the new University College of Ibadan at Ibaban. Ibadan University College graduated its first medical class in November 1960. Under a special relationship with London, thirteen students received the MB and BS degrees. Dr. Adelola Adeloye, the famed neurosurgeon and medical historian, was in this first group of graduates.[31]

Northern Nigeria, Islamic and once a separate protectorate from the Christian southern Nigeria protectorate until 1914 (when the two sections were amalgamated), had initiated its own medical school at

Kano in April 1954 with a most capable first class of twelve students. Officials planned to admit the same number each year, and Dr. M. O. Adeleye became known as its most outstanding graduate in surgery and midwifery during his years of practice in the Maiduguri hospital.[32] Following a fact-finding tour of January 1958, Professor R. B. Hunter of St. Andrews, England, recommended to the minister of health of northern Nigeria that the Kano Medical School be closed due to a number of negating factors. Hunter further recommended its replacement by a new and more comprehensive school to be opened in 1960 at Ahmadu Bello University at Samaru-Zaria. Those students already enrolled at Kano were to be allowed to complete their studies. The new plan entailed establishing a medical school that would produce and maintain a cadre of 1,000 doctors for northern Nigeria. While this would take about twenty years—until the school was in operation that long—the ratio of physicians to population would be 1 : 18,000, whereas in 1958 the optimum ratio of all doctors to the population at that time in Anglophone West Africa was considered to be 7 : 10,000. Until sufficient numbers of northern Nigerians could be trained, expatriate doctors would be employed in order to maintain service at then current levels. Hunter also indicated how the new school should structure its program in order to qualify for accreditation by the Royal College of Surgeons and the Royal College of Physicians.[33]

In southern Nigeria the independent government established the Lagos Medical School and Teaching Hospital on the mainland and at Suru-Lere in April 1962. Dr. Ralph Schram (MA, MD, Cambridge; DPH; DIH)—the noted colonial physician, medical scholar, and medical teacher—observed that this development was in contrast to the lack of similar establishments in other African countries (see figure 2).

By the 1960s most countries had not founded their own medical schools. For example, the Dakar Medical School served the vast region of Francophone Africa, Khartoum served the Sudan, and Makerere served East Africa. Ghana, Sierra Leone, and Gambia relied solely on the Ibadan facility to meet their needs for medical personnel. Ethiopia, Tanzania, and Kenya were only in the initial stages

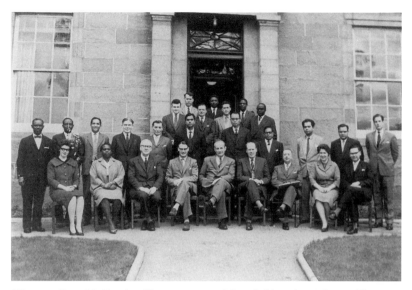

Figure 2. Drs. Ola During (first row, second from left) and R. Schram (first row, far right) during a training session at Queen's College, London, c. 1962–63. Courtesy of M. Aboko-Cole.

of developing their own training facilities. Liberia had certified only 2 doctors by 1955, in spite of the fact that it had been an independent republic since 1847. Schram noted that Monrovia's hospital was described as the "worst single sight. . . . More . . . [money] was being spent on brass bands than public health."[34] In Central Africa, Salisbury University of Rhodesia (now the independent country of Zimbabwe) was still only in the planning stages. The Congo, with only 12 university graduates at the time of independence in 1960 out of a population of 13.5 million, had not graduated a single physician by that same time. Similar to Dakar and Yaba, the Congo first produced only medical assistants until the 1960s. This country had 2 interracial universities: the Catholic University of Lovanium, founded in 1954, and the nonconfessional state University of the Congo in Elisabethville (now Lubumbashi), founded in 1955. Lovanium graduated its first 2 physicians in 1961, and the Congo graduated its first 5 physicians in 1963. The 3 Egyptian medical schools were of little use to sub-Saharan Africa, and the damage of apartheid policies in the Republic of South

Africa to African professionalism is all too well known, where, at the time of publication, the ratio of white South Africans to physicians is 1 : 326 and the ratio for blacks to physicians is 1 : 3,400. The Medical University of Southern Africa (Medunsa), founded in 1978 in South Africa, was the first medical school for the training of blacks.

The late 1960s onward witnessed a renewed interest in the development and planning of medical schools in West Africa beyond Nigeria. In 1967 the newly established Ghana Medical School had 100 students in residence at its teaching hospital at Korle Bu, and the first group of doctors graduated in 1969.[35] Despite the long history of Sierra Leone in the development of the professions described in chapter 3, it took 25 years of planning before the first Sierra Leone medical school was established in September 1988 with an entering class of 20 students. In 1988 Sierra Leone had some 273 doctors registered: 182 employed by the government, 4 on Secondment or on loan, and 29 on study leave, although some had not returned after an 8-year absence and indeed may never return to practice in Sierra Leone. The rest of them are in private practice. The country is not without specialists: there are 50 employed in government service, 12 in the provinces and 38 in Freetown. These numbers do not include specialists in mission hospitals and the Russian and Chinese teams in Magburaka and Rotifunk, respectively. Sierra Leone has the medical infrastructure and faculty to train medical support staff, physicians, and specialists. Facilities involved in training doctors include 9 government hospitals and 5 private hospitals in Freetown, and 13 government and 6 mission hospitals in the provinces.

Although a few other African countries are ahead of Sierra Leone in medical institutional development, Sierra Leone's priority health problems present a pattern similar to that found in other developing African countries. It has a high mortality rate, estimated at 138–225 per 1,000, resulting from mostly preventable diseases. Of all reported deaths, 55–65 percent are caused by parasitic and communicable diseases. Malnutrition is also a major public health problem, and is often a contributing cause of death as well as a factor in abnormal prenatal conditions and complications of childbirth. Children under 5 years of age account for 50 percent of the deaths. Finally, the life expectancy at birth is 46.9 years for males and 50.1 years for females.[36] (The life expectancy in developed countries averages about 72 years!)

African Physicians in North America

African doctors were also trained in significant numbers in the United States and Canada. British medical culture tended to work against the African doctor trained in the United States who wished to practice in West Africa. Our study first explores this issue in chapters 5 and 6, focusing on two Sierra Leoneans who graduated from Howard University. Aspiring doctors also went to Nova Scotia as well as other medical schools in Canada to qualify for the registration exam of Licentiate. On completion of their studies the African doctor trained in the United States had to go to England for further studies in tropical medicine, and a number of medical doctors chose this route in order to be employed in West Africa. In 1951 the West African Medical Directors introduced new provisional policy measures that mitigated these requirements.

In spite of the relaxation in requirements, Dr. Latunde Odeku, who remains the most famous African graduate of Howard University Medical School (class of 1954), and who, according to his biographer, "was the founding father of neurosurgery in black Africa,"[37] went to London, Ontario, to study at the College of Physicians and Surgeons of the University of Western Ontario in order to receive the Licentiate of the Medical Council of Canada (LMCC) in June 1955. Shortly afterward he returned to Nigeria to begin his distinguished practice in neurosurgery, which he maintained until his death at the age of 47 in 1974.

Independence Era: Decline of Medical Standards

In West Africa the transition from colonialism to independence was accompanied by a decline in medical standards in the government-sponsored hospitals. Europeans became concerned about their protected status as the colonial era approached its end, so the resultant exodus of foreign specialists was a damaging blow in some areas to health care. Let us take for an example the Colonial Nursing Association (CNA), which the Colonial Office established in 1896 for the crown colonies. European firms operating on the coast of West Africa insisted that whites who fell ill should be cared for in nursing homes, and the CNA was called upon to staff them. Freetown received its clinic in 1899. The Colonial Hospital in Lagos first employed European nurses in May 1896; the Gold Coast (Ghana) began to recruit them in 1897; and Nigeria got its first contingent in March 1898 for the West African Frontier Force. In time these nurses not only looked after the Europeans but also treated the African population. The CNA had the responsibility of training both male and female nurses to a standard acceptable to the Royal College of Nursing in Great Britain.[38]

The Nursing Sisters, as they were apparently called, performed a number of functions. As clinic and hospital officers they provided around-the-clock relief to the district medical officer who dealt with minor casualties, and they kept the resident doctor informed about serious new cases admitted to the hospitals and the critical cases in the wards. In addition, they operated the X-ray plant and assumed the duties of the anesthetists. Even more, the Sisters were responsible for the child-welfare and maternity clinics in the various districts. Their contributions were invaluable to the smooth functioning of the medical infrastructure, and newly trained African nurses lost a valuable source of collective experience with the exodus of the European nurses. Consequently, the nursing profession declined in effectiveness immediately following independence.

Toward the end of the colonial era, in the late 1950s, the dismantling of the Colonial Medical Services began. Medical departments throughout West Africa soon came to realize that the expatriate exodus was not their only problem. For experienced African doctors also left the government service to go into private practice. In some places the shortage of doctors became sufficiently acute to force some health centers to close. Others reacted by sending out invitations to their nationals abroad to return home in order to fill the void even before the 1950s. However, some European physicians with extensive experience did remain to facilitate the orderly process for the new African doctors.[39]

The new generation of African professionals began to experience job dissatisfaction throughout the government health service. Declining nursing standards and appalling conditions in the public hospitals were a significant source of discontent. Doctors with a strong preference for clinical work expressed little interest in being trained for administrative duties in public health, while others preferred to work for themselves. Such an example was Dr. M. A. Barnor of Ghana. He retired from the government medical service in 1958 and established his own private clinic as the Link Road Clinic, where he was later joined by Charles Odamten Easmon.

Physicians Face Off with the Government

Sierra Leone doctors employed in the government service responded to the declining medical conditions by threatening a general strike in 1965. A group of brilliant and dynamic doctors had returned to Sierra Leone from training abroad, including Dr. Walter Awooner-Renner, the first Sierra Leone doctor to be trained on the Continent and now established in private practice; Dr. Huxley Hubert Mauritz Knox-Macauley, who is now at Ahmadu Bello University Teaching Hospital at Samaru-Zaria; Dr. Mohammed Sorie Forna, a brilliant man who later became minister of finance and was executed by the government; Dr. Ibrahim Benjamin Amara, now a psychiatrist in Canada; and Dr. Daniel Josephus Olubami Robbin-Coker, now in private practice. These young doctors were aggressive and well trained. They had been exposed to modern standards of medicine in Cambridge, Durham, Aberdeen, Birmingham, Liverpool, Dunelm, Hamburg, and Basel, and they wanted to raise health standards because of the poor health care delivery conditions surrounding their work in Africa. They realized that collective action meant strength, especially after promises made by the government of Prime Minister Sir Albert Margai had not been kept. The doctors, now numbering thirteen, made plans for their strike in the residence of Awooner-Renner, then in charge of the Hill Station Hospital. Someone in the group, how-ever, became frightened about the proposed strike and leaked infor-mation to the government. Sir Albert threatened to recruit doctors from Ghana and Nigeria and to remove the Sierra Leone doctors from the Medical Register. Obviously, he failed to recognize that the Ghana Medical Association and the Nigerian Medical Association, both with influential links to their governments, would not have ap-proved such a request, and, in addition, that the conditions of service in Sierra Leone were not good enough to attract replacements.[40]

Nevertheless, the government doctors found themselves in a des-perate plight and entered into negotiations with the minister of health. The minister advised them of the need to yield to the govern-ment's recommendation of how their working conditions might be improved before their wishes could be considered. When the doctors agreed to hear what the officials had to say, the government backed out. Negotiations continued until an impasse arose. At that point some older doctors advised the rebels to back down, noting that the government had promised reforms. But when the young doctors yielded to the government's demand, they got nothing in return. It is said that their strength had been weakened because some of their members went over the government's side. The doctors soon came to realize that their conditions of service, when it suited the government, made them part of the Civil Service, so their views in opposing the government could not be pursued actively.

The medical profession was not related to politics in the same way as the legal profession or other marginal professions. Doctors in poli-tics diminished their public health integrity in the eyes not only of their peers but also the public at large. And failure to win in politics might have meant the ruin of a successful practice, especially once the doctor's political views became known. In the long run politics had a great deal to do with public health standards and with the conditions constraining the practice of medicine in the public hospitals.

More recently, Nigerian doctors have turned to striking as a means of seeking redress. The crisis, according to the physicians, resulted from the failure of the government to fulfill its commitment to devote not less than 5 percent of the national budget to the health sector in

1985. The government's procurement of $4 million from UNICEF for the hospitals in October 1984 was said to have lasted only four weeks, according to the doctors. The conflict between the doctors and the government began with a strike in September 1984, which apparently ended with an uneasy, makeshift compromise resulting in the next stage of escalation. Grievances concerning the quality of medical services were the root cause of the problem. It is said that various public servants were allowed free medical treatments, but a government order denied people who worked in the public hospitals the same privilege. The health care delivery system suffered; nationally, 85 percent of doctors in government employment failed to comply with the ultimatum and were summarily dismissed. Patient services were disrupted in both private and government hospitals; 120 patients in Ogun State alone were said to have died for lack of emergency treatment during these events. Further, the leaders of the medical associations were detained for security reasons.

On April 12, 1985, the federal military government of Nigeria banned—"with immediate effect"—the country's two major medical associations, the Nigerian Medical Association (NMA) and the Nigerian Association of Resident Doctors (NARD). *West Africa*, a major weekly periodical, reprinted a report on a segment of the government's statement, which read as follows:

> The Federal Military Government has noted that the record of the activities of the Nigerian Medical Association over the past five years shows that the association has consistently used any excuse for industrial action [strike] by doctors in the public services on which the government (Shagari regime inclusive) has demonstrated extreme goodwill in a spirit of compromise. Thereafter the association has exhibited unpardonable bad faith by making endless demands on matters which are exclusively the responsibility of the appointment boards, introduction of consultancy services in teaching hospitals and the ongoing cost reduction measures in the public service. These are policy matters which cannot be subject to negotiation. By their actions, members of the Nigerian Medical Association and the National Association of Resident Medical

Doctors have exposed themselves as a group of unpatriotic, selfish and callous professionals who have no regard for the serious economic predicament facing the country, and the much needed peace required by the Federal Military Government. . . . The Federal Military Government cannot tolerate or condone a situation in which an association of professional persons sets out to cause its members to withdraw their services without regard for prescribed procedures and in violation of applicable laws.[41]

These medical bodies, according to the government, had become subversive, and the statement stipulated that government doctors who did not comply with the order to return to duty immediately must vacate the residential quarters "within twenty-four hours" and be dismissed from the service.

On the one hand, doctors, too, were subject to allegations of malfeasance over the age-old central issue of private practice versus government medical service, which is dealt with in chapter 4. Doctors must be held accountable in resolving a conflict-of-interest pattern; that is, being employed in public hospitals and participating in the corrupt practice of diverting drugs, equipment, and patients to their private clinics. On the other hand, government employment and private practice represent an unresolved problem inherited from the colonial era.

But this is not the fundamental health problem facing the new African nations. Far more pressing are the economics of public health. Budget allocations for public health are a declining portion of total budgetary outlays, indicating a declining commitment to health care delivery for Nigeria and the other West African nations under study. This pattern is complicated by a number of factors: absence of financial accountability by governments; devaluation of the currencies in Anglophone West Africa through Western lending institutions, where the price of imports rise and the price of exports decline; and the decline of per capita income for sub-Saharan Africa that began in the 1960s, which now stands at maybe U.S. $400 and is predicted to decline through 1995. The average African, therefore, has less to spend on health care than at the time of independence in 1960.

And as long as this pattern persists, the truce between doctors and governments will remain an uneasy one.

Preventive Medicine and Primary Health Care

Nevertheless, the medical profession has an indispensable role to play in African health care development strategies. Under favorable policy conditions, practitioners can play a major role in the campaigns against diseases that affect mass populations. Preventive medicine and primary health care remain significant objectives of economic development. As the late Dr. B. B. Waddy, a colonial district officer in northern Ghana recognized, the medical profession must continue to give priority attention to the most significant public health measures that "increase the energy of the agricultural labour force at the planting season—the six weeks or so at the beginning of the rains—on whose productivity depends the amount of food that will have to last a whole year. It is during the early rains, when humidity rises, that the bone pains of yaws come on, the guinea worms emerge (and guinea worms can paralyse a village), and the annual attack of clinical malaria comes on. It is a long time since the last harvest, and energy is short. Epidemics during the dry season may have left the remaining population exhausted and dispirited."[42] Other diseases that attack mass communities are measles, polio, cerebrospinal meningitis, smallpox, and river blindness (onchocerciasis). Other approaches to improving the health of the labor force must also be considered in health planning. In West Africa, as almost everywhere else, nutrition must be taught because children suffer from malnutrition generation after generation. In all of these initiatives the medical profession at all levels of society must be involved.

Medical history can still play a role in current African development through research both relevant and useful to African governments. Ecology must receive renewed attention in light of the famines facing African societies. The forest region generally has been more advanced in food production, but for the Sahel-savanna region, "disease is history and history is disease."[43] Mali, the non-desert-edge medieval empire with its capital, Niani, along the banks of the Sankarani, was believed to have been wiped out by an epidemic of sleeping sickness. If the fourteenth-century Arab historian Ibn Khaldun is correct, King Mansa Djarta of Mali died of sleeping sickness in A.D. 1373–74.[44] Even today, sleeping sickness is one of West Africa's most dangerous diseases. It is a disease endemic at a low rate in the forest but endemic at a higher rate in isolated pockets in the savanna, from which the disease usually spreads elsewhere. The World Health Organization is making a gigantic effort to eradicate this disease and is also actively campaigning against onchocerciasis. In the past onchocerciasis had driven people away from the rivers. But droughts, overgrazing, and the cutting of trees for firewood further eroded the watershed, the drainage area that lies between the rivers, and, in a country such as Burkina Faso, people overcrowded the watersheds. Then, unable to find farming land, they returned to the infested rivers because they just did not believe that conditions could get any worse. This process repeated itself, whereupon the land became sterilized with continued erosion, causing population movements. We really should not need to be reminded about how these conditions with historical antecedents are causing problems for African governments and the world today.

The Medical Profession in Africa from Ancient Times to 1800

*I*n ancient times Africa itself provided for the education and training of its doctors. Some four thousand years ago Egypt was a major center for medical practice. The medical profession of this time was neither standardized nor supervised in the manner that developed during the nineteenth and twentieth centuries. The dissemination of medical knowledge was limited to a few families, so some secrecy prevailed. Practitioners almost always came from these families, although the system was not closed to outsiders without links to these families and where the talent for the medical art revealed itself. The physician's status was one of high esteem, and a person in the profession was sometimes referred to as *hakim,* denoting a wise man or philosopher.[1] Doctors had their own boats and traveled the Nile to treat their patients. Since Egypt did not have a monetary economy, trade was in barter and physicians received their pay in kind. The state had a large bureaucracy and served as the major consultant for these doctors. Rulers surrounded themselves with physicians to ensure their good health. But the noblemen and the wealthy also sought and utilized the clinical expertise of both state-employed doctors and those in private practice for their households, treating servants, serfs, and slaves as well. Medical cures ranged from the use of incantations or "magico-spiritual" elements to the more preventive and rational diagnosis based on ancient Egyptian medical practices, the later Hippocratic and other scientific traditions of the times.[2]

Imhotep, who was the contemporary of Pharaoh Zoser (or Djoser) of the Third Dynasty around 2700 B.C., was the first physician to stand out in the world of antiquity, and in time he came to be referred to as the "God of Medicine."[3] Additionally, three ancient medical treatises have survived from 1900 B.C.—the Gynecological Papyrus of Kahun on diseases of women—and from 1600 B.C.—the Papyrus Edwin Smith on medicine and the Papyrus Ebers on surgery. The author of these texts may never be known with certainty.[4]

The African physician was not only initially trained in ancient Africa but served beyond its continental boundaries. The medical expertise and materia medica of ancient Egypt flowed across the Mediterranean to Greece, Rome, and the rest of Europe, where it was modified over several millennia. New medical expertise came to coastal Africa by way of the European trading post, rather than from across the Sahara, enabling Sierra Leone to develop an indigenous corps of British-trained African physicians in the nineteenth century.

African Physicians in Antiquity

The late Henry Sigerist, for example, reported on the widespread acceptance of the African physician in antiquity. He wrote as follows:

Darius was not the only Persian King [522–486 B.C.] who appreciated Egyptian medicine. Before him Cyrus [c. 585–c. 529 B.C.] liked to be surrounded by Egyptian physicians. The reputation of Egyptian doctors was great all over the ancient world. We read in the *Odyssey* that "in medical knowledge the Egyptian leaves the rest of the world behind." Egyptian doctors were frequently called abroad or pharaoh lent his personal physicians to foreign rulers as a token of friendship. A court physician of Amenhotep II [c. 1450–1425 B.C.] treated a Syrian prince, and it would be easy to give other similar examples.[5]

The Old Testament also mentions the Egyptian physician. During the long sojourn of the Hebrews in Egypt 2000–1200 B.C., the Biblical verse reads as follows: "And Joseph commanded his servants the physicians to embalm his father: and the physicians embalmed Israel" (Genesis 50:2).

This did not mean, however, that medical innovation was absent. Several centuries later the Greek historian Herodotus observed the developing specialization among Egyptian physicians, and commented as if he were describing medical innovations in our own time: "Medicine is practiced among them on a plan of separation; each physician treats a single disorder, and no more: thus the [region] swarms with medical practitioners, some undertaking to cure diseases of the eye, others of the head, others again of the teeth, others of the intestines, and some those which are not local."[6]

In recent observations on African medical science, Charles Finch (MD) commented on this tradition:

> It is of interest that the Egyptians were alone among the nations of antiquity in the development of specialty medicine. In the Old Kingdom, the diseases of each organ were under the care of a specialist. In later epochs, the specialists disappeared as the Egyptian physicians began to function as generalists. However, during Ptolemaic times [367–30 B.C.; Roman Province in 30 B.C.], specialization came back in vogue, probably as a result of renewed interest in the archaic culture. Not until the 20th century did anything comparable in the sphere of medicine develop. Contemporary doctors are accustomed to believing that modern specialty medicine resulted from a progressive evolution of medical techniques and knowledge, hardly realizing that it is a throwback to the earliest form of Egyptian medical practice.[7]

If contemporary doctors are now aware of their indebtedness to ancient Egyptian medical practices, it is a recognition that exceeds the benefits that the African citizenry received who lived at the time of these innovations in ancient Egypt. Unfortunately, the other peoples of Africa did not benefit from these ancient medical advances by the Egyptians. The trade in material goods and culture and medical knowledge was only trans-Mediterranean, exclusively between North Africa and the European continent. The Hippocratics and Galen of Pergamon (A.D. 129–c. 199) were its immediate heirs.[8]

The physician's art in Egypt was never established in Southern Africa for a variety of reasons. Although the Egyptians rank as one of the oldest cultures in the world, ancient Egypt—in common with many other cultures of the same period—remained obsessed with the cyclical nature of time and the world of the past, and thus failed to develop what Robert Heilbroner calls "the idea of social movement, of aggregate betterment, of progress [in the future]."[9] The factor of external invasions after 661 B.C. caused officials to look northward rather than the south beyond Meroë in Nubia, and climatic change reinforced this tendency. With declining precipitation, the dry phase of c.2500 B.C. created the Sahara Desert and dispersed the aquatic Negroid cultures of Middle Africa. Their southward population movements isolated them from the scientific changes occurring in the Mediterranean basin.[10] Ethiopia was the exception to this development with its worldview and moral imperative based on prerabbinical Judaism dating back to 1000 B.C. and Christianity dating from the fourth century A.D.

Routes to Medical Training

The medical profession continued to make progress during the medieval era. Although sophisticated in a number of ways even by modern standards, it was still relatively unstructured. Medicine was highly advanced in the caliphates of the Middle East at the time and, even there, students could enter the medical profession in a variety of ways. Sons and daughters often learned the profession from the father, and medicine might become a family's major profession for several generations. There is evidence that people also taught themselves. Such students compiled a list of medical texts, which were then read until he or she was satisfied that their contents had been learned. However, few advanced into medicine in this manner until translations of Greek medical and scientific works with commentaries became accessible. The major pitfall of this method was that the omission of diacritical marks in the Arabic often caused students to misread the manuscripts. Gary Leiser, in a recent article from which much of this discussion is drawn, reports an instructive anecdote. *Tashwiq al-tibbi* (The Arousing of Medical Desire) is a book on medical ethics completed in A.D. 1072 by Said b. al-Hasan of Syria and Iraq. It contains many stories about self-directed medical training. One of al-Hasan's stories is sufficient:

> I encountered one of them who was carrying a whimpering puppy (jarw) in his sleeve. So I said to him, "What are you doing with that?" and he replied, "I want to make a medication for a friend." Then I said, "What are you going to do with the dog?" and he answered, "It will be made into medication." I then asked, "What is the medication?" and he handed me a text that he had copied and misread for there was written in it "dung (*Kh* urū) of a dog." So I said, "My good man, you have made a mistake. You have no use for this dog. You only need the dung of a dog." He then tossed the dog from his sleeve, cursed it, and threw a stone at it. Afterwards, he finally said, "My God, ever since I began carrying the dog, I was wondering how I was going to use it."[11]

This example indicates how difficult it could be to learn accurately through self-teaching, but successful doctors did indeed come from this tradition.

A third route into the medical profession was through classes in hospitals (*bimaristan* or *maristan*) or medical schools. Hospitals appeared early in the Islamic world and were highly regarded long before any such degree of sophistication was reached in the Christian

West, and they were open to practitioners of all faiths. The Umayyad Caliph al-Walid I may well have founded the first hospital at Damascus during the period A.D. 704–15, although the earliest documented hospital was built at Baghdad by Harun al-Rashid (786–809). The Baghdad hospital received its foundation support from the hospital and medical school at Jundaisabur, about one hundred miles northeast of Basra in Iran.

Just as medical expertise was passed on to the Greco-Roman world by the Egyptians, so the Muslim Arabs disseminated their medical knowledge throughout the Mediterranean during the seventh to the eleventh centuries. Unlike the Egyptians, the Arabs were trading within the African continent, beyond the shores of the Mediterranean, and the study of medicine followed into *Bilad al-Sudan,* or the land of the blacks in the western Sudan.[12]

Bilad es-Sudan: Timbuktu

With the exception of Christian and Judaic Ethiopia, nonliterate cultures predominated in sub-Saharan Africa until about the eleventh century A.D., when Islam introduced Arabic literacy into the western Sudan.[13] This region became both a literary center and one for the introduction of Arabic medicine. Michael Dols's recent work shows that the medical profession in medieval Islamic society was organized around a series of occupations of those medical practitioners who adhered mostly to the Greco-Roman medical theory and practice defined as Galenism. The study of Hippocrates, "the father of medicine," and Galen was a major component of medieval education, and some earlier practices used in Alexandria were adopted by the Arabs. Muslim students studied the classical Greek medical texts in Arabic translations, and in this way the Alexandrian canon of the twelve works of Galen could be consulted first-hand.[14]

Western Sudan, with Timbuktu as the intellectual focal point, became a center for the introduction of Arabic medicine. During a visit there in 1513, Leo Africanus—a Spanish Moor born in A.D. c. 1485 and whose real name was al-Hasan ibn Muhammad—observed the presence of the physician among other professions: "Here are great store of doctors, judges, priests, and other learned men, that are bountifully maintained at the Kings cost and charges. And hither are brought diverse manuscripts or written books out of Barbarie, which are sold for more money than any other merchandize."[15]

Even more, the curriculum at the famed University of Sankore at Timbuktu in the fifteenth and sixteenth centuries included courses on anatomy and other scientific subjects. The doctors of Sankore probably matriculated initially at the prestigious Al-Azhar University, which was established in Cairo as early as A.D. 974, and at the Dar-el-Hikma, the House of Wisdom, also in Cairo, which was built in A.D. 1005 and funded by the Fatimid rulers who governed North Africa. Both universities offered as part of their curriculum Quranic sciences, Arabic, astronomy, mathematics, chemistry, zoology, botany, mineralogy, medicine, and pharmacology. Scholars of high esteem received appointments, and education was free. Hence, scholars from the Sudanese empires of Mali and Songhai took advantage of the career opportunities offered at these science academies in Cairo and introduced their innovative practices to the Timbuktu community upon their return.[16] Unfortunately, Africanus did not provide us with more detail about the ethnic composition and origin of the physicians at Timbuktu. Nevertheless, the hajj (pilgrimage) to Mecca served as the mechanism for the voluntary diaspora; the consequences from this were the intellectual feedback process from abroad and the influx of ethnic diversity.

Elias Saad, who cites the Timbuktu scholar Al-Sadi Abd al-Rahman, notes the presence in that city of a doctor named al-Tabib Ibrahim al-Susi. Al-Sadi, who sometimes visited the city between 1600 and 1655, reported that al-Susi performed a successful eye operation on al-Sadi's brother, Muhammad Sadi. There are no historical references to an individual physician at Timbuktu, according to Saad, although Ahmad b. Abu Bakr al-Bartili, who was an eighteenth-century Walata scholar and physician from just north of the Senegal River, was praised as "the Tabib of his time" for extending his services to everyone, even to slaves.[17]

Timbuktu and Jewish Physicians

Although firm evidence is lacking, Jewish physicians may have been present in Timbuktu. It must be borne in mind that medicine was one of the most cosmopolitan professions in the Islamic world, in spite of its noncorporate nature. Jews and Christians were major contributors to Islamic medicine in its early phase of development, and their role in medical practice remained important in the early Middle Ages. The Muslim conversion of non-Muslims in the Fatimid period (A.D. 909–1171) led to the decline of Christians and Jews in Egypt and their earlier dominant role in medicine. The career of Ali ibn Ridwän's (A.D. 998–1068), a noted Egyptian physician remembered for his treatise in 1062 *On the Prevention of Bodily Ills in Egypt* and his debate in the treatise with Ibn al-Jazzar (d. 980), a Tunisian doctor, represented the ascendancy of a Muslim practice during the eleventh century in Egypt.[18] At the same time Muslim governments supported populist agitation in North Africa against Jews and Christians in the later Middle Ages, which found its counterpart in anti-Jewish ferment in Catholic Spain.

In medieval Spain Jewish doctors were, for a time, less excluded from the practice of medicine than elsewhere in Europe. These doctors were not only familiar with Hebrew and Latin but versed in Arabic, a facility that enabled them to study medical textbooks written by both Arabs and Jews in earlier times. When Spain finally succeeded in expelling the non-Christians—Arabs and Jews alike—in 1492, many of the Jewish refugees resettled in Northern Africa.[19] Africanus made note of their arrivals around 1513 and did not allow the presence of these Sephardic refugees and indigenous "oriental" Jews to go unnoticed, which further enhances our speculations on medical innovations in and around the Niger Bend at Timbuktu:

> The Iewes [Jews] increased afterwards in Affirick [Africa], when first Emanuell King of Portugal, put them forth of their dominions: For then many went over into the Kingdomes of Fez and Maroco, and brought in thither the artes and professions of Europe unknowne before to those Barbarians. In Bedis [Badis], Teza [Taza], and in Segelmesse [Siljilmasa] every place is full of them.

They passe also by way of traffick even to Tombuto [Timbuktu], although Iohn Leo [Leo's father] writeth how that King was so greatly their enemie, that he confiscated the goods of those that traded with them.[20]

In order to avoid hostility and persecution, Jews occasionally converted to the host religion in the Maghrib and elsewhere.[21] The mixed oriental-Sephardic population may have been granted *Dhimmi* status (membership in a protected community) and confined to a special quarter called *mellah,* in accordance with Islamic law, but it seems likely that there was Jewish interaction with Sudanese and Arab physicians at Timbuktu.

Songhai Decline and Scientific Interest

The Songhai empire, perhaps the strongest state organization that West Africa ever saw, abruptly ended with an invasion of the Moroccans in 1591. Its demise was a major factor in the reduction of scientific interest at Timbuktu. The Niger Bend that drew such a diverse mix of talents to its banks in the sixteenth century lost its attraction in the seventeenth century. However, scholars will continue to debate the vitality of the Islamic sciences and politics in the region during the seventeenth and eighteenth centuries.

It must not be forgotten, however, that the exiling of Timbuktu scholars by the Moroccans following the 1591 invasion was only one reason for major changes in the area. The probable catastrophic effects of famines and epidemics in the seventeenth and eighteenth centuries altered life in the region in ways that remain immeasurable. The famines occurred approximately every seven to ten years in the seventeenth century and approximately every five years in the eighteenth century. Two famines, one lasting from 1639 to 1643, and the other one from 1738 to 1756, were especially damaging to the loop society. Prolonged famines diminished the food surplus reserved to support the class of specialists and weakened the population's resistance to disease, resulting in epidemics of cerebrospinal meningitis, smallpox, cholera, yellow fever, and other diseases. The population's reproductive capacity was impaired for generations. In both centuries conditions were so harsh that even the rich were severely affected.[22] Even more, it appears that decades of lethal infections in the Bend created apprehension in the scientific community in the Maghrib, which may have further slowed travel to the region from North Africa. However, the physicians remained. During his travels from Fez to Timbuktu in 1787, Al-Hajj Abd Salaam Shabeeny noted the continued existence of "professed surgeons and physicians" with an abundant materia medica available for medical needs of the wealthy and the poor, the latter being the most likely to die.[23] But it was ultimately the African educated elite's response to Western incursions south of the Niger Bend that brought medical science from Europe rather than from the western Sudan into Anglophone West Africa in the nineteenth and twentieth centuries.

Medical Science and the Modern Era

Medical science based on the Western model almost certainly reached West Africa during the first explorations in the fifteenth century. These early frontier, and generally intrusive, contacts with the indigenous populations increased with intensity on the arrival of slave ships with surgeons on board to care for their human cargoes. News relayed through consecutive arrivals and embarkations led to the accumulation of knowledge in Europe about the enigmatic disease environment in West Africa. European explorers' and physicians' accounts in the 1790s and early 1800s attempted to mitigate the European morbidity and mortality that initially accompanied imperial expansion. As the French did in the same region, the British military brought its physicians along to treat its administrators and troops. But British doctors got sick too and required not only furloughs to return to England but extended periods of convalescence as well. The medical doctors in the health care services were in constant peril. Officials and missionaries sought a solution to this problem. Since Africans had immunities to some of the diseases and did not have to take leave from their territories, it was decided to train Africans as doctors to assist British doctors in the imperial system.

Imperial needs, therefore, led to the training of African physicians in the early periods: 1790s–1845, 1853–1880s, and 1880s–1900. The first such doctor with a distinguished career was from the African diaspora, namely William Fergusson (1795–1845) from the West Indies, who rose from the ranks of medical officer, to principal medical officer, and then to the governorship of the Sierra Leone colony.[24]

Many of the African doctors described in the following chapters had important experiences in the diaspora. As we have described earlier, a number—a somewhat more privileged group—returned to their homeland following periods of education and training elsewhere—in Europe, Canada, the United States, the former USSR, other Eastern bloc countries, and possibly the West Indies. A second group consisted of repatriated former slaves, who arrived in Sierra Leone as aliens eager to participate in a free society. Because they retained cultural and linguistic links to the homeland, these "Creoles," as they came to be called, moved readily into their new society, and by the 1840s the members of this group had become the first black professionals on the Western model in Anglophone West Africa.

Intraprofessional Conflict and Professional Struggles

CHAPTER THREE

The Sierra Leone Nexus

Freetown, Sierra Leone, was formerly described as the Athens of West Africa. The city was the most significant frontier medical community to develop in the region, and in time physicians there spread Western medicine beyond Sierra Leone to other countries in British West Africa. After the abolition of the Atlantic slave trade in 1807, Freetown, its capital, became not only a crown colony of the British but also an entrepôt for the settlement of slaves recaptured from ships en route to the Americas. These slaves, known as Liberated Africans, had originated from the Sierra Leone interior, Yorubaland, and elsewhere along the littoral of West Africa.[1] By this time the transportation of these human cargoes was in violation of the antislave trade law, and naval squadrons repatriated the slave cargoes captured in the Atlantic to Freetown and granted them freedom. Some of the repatriates had ancestral roots in the American colonies via Nova Scotia and the Caribbean, others came from Sierra

Leone itself, and yet others came from elsewhere in West Africa. In Freetown, now removed from their precolonial institutions, these youths responded to the new dynamics of risk, innovation, and individualism so characteristic of the West. The Church Missionary Society (CMS) and the British acted as the catalyst for this development. They promoted education for the "Creole" Africans, especially with the establishment of Fourah Bay College in 1827 and the rise of professionalism in West Africa.

As a result, Freetown became not only a cosmopolitan center in the nineteenth century but an enclave for the formation of a West African intellectual community. Martin Kilson shows that the rise of this type of community was determined to a large extent by where Europeans located their schools, plantations, agricultural extension services, railways, and other enterprises in the African colonies. The ethnic, regional, and religious groups that rose to the top first were based on their proximity to those facilities. Kilson stated his point as follows: "In Sierra Leone the fact that the initial settlement of the colony at the end of the eighteenth century was intended as a haven for freed slaves goes a long way to explain the large Creole representation in the new elite."[2] This new elite divided into multiple components that at the highest level became a distinct social class; in time it sought to elevate its overall position in society.[3] Within this community formal institutions arose and a set of rules was developed that provided the means for creative communication between individuals of varying social ranks, such as colonial administrators, church officials, medical professionals, repatriated Africans, and indigenous people. In time, the British imperial administrators and the missionaries realized that health care facilities would be needed before other goals—such as rescuing the slaves from the ships, setting up a college, promoting education, and professionalism—could be achieved.[4] The early history of the European presence on the West African coast provided ample experience for this realization.

Scientific medicine accompanied the initial European coastal expansion. The Portuguese posted a doctor-surgeon on the coast of West Africa as early as 1607. Spain, Denmark, Holland, France, and Great Britain employed licensed physicians to care for the health of their personnel in the various trading stations; these physicians also certified the health of the slaves prior to export to the Americas from Badagry, Lagos, and adjacent towns near the Niger and Cross rivers. In 1797 a young physician was appointed as assistant surgeon at Cape Coast Castle after having received only two years of training at a Glasgow hospital.[5] The Scots supplied two early explorers who were also physicians. Mungo Park (1771–1806), the first, not only introduced some form of health service to the region but also made known the directional flow of the Niger to the outside world. The second, William Balfour Baikie (1825–64), demonstrated in an 1854 expedition the first successful use of quinine against malaria. His successful ascent from the sea up the Niger and his subsequent return without fatalities not only opened the vast, wealthy interior of Nigeria for trade with Europe but also encouraged the Europeans to further exploration into the interior.

During the nineteenth century, however, the British Army Medical Service and the Colonial Office were the two main suppliers of doctors on the West African coast. The army had posted surgeons periodically on the Gold Coast since 1631. Sierra Leone had a total of twenty-seven surgeons in 1827, but the entire West coast had only one surgeon in 1842. Following the Baikie expedition of 1854, the total number of doctors rose to sixteen; Gambia had seven, the Gold Coast seven, and Sierra Leone two. Recruitment remained a problem until 1860 because of the lack of inducement. But to understand how all of this developed, we must review the last decade of the eighteenth century.

The Dispensary System and "Open System" for African Recruitment

The dispensary system, initiated in 1790, became the first training ground for the transfer of Western medical skills to the emerging African medical elite. Africans working as assistants in the colonial apothecary shops developed a familiarity with British pharmacopeia. With European doctors in short supply, colonial officials soon realized the practical advantages of training qualified West African medical personnel.

The European recruitment of Africans for medical service began in nineteenth-century Sierra Leone, although the Europeans adopted the system only because there was no other arrangement that was preferable. Missionaries recommended elite coastal Africans for medical training, and John Macaulay Wilson, the son of a chief, was probably the first to be selected this way. He was taken to England for medical training by the Sierra Leone governor in either 1794 or 1796. Upon his return he worked as an apothecary for the private Sierra Leone Company and later served under the auspices of the crown colony until 1815. Extant records do not show whether Wilson received a medical degree at Edinburgh, but he briefly served as surgeon of Regent village in efforts to control an epidemic of smallpox in 1817. Officials finally appointed him as assistant colonial surgeon at the hospital of Leicester. Among the Nova Scotians settling in Sierra Leone in 1792, John Easmon, who is linked to a long lineage of medical doctors well into the twentieth century, acted in the capacity as first dispenser. However, Alexander Bucknor, another Nova Scotian, may have obtained an MD. In 1826 Governor Sir Neil Campbell (1826–27) accepted in principle the policy of employing local medical men, and he posted two Maroons, who had settled there from Jamaica in 1800, to health care centers.[6]

The new policy change reflected the growing European image of coastal Africa as the white man's grave. British traders had been on the Guinea coast for over two centuries before Sierra Leone was established in 1783, but reforming society had to take into account the fact and reality of European mortality. In the late eighteenth century European newcomers to the coast died roughly at the rate of 300–700 per 1,000 per annum. As Europeans continued to arrive in Africa, they figured out better ways to manage the diseases that felled their predecessors and so their mortality rate declined. But the rate remained high enough—80–120 per 1,000—to make Europeans uneasy. Even the lower rate of mortality was several times higher than that for Europeans working in tropical America and Asia. These mortality rates were caused by a wide range of debilitating disease parasites. Malaria and yellow fever, sleeping sickness, Guinea worm, bilharzia, yaws, and dysentery were among the most common.[7]

Malaria was the most deadly of all the killer diseases in West Africa, a factor that made this region different for the British from the other tropical regions where the empire had commercial and political interests. *Anopheles gambia* and *anopheles funestus* are the most efficient vectors for transmitting plasmodial parasites from one human host to another, and in almost the whole of West Africa these vectors have a most conducive environment. *Plasmodium falciparum* is the most widespread form of malaria and probably the most dangerous of all malarial infections. The West African coast has a very dense population and therefore provides a more favorable environment for spreading disease.

Medical science could do very little to explain the disease environment of West Africa in the late eighteenth century, a region that was classified as hyperendemic for malaria. This classification was given because people rarely escaped an infection during a year-long stay in West Africa. The European high mortality rate there was in sharp contrast to the native West Africans, for whom the incidence of death from disease declined sharply after childhood. The problem of disease was exceedingly troublesome for the British, who were attempting to maintain military forces in the tropics. Despite the fact that tropical medicine had become an important component of British medical science, Philip Curtin reports further: "The germ theory of disease and the cellular structure of the body were unknown. Medical knowledge was still dominated by the tail end of humerol pathology, re-expressed through the eighteenth-century tendency to build medical systems. The essence of any of these systems was to see all pathological conditions as the result of a single set of causes. The humoral pathology considered all disease as an imbalance or impurity of the bodily fluids. Treatment therefore aimed at readjusting the balance by bleeding, purging, and the like."[8] If, however, medical science did not understand the multiple causes of disease, the British did initiate reforms in Sierra Leone that through time would enhance the overall professionalization of medicine in West Africa.[9]

Between 1790 and 1826 Edinburgh offered the most prestigious medical education in Great Britain, and Sierra Leone was one of its early beneficiaries. Prior to 1824, the MD course lasted for three years, and the curriculum consisted of such courses as anatomy, surgery, materia medica, pharmacy, the theory and practice of medicine, clinical medicine, midwifery, chemistry, and botany. Three months of study were required in two of the following areas: practical anatomy, medical jurisprudence, natural history, and clinical surgery. Since about 33 percent of the doctors served in the army, navy, and East India Company, military surgery was a necessary course of study as well. The medical faculty were of high quality, and students came from England, Ireland, Scotland, North America, Portugal, Brazil, France, Italy, Germany, Switzerland, and the West Indies for study. Graduates went on to excel in the medical sciences, teaching, the armed forces, and public health. For the period under consideration, 1790–1826, there were 2,309 medical graduates from the university, and the separate certifying body in Edinburgh, the Royal College of Surgeons, awarded 2,722 diplomas.[10] Dr. William Fergusson, who was born in 1795 in the West Indies, was among the Edinburgh graduates; he went on to an important career in which he notably advanced medical science in Sierra Leone.

Dr. William Fergusson

Fergusson was the first major Western-trained physician of African descent to participate in the imperial strategy in Sierra Leone. He obtained the surgeon diploma from the Royal College of Surgeons at Edinburgh in December 1813 at the age of eighteen. Soon certified by the Army Medical Board, Fergusson was employed as a hospital assistant to the armed forces, and in 1815, at the age of twenty, he arrived in Sierra Leone. In that year Governor Charles MacCarthy of Sierra Leone (1815–24) asked London to fill the post of second surgeon. Fergusson was serving as an army hospital assistant on the coast during this time. Governor MacCarthy believed that Fergusson would prove to be invaluable to the colony, especially in supervising medical services that the crown made available to the former slaves.[11] Fergusson, however, left the colony around November 1816 with half pay in order to take care of personal matters in London. He was apparently attempting to regain a large sum of money from a bankrupt estate in his native West Indies, and, in leaving the colony, he would have to reapply for a higher medical rank, if and when a vacancy became available.

Fergusson sought reappointment in a letter of October 18, 1822, to Whitehall. The position of second surgeon had become vacant once more. He reminded the officials that he was a mulatto, and that in the past his appointment was deemed consistent with the views of the African Liberated Institution to employ a person of color to interact with the "natives." Enclosures with his letter included appropriate documents from prominent residents of the colony in support of his reappointment. He emphasized further the advantage of his color: "from the experience I have had of the native Africans I am conscious that in my colour I project a rapport to their confidence which an European cannot have."[12] He thought that the appointment of educated people of color would make the children of the colony more inclined to accept a European education, and that the appointment further would indicate to them that scientific and intellectual knowledge were no longer out of reach but available to them all.[13] Colonized Africans too might begin to aspire to government positions, with profound implications for colonial policy.

Fergusson went on the full pay roster in 1823 and was appointed acting assistant surgeon to the Royal African Colonial Corps in 1824. A number of agencies competed for his expertise, and the name of the young doctor appears on the staff list of the Liberated African Department in 1826. Fergusson was also involved from early 1827 to August 1828 in assessing the health status of the ex-slave population of Sierra Leone, on which he reported to the health department. Lieutenant Governor Denham expressed satisfaction over the general health of the Liberated Africans, and attributed this improvement to Fergusson, who had been appointed as surgeon to the department in October 1827 at a salary of £150 per annum. Fergusson was in charge of the government hospital and the villagers in Kissy, regularly performing his duties without proper enumeration. The confirmation of the appointment was apparently delayed, and Denham attempted to speed the process so that Fergusson could be paid.[14] But the Liberated

Africans preferred the herbalist mode of treatment rather than Western medicine. Fergusson, it should be noted, was no stranger to these preferences, having observed them among the slave population of his native West Indies.

A near fatal smallpox epidemic hit Freetown in 1829 and Fergusson's medical skills were called upon again. Hospital returns show admissions of 560 patients; 285 died from this number, and 275 were summarily discharged. A plaque honoring Fergusson's work during the epidemic is displayed at St. George Cathedral in Freetown. It reads as follows: "During the fatal epidemic of 1829, He evinced superior skill, an Assiduity that was unwearied, and Humanity. . . . And were publicly And Gratefully Acknowledged By The Honourable Board of Council By valuable Testimonials From many of The Merchants And Inhabitants, And By The Home Committees of The Church Missionary Society."[15]

By 1830 the Liberated Africans numbered some 22,000, and their well-being was a subject of importance in the quarterly reports of the health department. Africans encountered different diseases as they traveled in slave vessels from the zone of capture in West Africa to the zone of freedom in Freetown. Hence, new repatriates brought with them additional health concerns. But colonial regulations were still in the process of being developed, further complicating the situation, and the needs of the military establishment took priority over the repatriates, depriving them of expert medical attention. Because Fergusson had to divide his time between the military, the European population, and the Africans at Kissy, William Brown, the Maroon apothecary, resided at Kissy as house surgeon until his death in 1831. Thomas Thorp, another Maroon, succeeded him but later was dismissed for malpractice. Ironically, Thorp departed for the Gallinas estuary, south of Sherbro, where some of the Mende lived, as a doctor to a Spanish slave trader in waiting to conduct a business now illegal.

Medical Standards in the Colony, 1830

An analysis of the clinical requirements from the Purveyor Stores, a central storage room for medical supplies, provides insights into the

medical standards of 1830 in the colony.[16] The stores allocated life ne-
cessities for repatriates and the European population. It is interesting
to note that some of these items available to patients in 1830 were no
longer obtainable in most hospitals by the early 1970s, according to
Dr. Walter Awooner-Renner. The requisites or inventories of 1830
show sheets in quantities of fifty each, along with one hundred shirts
of the long type, which could be used as either operating gowns or
dressing gowns. Patients in that period were even provided with slip-
pers. In colonial times provision for the indigent was made in Freetown's Hill Station Hospital and Connaught Hospital. Dress standards were maintained among the hospital staff, unlike today, where
people wear different styles and colors.

The list of pharmaceutical supplies suggests the emphasis was
upon mixtures during the nineteenth century. Various pharmaceutical ingredients were ordered by the pounds, which meant that the
physicians and druggists were highly dependent upon the old type of
European pharmacopeia. They mixed their own drugs and measured
them into dark-colored bottles to preserve their potency. The documentation additionally shows that the health centers were treating
large numbers of people. Huge quantities extracted from the dried
root of the Brazilian plant *ipecacuanha* were ordered to cure coughs, a
drug that remains one of the strongest ingredients in cough mixtures
even today. Opium was also widely used to cure the colds and coughs
caused by conditions at sea. But the Liberated Africans, many of
whom had never seen the sea, must have arrived with a lot of upper
respiratory infections. A lot of opium was used along with atropine,
an opium derivative.

Skin conditions such as scabies and dermatitis must have been
prevalent at the time because of the large quantities of zinc oxide
used. In September 1829 Fergusson ordered an entire group of returnees to shave their heads and to clean themselves thoroughly as a
means of eliminating lice. Muscular ailments appear to have been
even more widespread, for large quantities of liniments also appear in
the record.

The requisitions document of 1830, however, lists no drug for
smallpox, although the cowpox virus was discovered in the late

eighteenth century to make an effective vaccine against the dreaded disease. While drugs did not exist for immunization at the time, the traditional herbalist doctors offered some preventive measures against smallpox: for example, the Yoruba practiced immunization against the disease in some form. Smallpox at the time, however, was not very well known and not yet linked to a virus, and immunization was not a common practice. This process was introduced into medical practice through the work of Louis Pasteur (1822–95), the famous French scientist, in the 1870s. Physicians treated ailments systematically. Medical officers in 1830 may have known how to treat smallpox, but there is nothing to indicate it in the document.

Wounds appear to have been common, for large quantities of bandages are listed. No longer in use today but indispensable to medical practice of the 1830s were fracture boxes in which a fractured foot, for example, was placed for protection until it healed. Amputations were evidently done in large numbers, because wooden legs and crutches were listed in greater numbers than fracture boxes. Ligatures for suturing wounds appear on the list along with dental instruments for extractions. Ether is not listed in the document but may have been used in medical practice before its publicized date of 1840 as an anesthetic. It was used in amputations as an inhaled anesthetic. Doctors strapped the patient's hands and legs to a table. Then the anesthetist would come in and instruct the patient how to breathe, a porous mask was then placed over the face, and the vaporizing ether was applied as the patient fell asleep. The process was repeated until the operation ended.

Outside of attending to the medical needs of the military and the African Liberation Department, Fergusson also administered the medical certificates for Europeans in need of leave from the colony, and, in advising them on matters of health during their travels, he advanced medical science along the coast. Fergusson's correspondence from 1826 to 1843 indicates that the medical complaints of most individuals dealt with the obstruction and enlargement of the spleen and malarial fever, although he also describes the yellow fever epidemic of 1837, when a patient was treated for that disease. A return to England was usually recommended to British patients with chronic ailments peculiar to the tropics.[17] Fergusson advised the CMS in 1843 about how to provide for medical needs for a planned station at Badagry: "I have drawn out and herein enclose a list of medicines which I think will be indispensably required by the families about to proceed there. I would suggest that a supply of each of the articles, specified in the list, should be put up (for the sake of greater convenience) in two family chests, and the articles marked in the English language."[18]

In order to understand other aspects of Fergusson's career, we must go back a few years. Political changes underway in the colony allowed Fergusson to entertain ambitions beyond the medical profession. In August 1840 Governor Richard Doherty (1837–40) appointed Fergusson, who was then staff surgeon in charge of the colony, to be a temporary member of the Council of Government that ran the colony's affairs. In the move for confirmation, Doherty expressed the hope that neither Fergusson's profession nor his position on the military staff would interfere with an appointment on a more permanent basis.[19] Fergusson's favorite son status can be observed even more in Doherty's positive appraisal of his intelligence, long experience in the colony, and familiarity with its inhabitants. The Fergusson appointment was ultimately confirmed, and it paved the way for mobility into the civil establishment and legislative body of the colony.

William Fergusson and Medical Reforms

In spite of his changing political position, Fergusson did not lose sight of needed medical reforms. In a council meeting in March 1841 he drew attention to a peculiar disease of the eye that had been causing total blindness among the prison population during the preceding fifteen years. He described it as a contagious skin disease, which commenced at the mouth and spread to the nose, eyes, and eyebrows. Prisoners contracted the disease, he surmised, by sharing the same bowl while eating. Each prisoner dipped his hands into the dish, and the infection extended to all of them. Fergusson recommended to the council that each prisoner be allowed to eat with separate utensils and that those afflicted with the disease should be isolated from the other prisoners. The governor and the council agreed unanimously that these measures could not be adopted too soon, and since the Liberated African stores had an adequate supply of eating utensils on hand, the governor ordered that these items be immediately requisitioned and charged to the colonial account.[20]

Fergusson as Governor of the Colony, 1845

Fergusson's favorite son status and his continuing upward mobility were now challenged by the emerging West Indian factor in West Africa. First of all, morbidity and mortality levels of unprecedented intensity always left vacancies among the colonial administration, and the Colonial Office eventually decided to appoint officials of African descent, especially West Indians. The army had taken the lead in 1830 with the commissioning of William Smelie, an African West Indian, in the Royal African Colonial Corps. Now, in 1840, the West Indian contingent was bolstered further with the arrival in the colony of John Carr, a lawyer from Trinidad. He had studied at University College, London, was then called to the English bar, and now was appointed to the government of the colony as the queen's advocate. In July 1840 he took the oath of office and his seat on the council, just one month before Fergusson.[21]

Now two West Indians, apparently from different islands, contested for a position previously open only to Europeans following the death of Governor John Jeremie (1840–41), who had succeeded Doherty, in April 1841. Doherty had moved on to become lieutenant governor of St. Vincent Island in the Caribbean (1842–45). John Carr, who possessed a formidable memory for legal details, argued successfully that under the rules of the charter the acting governorship devolved upon him as senior member of the council. Fergusson protested that he had been favored by Doherty and Jeremie because of his long stay in the colony.[22] Nevertheless, Carr became the acting governor until September 1841, when the colony received a dispatch from the secretary of state with a commission for William Fergusson to be the lieutenant governor, a position that he held for four years.[23] In 1845 the new governor, Colonel George MacDonald (1842–44), was promoted to the Dominican Republic (which had been created the previous year), and Sir James Stephen, the undersecretary of state (according to Christopher Fyfe), being "convinced Fergusson's abilities outweighed any disadvantage attaching to his colour, had him appointed Governor."[24]

In accordance with a proclamation from the British government, William Fergusson became the governor of the colony of Sierra Leone and its dependencies on May 17, 1845, and the proclamation was announced at Government House on July 15, 1845. Fergusson was now the colony's principal medical officer as well.[25] He repeatedly petitioned the government's emigration agent to implement reforms that would improve the living standards of immigrants to the West Indian colonies to fill the labor shortage after emancipation in 1833, and as governor directed the queen's advocate to draw up a more comprehensive law governing living and working conditions of immigrants sent to the region as contract laborers on the sugar plantations. These laborers encountered other contract laborers, such as those of Chinese and Indian origin. Fergusson's concern was aroused because emigrants were being placed aboard ships where disease was rampant, particularly measles; young children were kidnapped; apprentices were taken without the consent of their masters; and even the aged and infirm were signed up indiscriminately for travel to the West Indies. But he hesitated with the West Indian legislative requirement that 33 percent of the emigrants be women to correct the existing low ratio of women to men in the colony. The colony census of 1841 had shown 23,863 males to 19,882 females, and the decline of the latter for Sierra Leone, he thought, might increase the mortality rate.

The Fergusson administration and its policies came under attack in July 1845. The governor of British Guiana had appointed W. S. Butts to carry out an enquiry into the "Prospects of the Emigration of Negroes from the West Coast of Africa to the West Indies."[26] Inasmuch as the secretary of state requested a clarification from Fergusson on several charges contained in Butts's report, Fergusson responded in a seventy-page dispatch from Government House on November 26, 1845.[27] The first issue concerned Butts's criticism of the separate educations then being given to Creole and newly liberated African children. Fergusson acknowledged that this had been the practice for several years. He explained that while the CMS had initially educated all classes together in the village schools that opened in 1824, the missionaries had complained that the brightest boys were leaving to become apprenticed to carpenters and masons. Instead, the missions intended to train them for employment as "native" agents for the general purposes of the mission. Further, the building maintenance strained the CMS resources. So around 1836 the CMS suspended its activities on behalf of Liberated Africans and ceased to offer free educational services. The children who could not pay were left to attend lower-quality government schools.

For its part, the Creole population was generally able to pay to have its children educated by the European teachers hired by the CMS, in preference to sending their children to the free Liberated African schools to be instructed by Africans with meager resources. Creole parents generally in the 1840s had moved into the colonial economy as merchants and in other vocations; this enabled them to pay for the education of their children. Fergusson argued that emigration and the exclusion from the CMS schools of Liberated Africans above the age of twelve resulted in a marked reduction in the numbers of scholars, a number that was lower than at any time in the century. Further, he warned that the Liberated African village schools were bound to become extinct if that pattern continued.

In time these divisions conferred important educational advantages on the Creole population. In the CMS schools of cosmopolitan Freetown, Creole children were exposed to European institutions and cultural practices, giving them a familiarity that later enabled them to work comfortably with the British, French, Germans, and Americans in trade, education, and particularly in the medical profession. Hence, the Creoles became the first major group of westernized elites, and by sheer numbers became the first recruits to study medicine in England. In time Africans from the English-speaking coast of West Africa took the road to Freetown for education in its schools.

Among the other criticisms in his report, Butts also noted the poor health of the repatriated slaves to Freetown, in Fergusson's charge, which he attributed to dietary changes following their arrival in Sierra Leone. Fergusson effectively rebutted this charge by referring to the Colonial Office abstract from the annual report, which, as principal medical officer, he had submitted to the director general of the Army Medical Department in March 1837. Fergusson successfully countered several other criticisms contained in Butts's report. Dysentery affected a large number of the Liberated Africans, Fergusson reported, but the malady had its origins in the slave ships or in places of confinement prior to embarkation rather than on shore, as Butts assumed. The disease often lasted for eight months following arrival and liberation in Sierra Leone, where attempts were made to treat those who were sick through dietary changes and other means. Dysentery, however, was rarely fatal; it appeared even among the Europeans and the natives born in the colony. Fergusson voiced opposition and added rejoinder to a number of other observations in the reports.

The Death of William Fergusson

Shortly after Fergusson's detailed reply to the Butts report, the governor assembled the council and explained, with regret, that on the advice of physicians he was taking a leave to go to England because of health problems. The council unanimously approved of a leave of absence and authorized his son, William Fergusson II, a writer in the civil establishment, to accompany him. The medical officers reported that Fergusson suffered from a severe digestive disorder, accompanied by acute pain, bowel obstruction, emaciation, and symptoms of liver disease. His stomach rejected all foods, even of the mildest type. The administration of the colony was transferred to the colonial secretary.

Fergusson set sail for England on December 27, 1845, aboard the barque *Funchal* and died at sea on Monday, January 19, 1846. After spending twenty-three years of his life in the colony of Sierra Leone, he was highly respected by his peers and colonial authorities. His achievements include the following: raising of medical standards that improved health conditions; increasing the life expectancy of the Creole and British populations; serving in an advisory role to travelers en route elsewhere in West Africa; providing an exemplary model for the mobility of Africans in the colonial service; stimulating commerce in the colony so that it was flourishing at the time of his death; and through his expertise providing a healthy, productive colonial treasury.[28] Charlotte Fergusson, his widow, filed a memorial requesting his pension on March 1846 but the request was denied by the colonial government. While the general rule prevailed against giving pensions to widows of civil servants, the pension fate of Mrs. Fergusson was, indeed, a saga in tragedy.[29] This occurred at almost the same time that the colonial government would consider the need for more trained doctors similar in competency to her late husband.

In the early 1850s the army medical staff began to note a shortage in medical officers on the Gold Coast and in Sierra Leone. In order to provide regular home leave for each British surgeon working in West Africa, a double staff of British physicians was required. This double staff did little good, however, since both convalescence and mortality of the doctors went virtually unchanged. The invalid and mortality rates of the medical staffs at stations in the Gold Coast, Sierra Leone, and Gambia show a loss of twenty-two officers from 1842 through 1852, out of a total of about seventy. Only four medical officers died in the healthier climate of the Mediterranean stations in the same period of a total of about thirty. A remedy was required for the West African situation and a recommendation was not long in the making.[30]

In 1853 Benjamin Hawes, a member of the War Office who had also served in the Colonial Office, proposed that a local medical corps be created and that Africans should receive training as doctors in England. Upon obtaining their medical degree, these newly trained doctors would return and serve in the ranks of British occupational forces in West Africa. Hawes broadened both the geographic origins of Africans to be chosen for study and the selection process when he wrote to the colonial secretary, the duke of Newcastle to inquire

> whether it may not be expedient to select two or more [African youths] for education [in Britain], who when qualified could be appointed to Commissions for medical service in Africa, or if ultimately found unqualified for medical service, might be employed in the civil service of the colony [of Sierra Leone]—the Governors

of Sierra Leone and the Gold Coast—might be able to select some youths whose parents, in consideration of the prospective advantages to be afforded them, would undertake to bear the expense of the maintenance of their sons while studying at the Hospital, the public providing [initial] board and education—and paying the fees necessary for passing through the requisite course of medical study.[31]

These recommendations paved the way for Africans to be trained as physicians, and may have also provided for the organizational framework for African recruitment to the civil service. The War Office was not unmindful of the successful precedent of William Fergusson in West Africa, and no doubt cited him as the model for the success of the project.

In June 1853 W. O. Marshall, an official in the War Office, warned that the new trainees might not be so well received in England: "They will, under any circumstances, have immense difficulties to contend with in the prejudice of this country against the Negro Race. As the sons of Merchants and treated by the Govt throughout as the sons of Gentlemen half these difficulties will be overcome."[32] The ability of Africans to adjust to the European climate also raised considerable concern. "From all that is known at present," one report noted, "the constitution of the Negro is less capable of undergoing transitions of climate, than that of any other race, the facts in this head are few, but they are sufficiently conclusive."[33] The same report held also that mortality from consumption among Negroes was indeed high even in North Africa. In response, Graham Balfour (MD), surgeon to the Royal Military Asylum of England, wrote to Benjamin Hawes in January 1854 that information on the impact of the temperate climate upon Africans was limited. However, he went on, Africans tended to show a high rate of mortality under conditions different from their place of origin. Balfour commented further: "the ratio of mortality among the white population of New York between the ages of 10 and 79 is 15 per 1,000 while that of the coloured inhabitants at the same period of life is 29."[34] The late W. Marshall, in his "Sketch of the Geographical Distribution of Diseases," states "that among Africans in

New York and Philadelphia the annual average mortality is 5.2 percent, whereas it is 2.5 percent among whites." African youths, Balfour continued, would have a higher mortality rate in England than the English population of the same age group, and he anticipated that consumption would take its toll, since no prevention had yet been discovered.

Officials delegated the task of selecting the African trainees to the missionary community. In general, missionary communities in Africa constituted cultural frontiers in ways that resembled the role played by the medieval city in feudal times; these communities were hubs of scientific and intellectual activity. Mission stations attracted people with skills useful for the diffusion of Western technology and, in the case of Sierra Leone, the repatriates and Liberated Africans began to transcend their former ethnic affiliations while residing in the mission stations. The Bible taught that all peoples belonged to one brotherhood. Roland Oliver describes the role of the missionary enclave in East Africa in terms analogous to West Africa:

> Within the enclaves there is no social ostracism to be endured for Christ's sake. There was no sorcerer to threaten with all too material injury the intending backslider from his vested interest. The ancestral spirits, whose power was purely local, could not pursue the delinquent to wreak their vengeance. There were no sexual initiation rites and no ceremonial debauches to inflame the passions beyond their normal vigor. Instead, there was a new social solidarity calculated to support the ethical doctrines of Christianity. Monogamy, the greatest stumbling-block, was a condition of residence, and polygyny in the new economic conditions lost much of its significance as the only means to wealth and power.[35]

It was, therefore, within this framework that African medical specialists surfaced in mid-nineteenth-century Sierra Leone. The Anglican Christian Missionary Society, which supervised the CMS Grammar School in Freetown, selected three young adult Africans for training in Scottish universities in 1854.

African Students as Doctors

It was not until 1855, however, that the most intelligent students were summoned "from the highest of the colored population of Sierra Leone." Samuel Campbell, a Woloff and the oldest, was a favorite student of the Rev. S. J. Koelle, a German missionary and linguist; William Broughton Davies, a Yoruba, passed up a teaching position in England for a medical career; and James Beale Horton, an Igbo, was the third student chosen for medical studies. These students were not sons of merchants but of manual laborers; they had grown up in an open-ended society in Freetown's population of 150,000, where one's color did not stipulate social status in society but social class, especially with access to Europeans who numbered only 150, was a factor. The students were well educated in music, mathematics, the Greek and Roman classics, and in geography. Their manners and intellectual habits were molded in accordance with those of the English middle class, and as long as they were treated fairly, without color becoming an issue, their chances of success would equal those of other students.[36]

The three students were admitted to King's College, University of London, where only three years were required in residence before being allowed to practice medicine; elsewhere in England the years spent in training varied considerably. Since the University of London did not award the medical doctorate under six years of study, it was thought that Edinburgh University should be the next stop for the trainees; here, a student could earn the medical doctorate after four years of training, three of which could be transferred from King's College. Under this arrangement, doctors could return to West Africa to begin patient care at least two years earlier.

The trainees experienced some difficulty in adjusting to both the climate and the medical routines. Apparently, they departed from Sierra Leone in the warm period and arrived in England at the onset of winter. Samuel Campbell had great difficulty with the fogs and cold in London, and at least in his case the health concerns expressed by the War Office for the Africans abroad proved to be warranted. By about the middle of 1855 he developed severe health problems and returned home; within a short time of his arrival back in Freetown, he died of bronchitis. Davies, too, fell ill but survived. Horton survived the climate change without difficulty. In order to make up for their lack of premedical training, the three were required to work a fourteen-hour day. Horton won top honors in his class, including a prize in surgery and five other certificates of honor in related fields of medical study. He soon became a member of the King's College medical society. Horton and Davies successfully passed the qualifying examination, earning membership in the Royal College of Surgeons in 1858 (MRCS), and both were admitted to practice (licentiate in medicine). They left for Scotland next: Horton to Edinburgh and Davies to St. Andrews, Fife, to qualify for the medical degree of MD. It was at Edinburgh that Horton registered as James Africanus Beale Horton, a name that linked him with his continent of origin. At that time the practice of Latinizing one's name was not unusual among scholars of rank, and Horton was acting in accord with a well-established practice.[37]

In October 1858 Davies received his MD from St. Andrews. Edinburgh University conferred their MD degree, which was at that time the first degree, upon Horton in August 1859. His qualifying thesis was titled, "The Medical Topography of the West Coast of Africa, Including Sketches of Its Botany." Horton further described himself as a "native of West Africa" on the title page of the thesis, and entered the new sobriquet "Africanus," which not only suggested a rising political consciousness but served as a harbinger of things to come.

In September 1859 Horton and Davies received commissions in the West African Army Medical Services as staff assistant surgeons for "duties only in West Africa." They returned to Sierra Leone in the same year that epidemics of yellow fever, measles, and smallpox had killed half of the European population. Doctors were among those who fell ill, creating a need for Horton's and Davies's services. However, the epidemics had stopped with the end of the heavy rains, and the government devised other plans for the two, despite petitions from leading citizens for them to remain in Sierra Leone. Much to their disappointment, the doctors were posted to the Gold Coast (modern Ghana) within two days of their arrival in Freetown.

At this time the Gold Coast colony had begun to eclipse Sierra Leone in importance. It received special government status in 1842, and in 1850 the British government separated the Gold Coast from Sierra Leone—the two colonies had been a single unit up until this time—and decided to give the Gold Coast its own governor and other governmental decisionmaking bodies. The Gold Coast had indeed lobbied for this new development, and the British had negotiated with the Fanti people for the imperial need to extend jurisdiction over the coastal area, resulting in some loss of independence for the Fanti. This agreement became known as the Bond of 1844. Having already acquired trading forts from the Danish and Dutch, the British next wished to control the hinterland trade in the north. They also wanted to divert that trade to the British coastal area of jurisdiction, but this objective required a commanding military presence. The British knew that the belligerent Ashanti of the interior was a formidable force, for the Ashanti had already defeated the British as early as 1824 and killed their commander, Governor Sir Charles MacCarthy. Now the West Indian regiment—troops from the West Indies—were garrisoned at Cape Coast under white officers. Hence the government felt that the talents of Horton and Davies could best be served with the medical staff in the Gold Coast.[38]

The posts on the West African coast were the least popular among the British military. The region was considered unhealthy, and the duty—commanding the West Indian regiment—was not prestigious. Some of the officers came out to escape creditors of family obligations and had little real interest in their duties.

The year 1859, when the first African doctors trained under government auspices joined the white medical establishment, also marked the beginning of a pattern of intraprofessional conflict that would persist through colonialism and into the independence era. The medical officers of the British middle class generally refused to regard the African doctors as their peers, and most resented their presence. While Horton's professional skill was never questioned, and he was never recorded as anything but a capable and diligent worker, attempts were made nevertheless to undermine his and Davies's authority with the troops. According to Fyfe: "An axiom of the European empires of race in Africa (and the British Empire during the nineteenth century grew steadily more race-conscious) was the belief that only a white man could command respect from non-white subordinates."[39]

White racial prejudices were reinforced by theories like polygenesis, which held that whites and blacks were not really of the same human species, having evolved from different ancestors. These attitudes remained an unrelenting barrier to upward mobility for the African doctors. Fyfe further reports that Horton's military superiors rotated him from one worn-down, damp station to another in efforts to humiliate him. For the most part Horton kept a low profile for fear that the government would not send other Africans to England to be educated, and went about his work quietly.

In 1872, shortly after the successful treatment of smallpox outbreaks at the Muniford station and in villages in the Windward district of the Gold Coast, Horton completed an application for the vacated post of administrator of the Gold Coast, and in 1880 he applied for the post of brigade-surgeon. He was turned down on both occasions, despite the fact that he had sometimes served in a number of significant civil and military capacities: in all sections of the medical department, as civil commandant both in the Gold Coast and Gambia, as commissioner of the justices of the peace, as military commandant in strategic posts; as the commissariat in large stations; and as superintendent of the medical department in Lagos. In this last position he was in charge of large sums of money, and no impropriety was ever alleged.

The training of more African doctors for service in the army, Horton thought, was the solution to the problem of racial prejudice in the medical profession. British acquisitions in West Africa required new stations, and Horton suggested that Africans should staff them. He made a fervent plea to the government to reinstate the arrangement by which he and Davies had received their medical training.

Horton also proposed local changes that would contribute to developing the West African medical profession. As early as July 13, 1861, he wrote to the War Office to recommend the establishment of a medical school in West Africa. In his letter Horton proposed the establishment of a small medical training facility in Sierra Leone. Attending it would be outstanding young men, not above the age of twenty, selected from the Church Missionary College and schools, with preference given to those demonstrating exceptional ability in Latin, Greek, and mathematics. (In a subsequent letter Horton suggested that the students should be drawn from Great Britain's four colonies and settlements—Gambia, Sierra Leone, Lagos, and Cape Coast.) The new school should offer a two-week program focused on certain preparatory subjects—anatomy and dissection, physiology, chemistry, African botany and natural history, hospital practices, and pharmacy—as well as some more traditional academic subjects. The director of the school should be African and should be given full authority over admissions and the management of the school, although in case of any doubt he was to consult the Church Missionary Society of Sierra Leone. Horton reminded the officials of the War Office that it was very difficult for a student to begin medical training in England without these preliminary courses, and suggested the benefits that would accrue to the country and its people if his program were implemented. The tone of his letter was conciliatory.[40]

Communications on the proposed scheme were forwarded to Dr. Charles O'Callaghan, the principal medical officer, and Captain J. F. Brownwell, commanding officer of the Gold Coast Artillery Corps. The director general of the Army Medical Department sent out a communiqué requesting advice on whether the "intended substitution, either wholly or in part, of native African for European medical officers is likely to be successful."[41] Brownwell commented on December 13, 1861, that the African assistant surgeons sent to his command were comparable to others in performing their duties, but that the European and African communities, the proposed patients for these African medical professionals, lacked confidence in them. The European surgeon was looked upon most favorably, not just among the entire civil community but among the African soldiers as well. O'Callaghan's letter of the same time echoed a similar tone but went one step further. The government had made a mistake, he submitted, in its dispatch of "native" medical officers to the director general: "The Freemen of the tribe of this Protectorate are a forward & high-bred race, & they regard the natives of Sierra Leone especially with a distrust & barbaric a version [*sic*] of which but a feint [*sic*] conception can be entertained in England."[42]

On June 19, 1862, Horton received his long-awaited reply. Secretary Sir George Lewis relayed the information that the War Office was discontinuing "for the present time" the training of Africans as medical doctors, thereby making the proposed scheme unnecessary.

Despite this setback, Horton continued to pursue his advocacy of an indigenous center of higher learning for West Africans. He and Davies had somehow gained access to some of the correspondence concerning the proposal, and they were incensed at the charges that Europeans and local Gold Coast residents had little confidence in their professional abilities. In November 1863, after a long delay caused by probable job rotation assignments and the need to gather more information, Horton wrote a lengthy letter to the Educational Committee of the War Office supported by ten testimonials from European officials and merchants and the principal indigenous merchants, most of whom he had treated. Horton submitted that it was ironic that the War Office would give so much credence to the fallacious statements of O'Callaghan and Brownwell, who had not only just joined the army but whose names in ink had not even dried on the Medical Register. It was doubtful indeed that the European population would give preference to individuals that they scarcely knew over a medical officer of color who had gained their trust. And to say further that the local population would prefer medical assistance from those "neophytes" rather than from well-known physicians of their own color was very doubtful.[43]

Horton argued that his proposal would save the British government money. Since the coastal climate was detrimental to the European medical officer, the government had to send out and recall such medical officers every year, a considerable expense. Eighteen medical officers were stationed on the coast of Africa altogether and at the rate of £80 for passage to England for each officer, the total yearly expenditure for this single purpose was £1,440, or £14,440 in ten years. Horton's scheme, therefore, would not only reduce expenditures but increase efficiency as well, a policy that the government had always espoused.

Governor Richard Pine (1862–66) commented that Brownell and O'Callaghan, with whom he was acquainted, appeared to have moderated their views in the intervening two years, and stated that he personally hoped that Horton's proposal would be implemented. Pine went on to say that the factor of racial prejudice, while admittedly troublesome, would likely diminish in time. He reminded Horton of the late William Fergusson and other Africans—especially Mr. Carr (West Indian), who was appointed chief justice of Sierra Leone—who enjoyed respect and acceptance in the pursuit of their professions.[44] Pine's supportive response leads us to speculate whether Horton would have met with greater success if he had proposed establishing his medical school in the Gold Coast!

Horton, however, discontinued his advocacy for a center for higher learning in West Africa for Africans. Moving toward a more global perspective of the scientific world, he warned that West Africa educated its youth in "the study of only scripture, history, geography, grammar and arithmetic," while the curriculum of science was only available elsewhere in the Commonwealth, such as Australia, India, the West Indies, Canada, and the Cape of Good Hope. In West Africa he asked: "Where are the schools for the study of botany, of mineralogy, of physiology, of chemistry, of engineering, of architecture, and of the other kindred subjects which are the fundamental sciences which elevate the mind and develop the intellectual growth of any race?"[45] Horton advanced the idea of a university of West Africa, suggesting that Fourah Bay College, which was founded in 1827, form the nucleus of such a development. This complex would be staffed by those equipped to teach and carry out research. While the university of West Africa idea was never developed, Fourah Bay College became affiliated with the University of Durham in 1876, beginning a pattern that other universities in West Africa would follow in the twentieth century.

African Physicians and Medical Achievements

Although Horton's initiative failed to gain sufficient support for the establishment of an indigenous African medical infrastructure, the degree of medical knowledge in tropical countries paralleled that in Europe. While physicians had indeed advanced their knowledge of diseases since the eighteenth century, more remained to be explored. The role of insects, bacteria, and viruses in the transmission of disease was not known; accepted medical strategy was still to treat symptoms of illness or the part of the body affected. Some treatments did more harm than good, and often patients were afraid to enter hospitals. One such treatment was bloodletting, a procedure that might remove as much as half of a patient's blood. This procedure was used to treat a disease like malaria, which produces anemia, so bleeding could have disastrous consequences. Calomel, a mercury compound used as a purge and also to induce salivation (seen as evidence that a fever had subsided), was another harmful treatment used against all fevers. Such treatments, in fact, share a major part of the blame for the high mortality rate for Europeans in tropical countries. As early as 1867 Horton explained that calomel and other mercurials were responsible for more deaths than fever, and warned that they had no curative power for malaria, exposing the body to two poisons rather than one.[46]

Horton advocated the integration of traditional and Western medicine in the treatment of diseases and probably he was among the earliest to do so. Horton's MD thesis of 1859 at Edinburgh discusses how bark from the mangrove tree was used in the treatment of fevers in Gambia and how the leaves of the castor oil plant helped to boost the secretion of breast milk among women of the Cape Verde Islands. In Sierra Leone Horton described how the citrus medicae was used to treat seasickness and that the unripe pawpaw (carica papaya) was useful in expelling worms. During his tenure as an army doctor in the Gold Coast, Horton reported how the use of tinctures from the herbal assafetida was useful in curing guinea worm infections.

In 1874 Horton published *The Diseases of Tropical Climates and Their Treatment.* This classic work was the first of its kind written by a West African, describing the accepted methods and treatments of his time. Curatives range from bicarbonate of soda to bloodletting, from olive oil to opium, and from turpentine use to numerous other recommended remedies. Considering that Horton lived in comparative isolation in West Africa, the text is remarkable indeed. Most of his statistics and sanitary and medical information came from his own publications, but he also drew upon such monographs as Budd's *Diseases of the Liver,* Charles Moorehead's *Clinical Researches on Diseases in India,* and from various journals such as the *Lancet,* the *Medical Report of the Army Medical Department,* the *N.A. Medical and Surgical Journal,* the German *Handbook of Historical and Geographical Pathology,* and the *British and Foreign Medical Chirurgical Review.* Horton's book was organized into three parts: part one dealt with fevers, part two with disorders of the gastrointestinal tract, and part three with general afflictions such as anemia, nutritional deficiencies, rheumatism, and parasites.[47]

A subject Horton did not write about was the steady migration of African Americans to West Africa in the nineteenth century and the harsh disease environment that awaited them there. The American Colonization Society, in particular, sponsored the resettlement of free blacks to Liberia beginning in the 1820s; its goal was the removal of the entire black population from the United States. Out of 4,571 emigrants sent to Liberia between 1820 and 1843, only 1,819 remained in 1843; malaria being the principal killer. Certainly, Horton was aware of the problem: he was raised in the repatriated society of Freetown, and his second wife, Selina Elliot, was an African American. E. A. Ayandele suggests a possible explanation for Horton's silence on the subject: "the nineteenth-century African educated elite and blacks in the New World did not form a monolithic unity in their ideas and vision to the extent usually assumed by scholars of African-Negro relations. The thinking, the points of emphasis, and the visions entertained by Negroes in the New World, or with the New World background, were never identical with those of their African counterparts whose ideas and hopes were determined essentially, quite often exclusively, by the African milieu and events on the African continent."[48] Horton's prolific writings on scientific and sociopolitical subjects may well have been motivated by the need to demonstrate to the world at large the intellectual capabilities of the African physician. In the world of Horton in nineteenth-century West Africa, researcher Edith Sanders shows that race was a hierarchical construct headed by the Teutonic and Anglo-Saxon peoples, and followed, in descending order, by the Slavs; the Hamites, who were introduced as a new "breed" and the representatives of European civilization in Egypt; and finally the "Negroes" (that also included Africans), who were at first the cursed sons of Ham. This "invention" of Ham was shifted after 1798—the year of Napoleon's conquest of Egypt and the foundation of Egyptology—to the cursed sons of Canaan, who were of the "southern nations" and black. Canaan's brothers Cush and Mizraim were not cursed. Egyptologists of 1798 held that Mizraim was white, and the "father of Egypt." Egypt next became a "white civilization" and so passed on into world history. The blacks, now of sub-Saharan Africa and of the diaspora by these "invented traditions," were at the lowest rung of this pseudoscientific racial classification.

Using the West as a measuring rod for achievement, Horton wished to raise the level of achievement for Africans. But as Horton's *West African Countries and People* shows, he was a black Victorian and middle class in his cultural view. As an adherent to the cyclical theory of history, he believed that nonliterate people had no history—"a Hegelian idea," an idea that African history of the last thirty years has virtually destroyed. Hence, Horton was provincial; his ideas for the development of the race were exclusively focused on West Africans and his British mentors, and he did not concern himself with the problems of blacks in the diaspora. For example, two African Americans—Ewing Glasgow and Robert Johnson—matriculated with Horton at the University of Edinburgh in 1858 during the apogee of slavery in the United States. Although both were politically active in publicizing the abolitionist cause, Horton remained indifferent to abolitionists. Frederick Douglass visited Edinburgh shortly after Horton's departure; our assessment of Horton on this matter might be different had they met. In contrast, Edward Blyden (1832–1912) was an educator and pan-African patriot, who directed his cultural nationalist messages to African Americans and Africans alike; the need for unity on both sides of the Atlantic between leaders of both groups remained his essential theme. Horton, on the other hand, might have lost some of his confidence in the civilized world had he lived to see the age of pessimism in Europe and the coming of World War I. However, he died from erysipelas in 1883 in Freetown at the age of forty-eight.

Physicians after James Horton

By midcentury other Sierra Leoneans were receiving medical training in Great Britain and making important contributions to their society. Robert Smith (MRCS, 1865, England; FRCS, 1871, Edinburgh) began his career in 1865, holding a position as deputy inspector of health and shipping and later becoming an able assistant colonial surgeon in charge of the Colonial Hospital, Freetown. Future doctors received their training from him in the dispensaries. Thomas Hamilton Spilsbury (MRCS, 1865, England) started his service at Banjul (then called Bathurst), Gambia, in 1872. Spilsbury was colonial surgeon for several years, the first African to head a medical department in the British West African colonies. Before he died in 1890, Spilsbury had been joined in Gambia by D. P. Taylor (MRCS, 1875, England). Of Yoruba descent, Taylor received medical certification at King's College, London. Shortly after graduation in 1874, he went off to Gambia and engaged in private practice until his death in 1904. John Farrell Easmon (MRCS, 1879, England; LKQCP and LM, Ireland; MD, Brussels, with distinction) emerged in the early 1890s as the holder of the highest post ever for an African in the Colonial Medical Service; he is the subject of our fourth chapter. William Renner (MRCS, 1880, England; LKQCP and LM, Ireland; MD, 1881, Brussels, with high distinction), who took the name Awooner-Renner in 1912, was assistant colonial surgeon from 1882 to 1913. He served on a number of occasions as principal medical officer to William Thomas Prout (BM, ChM, Edinburgh), a British medical officer. Joseph Spilsbury Smith (LSA, LRCP and S, 1883, Edinburgh), the younger brother of Robert Smith, served in the Gold Coast until his death in 1894. Sylvester Cole (MD, MS, 1883, St. Andrews) began service on the Gold Coast. Isaac Nicol Paris (MB, BS, 1889, Dunelm) served as medical officer in Sierra

Leone from 1892 until his accidental death in 1897. Other names could be added to this list of Africans who contributed in important ways to raising the medical standard of medical care in Sierra Leone, while demonstrating competence equal to that of the colonial doctors coming from the British middle class.

The Nigerian Medical Returnees

African doctors, whose parents had been repatriated to Sierra Leone after being recaptured at sea from slavers, also returned to their ancestral homeland, Nigeria, with medical degrees in hand. Sierra Leone had served as their initial center for education and preparation for medical training in Great Britain. Dr. Nathaniel King (b. 1847), however, was not only a product of the Sierra Leone connection, having been born in Hastings on July 14, 1847, but also a successful student in the early 1860s at the first premedical school established at Abeokuta in Nigeria. Under the auspices of the CMS in London and not the colonial government, medical missionaries founded the medical school and taught anatomy, physiology of muscle action, natural philosophy, chemistry, and materia medica to young boys in the mission. The school closed down in 1864 with the death of its founder, and King, with the help of a rich maternal uncle, returned to Sierra Leone to study at Fourah Bay College in 1866. In 1871 he enrolled in King's College, London, where he received his MRCS in 1874. He received the MBCM in 1876 and the MD from Edinburgh in 1879. The CMS aided in the funding of his medical training. Following his return to Lagos in 1879, he found the era's racial discriminatory policies restricted both the nature of his appointments and his salary. King participated in the early campaigns of environmental sanitation in the colony of Lagos and contributed to the development of modern medicine in West Africa until his death in June 1884.

Other notable African doctors included all the following men, whose qualifications and careers are briefly described. Obadiah Johnson (1849–1920), a Nigerian, (LSA, London; MRCS, 1884, England; MB, ChB, 1886, Edinburgh; MD, 1889, Edinburgh) was medical officer in Lagos in 1890 to 1897 and subsequently went into private practice. He wrote *The Therapeutics of West Africa* and rewrote and edited *The History of the Yorubas,* which was originally written by his brother, Rev. Samuel Johnson. Then there was C. J. Lumpkin (LRCS and LRCP, 1884, Edinburgh; MD, 1884, Brussels), who served as medical officer in Lagos until 1895 and then entered private practice. John Randall (MB, ChM, 1888, Edinburgh), a contemporary of John Farrell Easmon, was medical officer at Lagos from 1890 to 1893 and went into a thriving private practice there. Randall (1855–1928) wrote on guinea worm infestations and on the incidence of cancer among Africans. First known as Alexander Johnson Williams (1861–1935), Oguntola Odunbaku Sapara (LRCP, 1895, Edinburgh; LFPS, 1895, Glasgow) returned to Lagos in 1895 and held an unbroken record of service in the colonial medical department for thirty-two years. He received numerous accolades for the most meritorious and longest service of any Nigerian colonial surgeon of his time. Sapara displayed an unusual interest in lay medicine, and perhaps is best remembered for his destruction of the smallpox worshippers, known as the *Sopona*—the god of smallpox. He is remembered as well for numerous achievements in bringing modern medical technology into twentieth-century Nigeria.[49]

The Edinburgh Model versus the British Model

These achievements by the physician elites were remarkable indeed if one considers that the West African region as a whole did not possess a true scientific community in the nineteenth century. In fact, one might have to go as far as Scotland to find an example of a fully developed intellectual and scientific center at that time. An intellectual backwater in the seventeenth century, the Scots began to develop a reputation for medical excellence throughout Europe in the eighteenth century. Scottish medicine did not develop in isolation but as part of a general intellectual movement resulting from a number of factors. First, population growth and shifts to the cities led to the development of an urban middle class that demanded medical services. Edinburgh, Glasgow, and Aberdeen were the largest cities and the main centers for commercial and industrial growth. Second, the development of education was the most important factor producing the renaissance. In the case of Scotland, researchers Vern and Bonnie Bullough in 1971 showed that out of a total sample taken of 375 persons (364 men and 11 women) included in their data for the eighteenth century, 9 persons, 3 of whom were women, were known to have no formal education—(3 percent of the total sample); however, in 105 cases in the sample (28 percent) showed no degree of certainty about the type of education received at even the elementary level or how long; another 48 persons (almost 13 percent) were taught privately either by their parents, a tutor, or through other means. When the total sample is considered, 248 (66 percent) attended the university and only 78 (almost 21 percent) did not matriculate. The role of class in the Scottish urban setting and access to educational centers was significant in this unique development. Since prolonged schooling was expensive, most members of the sample (55 percent) were born into urban upper middle-class families, 8 percent into the upper class, 27 percent into the lower middle class, and 10 percent into the lower class.[50] The growth of medical achievement in eighteenth-century Scotland was dependent upon population increases in the upper-class families who consulted doctors and increased the need for more doctors to be trained. Even more, the general growth in scientific and intellectual literacy explains the emergence in Scotland of such medical practitioners as Benjamin Bell, Joseph Black, William Cullen, John Fothergill, Francis Home, John and William Hunter, James Lind, Alexander Monro, "primus, secundus, and tertius,"[51] Mungo Park, Benjamin Rush, William Smellie, Robert Whyatt, as well as numerous others in the intellectual fields, such as Adam Smith, Sir Walter Scott, Robert Burns, James Watt, David Hume, James Boswell, and James Mill.

Further, the major Scottish commercial and industrial centers had universities within their confines; Oxford and Cambridge, in contrast, were removed from such centers. Edinburgh had the most effective alliance of population growth, urbanization, prosperity, and opportunities for education. Its medical faculty dates from 1726, and standards for the medical degree were set by organized medical groups in Scotland. Edinburgh suffered from no dearth of students, for "the average number of medical graduates per year by decade is as follows: 1751–60, 11; 1761–70, 12; 1771–80, 21; 1781–90, 28; 1791–1800, 39; 1801–10, 40."[52] The achievements of these alumni made Edinburgh a household word in nineteenth-century West Africa. African elites were also attracted to Scotland because of its liberal tradition and tolerance for dissent. Since British colonialism was evolving in West Africa, the medical elite had something in common with the Scots, whose nationalism had already found expression against the British.

But West Africa's developing peripheral relation with the core of Europe in control of the world order meant a delay in the development of a medical and scientific community comparable to that in the core region. And as proto-nationalism rose in West Africa, the scientific needs of the region became more political. The British presence and the power of colonial authority meant that its model of scientific development rather than that of Edinburgh would be followed. The college would play only a partial role, if any, in the development of medical education and medical professionalism; and, as at Oxford and London in the nineteenth century, medicine would develop in isolation from the college. The African medical elite lost an opportunity to train more African professionals and to elevate its status because of the factor of intraprofessional conflict that was introduced by the English. And to the medical elite, university training provided for a more powerful lobbying position toward influencing the state. Medical training provided a way for the medical elites to distinguish themselves from, and seek preferential treatment over, their traditional competitors—apothecaries, grocers, barbers, and the lay African practitioner. As matters turned out, the colonial administrators did nothing to alter this situation—a legacy which still hampers health care delivery in independent Africa. They could (and should) have created more medical centers in the urban and rural villages with nurses and doctors to operate them. Two health systems prevailed; the emerging African elite patronized medical doctors in the cities, but in the urban slums and rural peripheries, folk remedies and the lay healer remained dominant. The shortened life span further diminished the likelihood of intergenerational mobility among the doctors, denied them of scholastic attainment, and denied them of the privilege of living long enough to update their work. While the medical profession was a status symbol to the aspiring African, success could also be marred by tragedy, as in the case of the Sierra Leone nexus in the Gold Coast in 1897. So we now turn to consider the third generation of African physicians and this tragedy in the colonial history of West Africa.

CHAPTER FOUR

The Easmon Episode

*T*he third generation of African physicians faced unusual challenges. Pseudoscientific racism permeated the colonial service in West Africa at the end of the nineteenth century. While Africans and West Indians had held high administrative positions in the earlier so-called "open phase" in the colonial service, the color bar became a fact of life in the 1890s as the British middle class began to monopolize top posts. Africans in all branches of the colonial service, many of whom had been educated in the same schools as their European counterparts, now found their careers blocked by racism and intraprofessional conflict.[1]

By the 1870s the Gold Coast colony was the most powerful center in British West Africa. Competing British stations along the coast were annexed in 1871 with the Gold Coast at the apex. This process restrained the unbridled expansionist interests of British trading companies. After 1874 the British and their African allies had broken the military power of the Ashanti in the interior and assumed protectorate rule. Existing British trade with the coast was now linked to the interior chiefs with more efficiency and with less cost to the government. The lure of gold and other commodities drew African merchants and European trading firms to the northern region because of more security under British authority. Domestic change was marked by the emancipation of slavery, which created a larger labor force available for wage-earning employment. The year 1874 also was notable for the publication of at least sixteen works on the Gold Coast and Ashanti affairs by British writers, who included soldiers, journalists, adventurers, missionaries, and colonial administrators. The British version of the Gold Coast past or imperialist historiography was the dominant focus of these books. This was disheartening to the African intelligentsia because the studies, unlike those of the Ashanti and Muslim kin of the northern groups, rendered them and their ancestors invisible or left them with only minor roles. These books served a multifold purpose: they distorted the past of the Gold Coast and extolled the acquisition of English cultural skills, values, and knowledge. But British colonial law made all Africans "natives" and subordinate to the British middle class. Secondly, the books became manuals for the British colonial administrators with the advent of a formal empire and the scramble to negate the past of the Gold Coast. (The African intelligentsia understood the need to dismantle the imperialist historiography and began to do so from the 1890s onward through publication of their own books.)[2] Lagos, a coastal state until 1851 when the British imposed protectorate status in order to suppress slavery and create a site for a consulate (in 1852), was first administered from the West African station at Sierra Leone. Still tied to Sierra Leone, Lagos became a crown colony in 1862. This status changed again in 1874, when Lagos was transferred to the authority of the Gold Coast. This relationship persisted until 1886, when Lagos became a separate colony.[3]

These developments in the colonial infrastructure, however, created a demand for African personnel. Just as it had earlier in the century, Sierra Leone continued to supply British needs from Freetown—the center of recruitment and posting for the British colonial apparatus in West Africa—but this did not help Sierra Leone's development. K. A. B. Jones-Quartey described this brain drain in the following manner: "For generations in the early days of the opening up of West Africa, involuntary Sierra Leonean expatriates were sent out to the Gambia, Nigeria, the Gold Coast, Dahomey, Fernando Po, and elsewhere by Government, the Church, and the trading firms; . . . they went as accountants, clerks, teachers, ministers, and even top administrators, without whom no modern processes or installations in those countries could have been worked."[4] However, the use of quinine against *falciparum* malaria permitted the gradual increase of the European population on the coast, and the Berlin Conference of November 1884 and February 1885 signaled the end of the informal empire, the first phase of the European presence in Africa marked by commercial ambition and the establishment of trading posts. The Berlin Conference represented the beginning of formal empire, the phase characterized by political ambition, guns, and steamships, and the partitioning of Africa into territorial boundaries that led to the creation of the colonial states. These boundary groupings respected the rights of an emerging centralized control for each of the separate European powers in Africa such as the British, French, German, Portuguese, Belgians, and Italians. But these developments created problems for the African elite. Since the African medical elite held some of the highest posts under incipient colonialism, they were the first to experience career constraints under the new forms of domination. As the chief medical officer (CMO) in the Gold Coast, John Farrell Easmon was the highest ranking African in the colonial service from 1893 to 1896. His duties as CMO included the supervision of medical officers under his charge; responsibility for medical attendance to the European and African officials in government employment; the direction and supervision of the sanitary needs of the colony; the welfare of and attendance upon the poor in the dispensaries and hospitals of the colony; and in the governor's absence, he occasionally became the acting governor. His dismissal from high office serves as

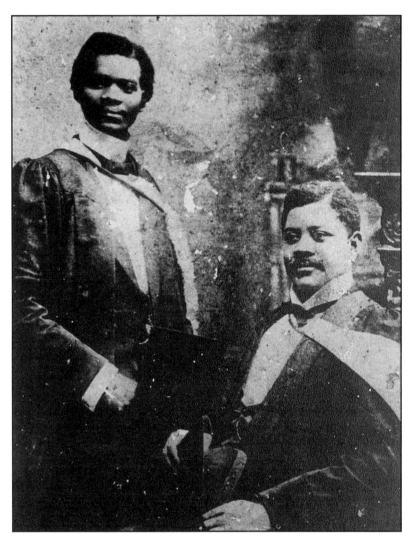

Figure 3. Drs. Albert Whiggs Easmon (standing) and John Farrell Easmon, Ghana, Gold Coast, c. 1896. Courtesy of R. S. Easmon.

the most appropriate paradigm to analyze intraprofessional conflict and the changing status of the African medical community in the Gold Coast.

The 1880s witnessed a new generation of African doctors in West Africa who did not owe their training to the colonial government. The doctors of the 1880s, like the earlier ones, studied at Freetown in the secondary schools and at Fourah Bay College, but their merchant parents and relatives of means usually paid for their medical training in England, Scotland, and Belgium rather than the government. Sierra Leone and Nigeria continued to supply most of the doctors during the nineteenth century because the Liberated Africans were the first to be sponsored by the CMS for medical education, and by the 1880s intergenerational mobility paved the way for others. Since the Gold Coast supply of Liberated Africans was zero, the impact of the CMS and its educational opportunities bypassed Africans in the Gold Coast. This is the reason why only two doctors came from the Gold Coast in the latter part of the nineteenth century.

To the financial independence of some of the third generation of Sierra Leone doctors was added another important element: a tradition of independent thinking, particularly among the doctors of Nova Scotian descent. Deprived of the land promised to them by the British for their loyalty in the American War of Independence, they retained a mistrust of the British and a habit of relying on their own resources.[5] Davidson Nicol sums up some of the salient characteristics of the early Nova Scotians: "Their social exclusivity from the Maroons, the Liberated Africans and the indigenous communities alienated them; they were largely snubbed by the Europeans. . . . By the middle of the nineteenth century when they started intermarrying with the others, they appeared to have lost their social and economic dominance to the Liberated Africans. . . . But their political influence of radicalism and of fighting against white supremacy and whatever they considered to be unjust, remained."[6] John Farrell Easmon (see figure 3), who distinguished himself in the world of medical scholarship, proved to be the most formidable representative of the Nova Scotian tradition in the new generation of African doctors.

Dr. John Farrell Easmon: Medical Rebel

John Farrell Easmon was born on June 30, 1856, in Freetown, Sierra Leone, of a Nova Scotian settler family, who had first come from the United States via Nova Scotia in 1792. There were 1,131 in their settler group. His father, Walter Richard Easmon, married three times; John Farrell Easmon's mother was Mary Ann MaCormack, the second wife. Born in Londonderry in 1794, she was the daughter of John Ma-Cormack, a scion of a renowned Northern Ireland medical family. MaCormack arrived in West Africa in 1813 and developed a thriving timber business for export, which, it is said, was the first major export business from the crown colony of Sierra Leone. MaCormack went on to hold several offices in the colonial government; an influential man, he involved himself in peacemaking in the interior and at times represented the governor in treaty negotiations. He returned to Great Britain in 1864 and died in London in 1866. But John MaCormack had kept his grandchildren in Africa in mind; upon the settlement of his estate, Easmon inherited £400.

John Farrell Easmon first matriculated at the Roman Catholic primary school in Freetown and attended the grammar school under James Quaker in 1868 for his secondary education. There, some of his peers were William Awooner-Renner, Obadiah Johnson, Joseph Smith, and John Randall, all future doctors; future barristers Abraham and Jabez Hebron and Peter Awooner-Renner; and others such as Principal Moore, Solomon Farmer, and Matthew Marke. Joseph Smith was the first in Sierra Leone to obtain the FRCSE (the highest specialist surgery degree in Great Britain), and Easmon was allowed to serve under his tutelage as apprentice dispenser and nurse in the colonial hospital. Easmon abruptly departed for medical study in London in 1876, taking with him his inheritance.

Easmon enrolled in the University College on Gower Street with a self-imposed allowance of £8. 6s. 8d per month. Qualification required four years of study, and in 1879 he earned the MRCS, following a distinguished academic career. In his final year Easmon took six gold and silver medals, and the Sierra Leone newspapers published several laudatory accounts of his accomplishments. After London he studied in Ireland, earning the LM and LKQCP. Following that

Easmon went on to Brussels to earn his MD, the most popular degree from the 1840s to the 1880s,[7] with distinction.

Opportunity beckoned again from a distant cousin of the Irish branch of the MaCormack family. Sir William MaCormack, president of the Royal College of Surgeons, senior surgeon at St. George's Hospital in London, surgeon to Queen Victoria, and perhaps the most decorated physician in Europe at the time, heard of his cousin's success and offered Easmon an appointment at St. George's as house surgeon, a position that would ultimately lead to an assistantship. This was the first such appointment ever offered to a West African but, for reasons unknown to this writer, Easmon spurned the offer and returned to Freetown instead.

There he set up his practice at 2 East Street, and he was quickly sought out by settlers in need of medical treatment. Observers noted how he dressed in the proper English medical attire: a silk top hat, a frock coat, and striped trousers. Thus, John Farrell Easmon became the first in a long line of distinguished medical practitioners (see figure 4).[8] The medical family tradition, however, was not the only route to distinction in West African social history.

Through time his success allowed for the concentration of diverse resources in the hands of a small number of elite families. It brought together couples with the best educations, those familiar with colonial rulers and their institutions and culture, and those individuals

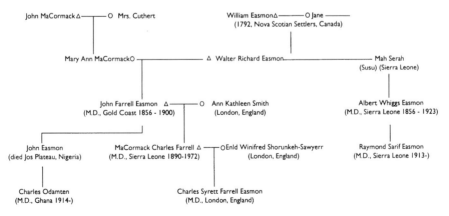

Figure 4. Easmon family genealogy.

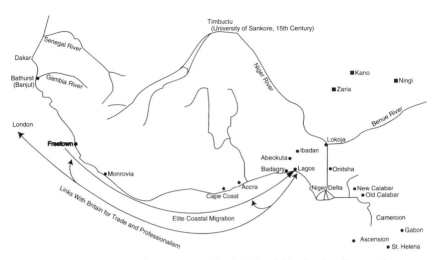

Map 3. Sierra Leone expatriate communities in West Africa in the nineteenth century

pragmatic enough to recognize the advantages of consolidating non-material assets. In addition, the web of relationships—conjugal and affinal—operated through extensive networks in the schools (both at home and abroad), at work, in the financial institutions, and within the colonial bureaucracy. Even further, as Kristin Mann has shown, individuals who in the precolonial era had been part of extensive lineages of corporate descent (that is, members of the general same group), transferred their allegiance to a different type of group, one united by a common identity and goals and based on the elite social class invention of new traditions.[9] Over the course of his life Easmon developed an array of connections with prominent families all along the West African coast—in Bathurst (Banjul), Freetown, Cape Coast, Lagos, Calabar, the Cameroons, Fernando Po, and Gabon—mutually beneficial in various ways for reinforcing and extending their elite status (see map 3).

Easmon in the Gold Coast

Easmon decided to leave his private practice in Sierra Leone and applied for a job in the Gold Coast Medical Service sometime in 1880. The need to increase his income may have prompted the move. On orders from the secretary of state for the colonies, Government House of Sierra Leone informed Governor H. J. Ussher (1879–80) in the Gold Coast of Easmon's appointment as assistant colonial surgeon on September 10, 1880. Easmon was to receive a salary of £400, rising by triennial increments of £50 to £500 a year; free quarters or an allowance in lieu of them; and the right to private practice. On October 9, 1880, Easmon received an advance of £50 and proceeded by steamer to the Gold Coast.[10]

From 1880 to 1882 Easmon was posted at Kwitta (Keta), Awuna District, in Ewe territory, where he was temporarily placed in general charge of the district, including the additional assignment of suppressing smugglers at Affonhoo. He received a commendation from the secretary of state for a job well done. From 1882 to 1883 Easmon was in Accra; he went to Lagos in 1883; and returned to Accra in the same year. There Dr. Joseph Jeans, the colonial surgeon, appointed him to administer the medical department in his absence. Akim was his next assignment, where he served on the Assinee Boundary Commission from 1883 to 1884. Fyfe reported that Easmon produced the first original contribution to European medical science ever written by a West African physician.[11] This assessment requires qualification because of Africanus Horton's earlier scientific studies. His magnum opus was *The Diseases of Tropical Climates and Their Treatment* (1874), based on more than a decade of medical experiments in the region.

On the other hand, the archival data support T. S. Gale's and Fyfe's findings and show the uniqueness of Easmon's contribution. Gale notes that "The term 'blackwater fever' was coined by Dr. J. Farrell Easmon in the Gold Coast in 1884 and thereafter it became the local name for hemoglobinuric fever. [In brochure form in 1884] Easmon wrote the first clinical analysis of the symptoms of the disease in English [J. F. Easmon, *Blackwater Fever,* London 1884]."[12] Easmon wrote this while administering the medical department in Accra in 1884.[13]

In Easmon's time hemoglobinuric fever was the most severe and yet least understood complication of falciparum malaria in West Africa. It struck many Europeans, but it was rare among the indigenous people, who had developed genetic resistance to malaria. It was recognized as a distinct syndrome in 1864, but Easmon's analysis in the Gold Coast was the first to show its most important symptoms to be severe anemia and excess hemoglobin in the urine. It struck people whose constitutions had been weakened by frequent bouts of falciparum malaria, and the mortality rate could reach 50 percent. The preferred treatment in the clinics and hospitals was a sizable dose of quinine. The Gold Coast governor forwarded Easmon's *Blackwater Fever* clinical brochure to the Colonial Office on December 15, 1888. On April 24, 1889, the Royal College of Physicians noted receipt of materials on blackwater fever from Easmon and other medical observers, thereby providing data on the disease that would be valuable to other colonial medical officers.[14]

Proper acknowledgment for Easmon's role in this discovery was long in coming, for several possible reasons. Although the data show that Easmon proved the relationship between blackwater fever and malaria, other medical researchers may have been careless in reviewing the medical literature and missed his study. Nevertheless, in *Tropical Medicine* (1913, second edition), the authors Castellani and Chambers refer to Easmon's first use of the term "blackwater fever."[15] Nevertheless, many colonial medical authorities refused to recognize blackwater fever as a separate syndrome and its relationship to malaria until around World War I.[16] However, in about 1917 E. W. Wood-Mason qualified for the degree of MD with his thesis "The Relationship of Blackwater Fever to Malaria" at the University of Aberdeen; in his review of the literature and bibliography, there is no reference to Easmon's groundbreaking work. By 1922 the Wood-Mason thesis had been sent out by the Colonial Office to Sierra Leone for circulation among members of the West African medical staff. Prior to this general circulation, Dr. E. H. Tweedy—evidently ignorant of Easmon's earlier findings—made the following remarks in a memo to the colonial secretary in October 1917: "I have carefully read this essay which reflects the greatest credit on the Author and shows that Dr. Wood-Mason has a thorough grasp of this most interesting subject. Dr. Wood-Mason has put forward a strong case and certainly to my mind has proved that there is a direct connection between the two diseases."[17] It is remarkable that Easmon published a brochure in

London in 1884 about blackwater fever, and yet this appears to be regarded as a new discovery in 1917. (One might understand if it had been originally published in Africa, but Easmon was not a figure of admiration in colonial circles even in 1917—this is elaborated on in chapter 6—and this colonial attitude was used to impede the employment of his son. This possibly explains Tweedy's omission of Easmon's finding. Another possibility was that the publisher went bankrupt and failed to distribute most of the copies of Easmon's brochure.) Nevertheless, this episode was just one among many in which white colonial officials demonstrated an insulting lack of regard for the intelligence and abilities of their African counterparts.

Easmon's reputation soared in the Gold Coast as a result of his official brochure on blackwater fever, and Easmon went on to hold other administrative posts. While he was stationed at the Accra General Hospital in early 1885, Easmon's treatment of the indigenous people aided in diminishing their suspicion toward Western medicine and expanded its sphere of acceptance among the African population. While the herbalists maintained their attraction for many people, a single day's records show 53 inpatients and 106 outpatients treated at the hospital during Easmon's stay. He was indeed responsible for attracting more African patients.[18]

In the 1880s public sanitation was still a significant problem in Accra. David Patterson reports that government gave only scant attention to sewage and trash disposal, or to the pigs that ran freely in the streets. In 1896 Easmon still described Accra as "a sink of filth."[19] Even more, it was a common practice for the government to move its doctors on short notice, and the government had Easmon in almost constant rotation. He was a comparatively low-level medical officer during these years, one who was moved around in response to medical need and one who might not have the authority to make a significant difference, for example, in the way Western medicine was accepted by the indigenous population or in sanitary practices. Apparently, he moved next to Akim to take charge of the medical department for an additional six months in 1885. As an indication of his rising importance in the Akim community, located in the eastern region, he became president of the executive committee of the Colonial and Indian Exhibition, Gold Coast section, which involved collecting, packaging, and transmitting the Gold Coast exhibits to England. These exhibits were a showcase of Africa's products and they facilitated trade in a wider world. Easmon continued to receive a wide variety of assignments during the remainder of the 1880s and into the 1890s. He worked in Accra, Salaga, and Winneba during 1886 and 1887 as the medical officer and district commissioner. In 1888 he was in Cape Coast and Accra as acting CMO. During his stay there he accompanied Governor William Brandford Griffith (1885–95) on inspection tours of Windward districts and on the Akim/Sarteh expeditions. Between 1889 and 1890 he was the acting chief medical officer for the Gold Coast colony. In these latter years he also served as the honorary secretary of the Agricultural, Commercial, and Mineralogical Society of the Gold Coast colony, whose membership included British firms in search of minerals; and secretary/president of the Census Committee[20] of the country's first census of 1890.[21] Easmon was still a doctor and these assignments, rather than being interruptions, represented an agenda that linked him closer with colonial power politics and future promotion.

In 1892, during his thirteenth year of practice (twelve in the Gold Coast), Easmon heard that Dr. Donald Ross, the colonial surgeon, would be leaving Sierra Leone for Jamaica. (Ross subsequently received the Nobel Prize for his discovery that the anopheles mosquito was the carrier of the *plasmodium* parasite that causes malaria.) At the time Easmon worked as a senior assistant surgeon, so he decided to apply for the vacant position. He may have known of Ross's criticisms of the colonial medical apparatus and his statement that "all the native Assistant Surgeons should be placed on the same footing,"[22] presumably with European medical officers. He may have hoped that Ross would exercise his influence to have Easmon promoted to the vacant position. However, the position was given in 1895 to Dr. William Thomas Prout, who had previously served in Mauritius. Although Prout had extensive experience with tropical diseases, he had less seniority than Easmon. Nevertheless, there is reason to believe Easmon had another goal in mind and was not disappointed at being passed over.

Governor Griffith: A Powerful Ally

Easmon's real objective may have been a promotion in the Gold Coast, where his success would be more likely because of his eight-year friendship with Governor Sir Brandford Griffith. Griffith, in fact, had refused to recommend Easmon, who served as his personal physician and confidant, for the appointment as colonial surgeon in Sierra Leone, feeling Easmon to be too valuable to the Gold Coast colony. Easmon had high recommendations from the CMO extending back to 1890, and in June 1892 the governor wrote to the Colonial Office, explaining that Easmon was indeed well qualified for the job he sought but that his removal from the colony would constitute a misfortune for not only the inhabitants of Accra but to each European, official and unofficial, at the colonial headquarters. He reminded the Colonial Office further that "Dr. Easmon's wonderful skill as a physician, his successful treatment of local diseases, his frequent visits and unremitting attention to his patients, his courage in difficult cases,—combined with gentleness as a nurse and a singular power of raising the spirits of his patients and making them more and more hopeful each time he visits them, are qualities which have attracted and attached people to him, and are invaluable at Accra where the European population has increased so much of late."[23] The motive for denying Easmon the promotion was not a selfish one, the governor went on, although it might appear so, but because of the general disappointment that his departure from the colony would create. For that reason, he just could not bring himself to recommend Easmon's promotion to Sierra Leone. Nevertheless, his demurring constituted a resounding endorsement of Easmon's skill from the highest level of colonial government at Christianborg Castle, a former Danish fort and then purchased by the British in 1850.

Easmon, however, had left himself an out. In his letter of June 1892 seeking the Sierra Leone appointment, he suggested that should the exigencies of public service in the colony prove inimical to his promotion, the colony should ask him to be considered for future vacancies of an administrative nature. He included a summary of his medical achievements from university days to 1892.

When J. D. McCarthy, the CMO for the Gold Coast colony, announced his retirement late in 1892, Easmon promptly applied for the position. F. M. Hodgson, the Gold Coast colonial secretary, confirmed Easmon's appointment. Easmon's outstanding professional skill was again borne out in testimony, and his salary, then at £600 per annum, rose to £800 with the promotion, with annual increments of £50 to the ceiling of £1,000 per annum, the salary then enjoyed by McCarthy. There were conditions, however, among them that Easmon was to be barred from private practice except "when it may be necessary that he should assist at 'consultations.'"[24] On May 17, 1893, Easmon assumed his post. Not since the appointment of William Fergusson, a West Indian, as principal medical officer and later governor of the Sierra Leone colony in 1845, had an African medical officer received such an important promotion in such an important colony.

Easmon accepted the appointment in a letter to the colonial secretary on June 1893, expressing appreciation to all the officials who supported him for the position. He did not, however, agree to all the conditions accompanying his appointment, especially the discontinuance of private practice. "With the reference to the conditions of the appointment," Easmon wrote, "I shall address you in a separate and distinct communication."[25]

The private practice issue was one of continuous vexation in the British Empire in West Africa. African doctors did indeed exercise the option of entering private practice, which enabled them to avoid the British and colonial regulations altogether. The small number of consultant patients put would-be competitors at a disadvantage in seeking private practice. Employment in the Colonial Medical Service plus private practice provided two sources of income, and some African patients began to believe that African doctors' medicine was better because of their association with the British or something white, rather than autonomous African medical practice or something black. Easmon noted that he had never fully accepted the terms of his appointment as CMO of the colony, which meant that he planned to continue his private practice. Although he promised to write further about the conditions of his appointment, he never did.

Consultation required either one or two medical officers present with the CMO in the treatment of patients, but it was almost impossible to have this number present because there were only two medical men at the Accra station. More often than not Easmon worked the station alone. When Governor Griffith had earlier been pressed about the conditions of employment, he had replied: "Doctor I heartily congratulate you on your appointment, but, recalled, whether you are Chief Medical Officer or not, I will always require you to attend me personally. I hold you personally responsible for the care of all my European officials; you must look after the European ladies, the wives of the officials; wait until the question of your private practice is raised."[26] At the same time Easmon reminded him of his very large clientele, which consisted of almost the whole private practice in Accra, the place where his reputation as physician and surgeon had been established. Many of the clients were personal friends of his and some patients had been under his care for years. Hence, it was not feasible to suddenly halt the private practice. Easmon promised to give up the private practice gradually, which he had done. The classes of patients attended, however, consisted of those in consultation with other medical officers, personal friends, old patients with diseases that required long treatment, wives of fellow officers not eligible for gratuitous medical aid such as all the English ladies, and former paying patients whom he often treated at his own expense.

Colonial medical doctors were not supposed to see private patients without the approval of their superiors, especially while on official duty, nor ever sell drugs from the colonial pharmacy to private patients. Obviously, some colonial doctors were very popular with European firms and the African elite whose members sought them out for consultation; if unregulated, this could become quite profitable and create jealousy among unpopular doctors, whether in government or in private practice. It is well known that as a former senior assistant colonial surgeon, Easmon had a sizable private practice. McCarthy, the retired CMO, may also have engaged in private practice while holding the position.

Easmon became CMO of a medical establishment whose budget was £15,621 by 1896, and with approximately twenty-two medical officers under his control. These included one chief medical officer, one colonial surgeon, two senior assistant colonial surgeons, and eighteen assistant colonial surgeons.[27] Besides Easmon there were three other African medical officers, Drs. Spilsbury Smith and J. O. Coker, both of Sierra Leone, and B. W. Quartey-Papafio of the Gold Coast, and a West Indian, Dr. Derment Waldron. The death of Smith in 1894 while serving as district commissioner at Tarkwa created a vacancy at the senior assistant surgeon level. However, Easmon's first appointment to fill the vacancy proved to be his downfall in the Gold Coast medical service.

Dr. B. W. Quartey-Papafio and Promotion

Easmon appointed Dr. Walter Murray to the vacant position on February 26, 1894. Murray was a British medical officer who had most recently acted as senior medical officer with the Hausa expeditionary force at Attabubu. In making the recommendation to the colonial secretary, Easmon said of Murray that he entered the colony as assistant colonial surgeon on May 17, 1890, and had displayed all the attributes of a qualified professional in the exercise of his duties. Easmon acknowledged that B. W. Quartey-Papafio (MRCS, 1886, England; MD, 1896, Edinburgh; see figure 5), assistant colonial surgeon, was senior in service to Murray, for he had been appointed on March 14, 1889, but Easmon was unable to recommend him for promotion due to lack of loyalty that was indispensable to the smooth functioning of the medical service. Further, Easmon reported, Quartey Papafio's professional skills had not generated confidence among his colleagues. The private secretary commented in the minutes to the marquis of Ripon, secretary of state for the colonies, concerning the approval of Murray's promotion to the higher grade: "Dr. Papafio is a native [he was a member of the Ga ethnic group of Accra] but Dr. Easmon does not hold any tenderness toward him. Request might be expressed that Dr. Papafio's service has not been such as to warrant his recommendation for promotion to the higher grade."[28] Approval for Murray's appointment was granted in a letter on April 6, 1894.

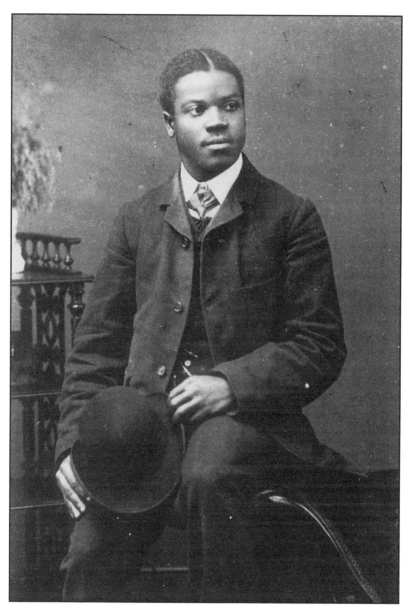

Figure 5. Dr. B. W. Quartey-Papafio, St. Bartholomew's Hospital, London, c. 1885. By permission of the Archives Department, St. Bartholomew's Hospital.

The disappointed Quartey-Papafio was the son of a merchant trading family. He attended the CMS Grammar School in Lagos in 1876–78, transferred to the CMS Grammar School, Freetown, in 1878, and studied at Fourah Bay College in 1880–82. He then went to Durham, England, where he was honored with the Hospital Prizeman Award in 1883 and wrote his medical thesis, "Malaria Hemoglobinuric Fever" (the so-called blackwater fever of the Gold Coast), in perhaps 1884.[29] He was the first doctor born in the Gold Coast in the nineteenth century. Gold Coasters had limited access to the CMS schools of Freetown, such as Fourah Bay College, and were not members of the Creole ethnic group that held a quasi-monopoly on African appointments in the colonial service.

Though the medical bureaucracy was controlled by outsiders, Quartey-Papafio had support from his prosperous family and the Ga ethnic group. In June 1894 he began to press his grievance against Easmon for passing him over for promotion. Writing from Akuse in the Volta River district, he forwarded a petition against the promotion of Murray on June 30, 1894, to the marquis of Ripon. Since the petition went through channels in the Gold Coast, Governor Griffith delayed its transmission and informed Easmon. The petition, which the governor described in reference to the paper as "Foolscap," contained forty-two pages of enclosures that included data on the appointment, information alleging previous instances of favoritism shown to Murray, correspondence, a summary of Quartey-Papafio's previous appointments, and quotations from testimonials and communications from public officials and patients whom Quartey-Papafio had treated. The section that dealt with his list of appointments and years of meritorious service is instructive.

Quartey-Papafio made an explicit charge of Sierra Leone ethnic bias against other Africans: "Before concluding, your Lordship's petitioner would with reluctance direct attention to the feeling of strong antipathy and dislike which unfortunately exists between the aboriginal natives of the Gold Coast and the very small colony of natives of Sierra Leone residing amongst them. Your Lordship's petitioner is himself not at all in sympathy with this strong feeling which he very much deprecates and to which he refers with regret, in as much as it has not worked for the mutual benefit of the parties concerned."[30] If one is persuaded by Quartey-Papafio's case, his petition refuted every charge made by Easmon; it further revealed the travails and triumphs of an African medical officer in conflict with a fellow African in the colonial state. African medical officers had already written about their lack of mobility at the hands of European medical officers. And now the Easmon decision not to promote Quartey-Papafio had left the Ga people with profound resentment against him and possibly against Sierra Leoneans in general. And with no apparent redress, they resorted to the media.

The Papafio family was part owner of the *Gold Coast Chronicle* (*GCC*), an important newspaper published in Accra, in which they initiated a scathing attack on Easmon in an article entitled "The Gold Coast Medical Service" on June 23, 1894. In an unsigned editorial the paper announced the promotion of Murray and argued at considerable length on behalf of Quartey-Papafio, while denouncing Easmon for his decision. It concluded with the hope that the colonial secretary would rectify the injustice and promised to keep readers informed on the case. That Easmon had been unfair to Quartey-Papafio ever since the latter's arrival from England was alleged by many persons. On the other hand, Quartey-Papafio was a victim of his extraordinary popularity, not only with the people of Accra but also with all the communities of the numerous stations in the colony. How could the governor approve the promotion without the consent of the secretary of state, the paper asked? It was the acting governor who not only referred the question to the secretary of state for his decision, but who found it regrettable that Quartey-Papafio was passed over.

The *GCC* stated that it had observed Quartey-Papafio ever since his return to the colony in 1887 and took much pride in his accomplishments. First, his popularity was due to his medical skills and had led to a monopoly of his private practice in Accra, to the envy of other doctors. In order to be promoted into the service, the paper reported, Easmon was more anxious than all the other doctors—McCarthy, Waldron, and Metherel—that Quartey-Papafio accept the appointment to Akim and the subsequent rotations away from Accra. Obviously, his professional skills were further evidenced through his successful promotion of European medicine in areas under the centuries-old dominance of traditional healers. Hence, the paper argued, if Quartey-Papafio had erred in the discharge of his professional duties, his opponents would have broadcast them throughout the colony. Doubts had been raised about the appointment of Easmon himself, the paper reflected, by everyone with considerable knowledge of the issue about whether a physician "who, besides his appointment as Chief of the Staff with a salary of £800 to £1,000 per annum, required to be permitted to take private practice, contrary to the usual rule."[31]

The Sierra Leone response took some time, until a rival newspaper could be organized. Published in Accra in 1895, their paper was the *Gold Coast Independent* (*GCI*). The editor, Bright Davies, was one of the ablest journalists in West Africa. The *GCI* published an unsigned article on August 3, 1895, entitled "Employment of the Native Doctors in Colonial Service." Less an attack upon Quartey-Papafio (for his name was not mentioned) and more a rejoinder on the private practice issue, the article opened by noting the concern expressed by the Liverpool Chamber of Commerce over the number of British and native doctors in the Gold Coast colony. The Chamber of Commerce had written to the secretary of state for the colonies in this regard on April 5, 1895, and their correspondence appeared elsewhere in the *GCI*. The paper purported to recognize the importance of the health issue among the Europeans residing in the colony but remained vague about what had prompted their interest in the correspondence from Liverpool. The paper further noted, with utmost satisfaction, the case in which the Miller brothers of the African trade section of the Liverpool Chamber of Commerce had attempted to defame the character of the native professional men. In a telegram to the secretary of the Colonial Office, Miller commented: "My Coast agent just home complains bitterly about coloured doctors employed by Government. They stand climate better than Europeans, thereby seniority gives advantage, and the lives of Europeans are at their mercy.

Possibly you may influence change."[32] The secretary of state, however, did not favor this request, and expressed satisfaction with the
African doctors in government service, the *GCI* observed.

The *GCI* then moved onto a collision course with the *GCC* and its
final allegations: "And it is clearly laid down that these officers are entitled to private practice, but now here it is established either in the
agreements signed by the respective medical officers, none by any executive acts found necessary subsequent to the employment of such
officers, as can be gathered from the published department's regulation of the medical departments of the Colony, that such medical officers are bound to attend any given class of patients outside the limits
of their official sphere of duties no matter what the hue of skin, or
twist of hair may be."[33] The article shared the general belief that medical officers should treat all of their patients, regardless of color. The
article concluded by arguing that Africans should determine their
own destinies and that the representatives of the civilized world
needed to have this principle impressed firmly upon them. Given the
Berlin Conference of 1884, in which Africa had already been parti-
tioned among the competing colonial powers, this was a bold statement indeed. Having issued this challenge, the Sierra Leoneans now
had to confront a new colonial governor who was not friendly to their
highest appointee.

Governor William Maxwell: Nemesis to Easmon

William Maxwell (1895–97) succeeded Sir Brandford Griffith as governor of the Gold Coast colony in 1895. With Griffith's departure, following ten years of service as governor, Easmon lost a powerful ally.
Maxwell, who was educated at Repton and began his career in the
colonial service in 1865, arrived in the colony with an impressive employment record. He had served twenty-four years in Oceania as legal
adjudicator and administrator at such places as Penang, Malacca,
Perak, and Singapore. He had been acting governor of the Straits settlements before his appointment to the Gold Coast, a region hereto-
fore unknown to him. As a member of the Royal Asiatic Society and

Anthropological Institute of Britain, Maxwell was exposed to the ideas of pseudoscientific racism at a time when the study of race was in the hands of scientific and behavioral specialists.

Following a year's residence in the Gold Coast, Maxwell returned to Liverpool to deliver an address before the African trade section of the Chamber of Commerce on July 1, 1895. The address, which was titled "Affairs of the Gold Coast and Ashanti," described Maxwell's own image of Africa and his perspective on the development of societies in history. Commenting on the need to reduce the European casualty rate from malaria in West Africa to a level comparable to that in Eastern Asia, Maxwell stated:

> The disadvantages on the side of Africa are manifold. Instead of being surrounded, as the Englishman is in India and China, by natives who have attained a high degree of civilization, who have a history, a literature, and an acquaintance with arts and industries, the European who goes to the Gold Coast finds himself among negroes of a low order of intelligence, who know nothing of value that they have not learned from the white man. His house is an inferior one, because the ignorance of native workmen and the difficulty attending the transport of materials make building terribly expensive. Its surroundings are very possibly insanitary, because Englishmen in West Africa have not yet learned to establish their residences at a distance from towns, the almost invariable practice in India.[34]

Even more, Maxwell reminded his audience, West Africa suffered from "the absence of progress and improvement," and that these conditions bound the European to an "apathetic and despondent" state of mind. Since Eastern Asia owed its development to the importation of "energetic native traders from Arabia and India, who brought with them their arts, manufactures, and handicrafts," Maxwell believed that the importation of labor from this region to West Africa would increase the output from the gold fields and improve the living standards for European residents.

A complete breakdown in communication between Maxwell and

Easmon had occurred by at least August 1896. Maxwell, according to the late Dr. M. C. F. Easmon (1890–1972), the son of John Farrell Easmon, "did not like having an African as head of the Medical Department and on his Council."[35] Generally, the CMO rotated the medical officers. But Maxwell began to change a number of assignments that Easmon had already made, thereby eroding Easmon's authority. On the other hand, Easmon was not without blame in the growing rift between himself and the governor, who warned the colonial secretary in December 1896 that "I see that the Chief of Medical Officers has made a marginal comment on my minutes of the 21st and that you have permitted this rudeness to pass unremarked. Please request Dr. Easmon to remove his additions by erasure."[36] In January 1897 the governor canceled a station change, again going through the colonial secretary rather than dealing with Easmon directly: "Inform the Chief Medical Officer that I consider it to be undesirable to place Dr. Waldron [the African–West Indian] at Accra or, as the sole physician, at any station where a European lady is resident and that this view is to be acted on in determining his destination when he returns from leave."[37] (In other words, a white woman was not to be treated by a trained black doctor under the new imperial order.) Correspondence followed between the colonial secretary and the CMO until the governor wrote concerning one of Easmon's letters, stating that it was "improper in tone" and should not have been mailed. By now the conflict between Easmon and Maxwell was obvious.

Maxwell began to gather information against Easmon concerning events that occurred in the Griffith administration. Public officers were prohibited from involvement in other occupations, such as trade or other commercial undertakings, without proper authorization. The governor directed the colonial secretary to inform Easmon of the charges leveled against him on February 18, 1897, requiring a reply in writing on or before February 25, 1897. Easmon was alleged to have connections with Gold Coast Publishing Company and its paper, the *Gold Coast Independent.* Easmon, the charges held, was a paid public officer who had actively engaged himself in the management of the *GCI,* as well as having written many of its articles, even though they were unsigned. Worse, some of these articles commented upon government measures and in doing so exceeded the bounds of objectivity.

Easmon responded on February 26, denying all the charges against him. He acknowledged authorship of an article on public health, which seemed justified by the enormous mortality rates then being suffered by the European community. He admitted that he had supplied some letters to his half brother, Albert Whiggs Easmon, for possible publication under Albert's name; it was not his fault that the letters appeared as editorials. After all, Albert was among the shareholders of the *GCI*. Another essay on a triumphal tour of the governor seemed harmless. Maxwell probably surmised that Easmon's letters published under Albert's name were not an innocent matter.

After responding to other charges, Easmon reminded Maxwell that his loyalty to the government had never before been questioned in sixteen and one-half years of service. He suggested that any further inquiries should be conducted in court, the only forum in which his reputation might be cleared.

Easmon got his wish. On March 3, 1897, the governor ordered an investigation of the charges by Justice Richards of the Colonial Court. Three days later Easmon was notified that in view of the evidence against him he was being relieved of his duties as chief medical officer.

Acting through the governor, F. M. Hodgson sent what must have seemed to Easmon an eviction notice: "I am accordingly to inform you that you are interdicted from duty with stoppage of half salary. You are to hand over charge to Dr. Henderson and you are, I am to state, to vacate the Government quarters which you now occupy within one week from this date."[38]

A commission of inquiry met between March and the end of May 1897 to investigate the case against Easmon, which now included nonprofessional allegations and charges. For example, Mr. Money, the acting attorney general, shortly thereafter began canvassing Easmon's patients and raising questions about his sexual intimacy with certain females throughout the coastal region. Persons who refused to cooperate were threatened with a summons. Thirty-two witnesses were called in the proceedings.

Commission of Inquiry Against Easmon

The crown was represented by T. Hutton Mills, an African who was the acting attorney general and a former patient of Easmon, while Easmon was represented by African barristers Peter Awooner-Renner and C. J. Bannerman. Easmon evidently had able counsel, but his attorneys were hampered by disadvantageous procedures imposed ad hoc by the colonial authorities. The colonial secretary and the registrar were the first two witnesses called and Awooner-Renner cross-examined them about Easmon's service and character.

On May 19, 1897, Awooner-Renner and Bannerman submitted an itemized brief of the charges against Easmon. First of all, they argued that no evidence appeared before the court that warranted the conclusion that Easmon had commercial undertakings or involved himself in trade of any kind. Second, he took no active part in the management of the *GCI*, and in fact there was abundant evidence that he disassociated himself from such activity. Third, Easmon never submitted an unsigned article to the *GCI*, and his essay "Weather and Health" was written in accordance with his right as CMO and sanitary officer, and therefore did not contravene colonial regulations. Next, it was not within the authority of any officer to alter the wording in the colonial regulations as the governor had done. Several other issues were raised by his lawyers that Easmon would later reiterate abroad. His defense stated that all the charges against him were based on colonial regulations 76 and 79.

In the first hearing of March 26, 1897, Awooner-Renner and Bannerman once again requested clear rules on how the proceedings would be conducted. The commissioner refused, and had informed the defense counsel that witnesses could be examined and reexamined upon any subject pertinent to the enquiry. This meant that the commissioner might question the witnesses about any charges, whether related to the case or not. The defense, however, was not allowed to open or review the evidence to which the commissioner had access. They were denied prior knowledge of the witnesses summoned before the court or the nature of the evidence on which they were to testify, and the commissioner supported the crown counsel in every respect. Hence, the inquiry was always conducted on a surprise basis and was far from impartial.

Commenting some eighty-eight years later on the brief presented by Bannerman and his grandfather (figure 6), attorney Raymond Awooner-Renner noted in 1985 that the "brief was not a proper defense."[39] He noted significant problems that should have compromised the legality of the inquiry. First, the rules of the inquiry could be altered by the commissioner, in contrast to the court, where the rules are strictly followed. For example, the word "habitually" as embodied in regulation 76 ("habitually exceeded the bounds of fair and temperate discussion in commenting on the measures of government") was not allowed by the attorneys in Easmon's case. Under this provision the government should have shown that Easmon acted "habitually" in order to build a just case. An inquiry, therefore, was a fact-finding tribunal. A commissioner could be empowered to make recommendations or to act in various ways as if empowered to make recommendations, or to act in various ways as if constituted with the powers of a high court, such as to issue subpoenas, to gather evidence under oath, and to punish for contempt in certain cases which could be referred to the minister of justice for appropriate action in the colony.

The government issued its report on the inquiry on May 22, 1897. Easmon was judged to be guilty of all charges with the exception of the direct involvement in the management of the *GCI*. Easmon appealed the decision around June 2, 1897.

The executive council met the day after receiving Easmon's letter. The council reviewed the charges as reported in the report of the commission of inquiry and shortly called Easmon in for further interrogation. The council adjourned and met again on June 8, 1897; Easmon was again required to be present and was questioned further. The council then informed him that it would notify him with regard to any future proceedings requiring his presence. On June 10 the council met again and deliberated more on the inquiry.

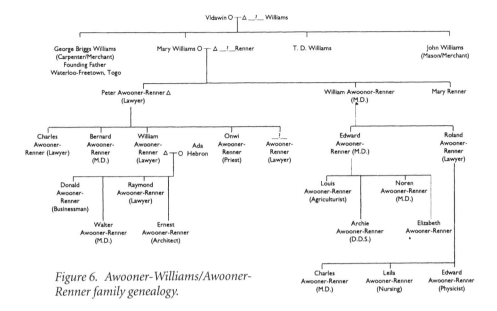

Figure 6. Awooner-Williams/Awooner-Renner family genealogy.

The council refused to believe that Albert Whiggs Easmon, then a medical student in Great Britain and financially supported by his older brother, was a bona fide shareholder in Gold Coast Publishing Company. It held that Albert's name on the list of contributors was a mere proxy intended to conceal Dr. Easmon's involvement in the *GCI*. It concluded also that Easmon's Sierra Leone witnesses had suppressed much of the evidence during the proceedings of the commission. Even more, M. S. Thomas, the printer, was accused of perjury for withholding additional information linking Easmon to the management of the newspaper. In addition, the council concluded that Easmon's response to the charge of contributing unsigned articles to the newspaper was unacceptable and in fact confirmed the validity of the charge. Easmon, the council continued, published articles in 1896 attacking the government and had therefore committed an error in judgment. It additionally stated that the charge of private practice both in Accra and Cape Coast had been proven and also alleged that the income from this practice exceeded the £100 to £120 a year as Easmon claimed—in fact, that the amount must have been several hundred pounds instead. It said the practice should have been shared by one or more of the medical officers in the government service, and even though Easmon claimed that the practice was now in the hands of Dr. Albert Easmon, his younger brother, the council believed that Easmon was still involved. Finally, the council found that he was unfit for the office of chief medical officer and recommended his suspension with ultimate removal from the Colonial Medical Service.

Easmon promised a protest appeal to the secretary of state for the colonies. However, its transmission had to be in line with section 218 of the colonial rules and regulations and go through the Gold Coast chain of command.

Several factors must be borne in mind regarding Easmon's problems. At the heart of the matter was the unwillingness of colonial officials to allow expressions of independent opinion and the exercise of independent action by the Africans in the colony. (Indeed, the British could behave no other way, for they had the power and were in charge. They continued to maintain control over the colony and behaved just as colonizers felt they must.) Easmon saw himself as the equal to colonial authorities and not one that should be their subordinate. We can only guess that Easmon felt that, with his British education and elite status, he had more in common with British than with many of the Africans who were his own countrymen; that the refusal of the British authorities to treat him as a peer was hurtful; and that perhaps he did not have the political shrewdness or savvy that would give him a cold and unemotional understanding of the whole situation. On the other hand, his links to the newspaper suggest an interest in political matters; perhaps he knew exactly the rules of the chess game he was caught up in. Perhaps that is why he kept struggling so long to redeem himself, even though he was able to do far better in private practice than pursuing a public career.

Joseph Chamberlain Supports Inquiry

While Joseph Chamberlain, secretary of state for the colonies, supported the findings of the commission of inquiry, he did not overlook Easmon's long and meritorious service to the government, nor "the good opinions which you have earned in your professional capacity."[40] He offered Easmon the post of colonial surgeon in the

Gold Coast at a reduced salary; Easmon accepted the offer and was on his way home when word reached him that Governor Maxwell wished him to be immediately assigned to an obscure interior post and that this and subsequent assignments might be of short duration. Easmon was not even to return to Accra, however briefly, to settle his affairs there. It is likely that Maxwell knew these terms would be unacceptable to Easmon, and in fact Easmon responded that, without a permanent assignment, he could not assume his duties as colonial surgeon. Not waiting for a reply, he proceeded to Accra. This decision was communicated to Maxwell, who was said to have replied: "either Easmon goes or I go."[41] These actions, the governor promptly wrote to the secretary of state, were tantamount to a resignation, and this time the colonial authorities, after some debate, agreed. Maxwell, who was born in 1846, died at sea soon thereafter on December 10, 1897.

Following his departure from the colonial service, Easmon, who was about forty at the time, moved into private practice in Cape Coast. The Cape Coast merchants immediately offered him a retainer with a minimum of £1,000 per year, equal to or more than his salary as CMO. Easmon died on June 9, 1900, aged forty-three, of injuries received from an apparent fall from a horse in Cape Coast, and he was buried there.

His early death prevented him from making adequate provisions for his children; MaCormack Charles Farrell Easmon was only ten, and Kathleen was eight at the time of his death. Easmon, however, had laid the foundation for a medical dynasty. Following the death of his own father in 1883, Easmon had acted as the family patriarch and provided his relatives with financial support.

Meanwhile, Dr. William Robert Henderson, a British officer, had replaced Easmon as chief medical officer. Murray, whose preferment over Quartey-Papafio had initiated the conflict, continued his rise in the Colonial Medical Service; he was promoted to colonial surgeon on Easmon's resignation. Quartey-Papafio got nothing for his campaign against Easmon; the Colonial Medical Service continued to bypass him. He filed a new protest upon the promotion of another European medical officer over himself. The acting governor took note that Quartey-Papafio was an efficient and diligent officer, but it was not the time for such a large group of European medical officers to be under the authority of an African.

David Kimble's observation that in the late nineteenth century "the doors of African opportunity were closing fast"[42] appropriately describes what happened to Easmon. Steven Feierman adds, "African doctors like Easmon would have been squeezed out sooner or later no matter who was the governor of the Gold Coast."[43] From that time on a new rule stipulated the "native medical officer" was to become the designated title for an African in the service, and NMOs would no longer be eligible for promotion beyond the rank of senior assistant colonial surgeon and could fill only one post out of two in that category.

The fate of Easmon, however, at the hands of Governor Maxwell gave his half brother Albert Easmon a profound disdain for the Colonial Medical Service—Albert worked in private practice all his life. In 1900 he returned to Freetown. Easmon's experiences were also bitterly remembered by other African doctors in years to come. The Easmon episode marked the gradual loss of prominence of African practitioners in the Colonial Medical Service of Anglophone West Africa. By 1900 many Africans' interest in medicine had declined, and they began to study law instead. The law required fewer years of study than medicine, and African lawyers experienced more autonomy and political leverage in colonial courts than was possible in the medical profession. The Colonial Medical Service remained important in providing employment opportunities for African medical professionals; for not everyone went into private practice as did the Easmon brothers. Yet private practice was increasingly becoming more profitable to African doctors in the twentieth century than it was in the nineteenth century. Indigenous people had more faith in Western medicine because of the colonial presence and its employment of African doctors; this factor meant more consultant patients in a new money economy. Private practitioners benefited further from the demographic growth of the African elite and from members of European trading firms willing and eager for personal consultation.

CHAPTER FIVE

Colonial Medical Union and African Reaction

*B*y 1900 the progress of colonialism was evident on several fronts in Anglophone West Africa. The British had driven out their European coastal competitors—the Danes, Dutch, and French—and had almost completely consolidated their control over the coastal and interior regions. By the 1890s, for example, European merchants had already become influential enough to competitively reduce the number of African merchants in the new colonial states, and some of these African merchants were very wealthy. In Sir Joseph Chamberlain, the scion of a manufacturing family in Birmingham, who also served as secretary of state for the colonies (1895–1903), the British colonials had a new official at the helm sympathetic to their initiatives. Chamberlain believed that the successful eradication of disease was indispensable to colonization, and that this process could best be served by migrant professionals from Great Britain manning the various posts and departments on a contract basis. Scientific discoveries allowed for not only better health and improved sanitary conditions—compared to the nineteenth century in Africa—but also made for a more positive image of West Africa abroad.

As almost full-fledged partners alongside their British counterparts, African physicians had left a legacy of medical achievements in the Colonial Medical Service from the 1860s to 1900. They understood the changes needed to make West Africa better for Europeans and Africans. A healthier environment was the outcome, which led to the increase of British middle-class officials and members of leading merchant firms in Africa, and they occasionally took up residence there with their wives.

In addition, West African intellectuals had left their mark on this period. Africanus Horton published his perspectives on African government reform in three major works: *Political Economy of British West Africa* (1865), *West African Countries and Peoples* (1868), and *Letters on the Political Condition of the Gold Coast* (1870). He argued that the Euro-African elite and the traditional elite should borrow selectively from Western philosophy and science in order for Africa to advance in the modern world.[1] Casely Hayford, a Gold Coast champion of the cause of African development and self-government, was a barrister. His efforts spanned several decades at the end of the nineteenth and into the twentieth century. An astute observer, he had inherited the protest tradition and sense of organizational structure from the much heralded Fanti Confederation of 1868, which met at Mankessim. Formed out of the states of Mankessim, Abura, and Gomuah, this body became known as the Fanti nation and wrote its famous Mankessim constitution in 1871. The Fanti, at least for a while, successfully resisted British efforts of establishing a formal empire in their region, but in Casely Hayford, the Fanti and African physicians had a spokesman to represent them.[2]

Journalism also flourished in West Africa, independently of the colonial state. Africans controlled and published their newspapers, and they exerted leverage against the British by publicizing African grievances against them. In this manner their editors and writers also became advocates of African nationalism and were indispensable in mobilizing African opinion. For example, Fyfe shows that twelve newspapers circulated in Freetown alone in the 1880s. Although they were very efficiently produced, all except the famed *Sierra Leone Weekly News* were dissolved by 1889. The newspapers in this group were the *West African Reporter, Watchman, Methodist Herald, Sierra Leone Church Times, Commonwealth,* and *Artisan;* the trade papers were the *Freetown Express,* and *Christian Observer;* those for agriculture were the *Agency,* and *Sierra Leone Farm and Trade Report;* and there was also *Sawyer's Advertising Medium.* Lack of public support, however, caused these newspapers to go out of business, while the *Sierra Leone Weekly News* survived by making its subscribers pay in advance of delivery. This paper, and others similar to it in the Gold Coast and Lagos, published articles on the sensitive issue of African doctors' employment in the Colonial Medical Service. While these newspapers were read at home, the African elite kept compatriots informed abroad through their circulation.[3]

Following John Farrell Easmon's unsuccessful battle with the Colonial Medical Service in 1897, most African physicians viewed the coming of the twentieth century with apprehension. Even those who did not admire Easmon recognized that they would have a subordinate position in the new European schema, and British merchants and policymakers, who had conducted a survey of British and African medical officers in the Gold Coast, did little to assuage their fears.[4] In addition, 1901 brought a new round in intraprofessional conflict.

Colonial Medical Reforms, 1901

The momentum for medical reform in West Africa could not be constrained. The British Medical Association (BMA) was founded in 1832 and became the representative body of certified doctors in Great Britain and the colonies; it published the *British Medical Journal,* which assembled statistics and health issues for its members. The BMA further served as consultant to the Crown Colonies and Protectorates Medical Service Committee. This committee submitted its preliminary report at the annual meeting at Cheltenham in August 1901. The committee pressed for the unification of the Colonial Medical Services and recommended that existing regulations in the outlying regions, meaning those of the legislative councils, should not supersede the unification objectives. Other recommendations stipulated that (1) the service be titled the Colonial Medical Service; (2) that candidates for appointment should hold qualifications registrable in Great Britain, "or such other medical qualifications as may hereafter be determined and approved"; (3) that competitive examinations given in London, under the supervision of the Colonial Office, should be required for admission into the service; (4) the age limit of thirty was set as the maximum at the time of appointment, which would exclude older African doctors already in the service; and (5) before the assumption of appointments, candidates were required to take a course in tropical medicine with evidence of proficiency.[5]

Further development was required in the colonial infrastructure to support these new medical initiatives in the empire. The London School of Tropical Medicine, whose doors opened in October 1899, and the Liverpool Medical Institution, which had a much longer history but officially included the study of tropical diseases and pathology in the same year, were the first centers for tropical diseases to serve the colonial enterprise in West Africa and beyond.[6] The London school staff consisted of notable medical professors. The session of October–December 1899 shows a list of twenty-seven European doctors with impressive credentials, and it constituted the medical vanguard for European health at the periphery of the empire. The school offered a wide-ranging curriculum pertaining to the illnesses physicians would be exposed to within the imperial system, including training in the examination of the blood and microscopic analysis, the study of the life phases of the malarial parasite, hemoglobinuric fever (blackwater fever), Mediterranean fever, Japanese river fever, yellow fever, cholera, dysentery, bilharzia, intestinal parasites, venomous snakes, poisonous arrows, and tropical hygiene. The Royal Victoria and Albert Docks, and the London and Liverpool docks served as laboratories for medical students studying the various diseases in the tropics, because arriving ships were laden with the sick, the convalescing, and the dead.[7]

The committee of 1901 recommended the establishment of a uniform ranking system in the Colonial Medical Service. An assistant colonial surgeon should have one to five years' prior service for appointment to this position; a colonial surgeon needed five to eight years; the senior colonial surgeon ten to fifteen years; and the principal colonial surgeon fifteen to twenty-five years. The Colonial Medical Service also imposed deputy ranks for administrative purposes; the position of deputy inspector general required experience of twenty-five years and upward. With years in the service exceeding the deputy rank, the inspector general held the top post and was responsible for the administration of the medical service in each crown colony and protectorate under the colonial secretary. Salary was essential for medical officers and should not be less than £350 at commencement. This was not the only attempt to link a salary to rank but showed that the committee worked systematically toward rationalizing the entire medical hierarchy. Physicians whose names appeared on the Medical Register in Britain and who served overseas were entitled to membership in the British Medical Association.[8]

The new Colonial Medical Service was to serve the colonial population. The European average annual mortality rate had declined from 43.7 per 1,000 in the period between 1891 and 1898, to 15.3 in 1903, and to 8.1 per 1,000 by 1907. Raymond Dumett shows further that the invalid rate dropped to 60.3 per 1,000 by 1903 and to 25.2 by 1911.[9] Philip Curtin and others show after 1922, "during the high noon of the colonial period . . . health conditions in Africa were far better for Europeans than they were for Africans and were only marginally worse than those prevailing in Europe."[10] An improvement in health conditions allowed for more productive economic pursuit and transference of medical technology to the colonials.

Hence, the ideology of professionalism was transmitted from the core of the empire and directed through its institutions and professional associations to the periphery. The moving frontier or penetrating stages of British colonialism in the mid-nineteenth century occurred at about the same time as the rise of professionalism in Great Britain. Both developments—colonialism and professionalism—

were offshoots of what Magali Sarfatti Larson describes as the "great transformation" that affected European societies and their overseas appendages. Reorganization of the economy and society around the market was crucial to the transformation. In the ongoing process of professionalism, providers of special services sought advantage in the market by controlling the use and availability of their expertise. A result of these collective assertions was the emergence of new ways of measuring social status and the possibility of upward social mobility. This development introduced new rungs on the ladder between elite, merchant, and peasant. Therefore, the rise of professionalism in the nineteenth century inaugurated unique inequalities within the occupational hierarchy, and—in order to maintain scarce resources, a foundation of the process—the instinct toward monopoly of expertise and status arose in the era of laissez-faire capitalism in modern societies. The type of education received and credentials acquired generated tensions and contradictions still unresolved in the contemporary model of professionalism. The most prestigious institutions that groups attended—or ones that were specified by the colonial government—determined the controllers of the market, whether this made them better providers of services or not. Nevertheless, these factors became the controlling variables in the market and social mobility within the professions.[11] The British Medical Council and its subsidiary the British Medical Association followed this ideology by imposing various forms of occupational control acceptable to officials of the empire.

West African Medical Staff

Sir Joseph Chamberlain, secretary for colonies, was very much aware of the vexing issue of how Africans could fit into the medical service, especially following the demotion of John Farrell Easmon in 1897. He had appointed a committee to inquire into the matter of African doctors being included in the new consolidation scheme. In 1901 the committee consisted of men from the British middle class, including H. J. Read, from the Colonial Office as chair; Dr. W. R. Henderson, who took over Easmon's job as chief medical officer and was now principal medical officer for the Gold Coast; Dr. R. Allman, principal medical officer for southern Nigeria; Dr. D. K. McDowell, principal medical officer for northern Nigeria; and E. H. Marsh of the Colonial Office. Gambia and Sierra Leone were not represented for reasons not explained.[12] Commenting upon the committee later, the Gold Coast auxiliary of the Anti-Slavery and Aborigines' Protection Society (ASAPS, see chapter 6) objected that the senior medical officers of the committee were colleagues of African doctors who had been in keen competition with them over consulting patients in private practice.[13] Dr. Oguntola Sapara, a Nigerian, in his report to the ASAPS on "Colonial Medical Appointments in the West African Colonies," said that European medical officers, most notably in Sierra Leone and the Gold Coast, had expressed concern for some time over their rank as juniors to African doctors. Several of the committee's members, Sapara held, had described this hierarchical listing that subordinated British medical men to Africans as "this indignity."[14] Such an approach may well explain Chamberlain's response to the amalgamation issue: he said that it was "pretty clear to men of ordinary sense . . . that British officers could have no confidence in Indian or Native doctors."[15]

The British medical professionals from West Africa had clearly won Chamberlain over to their side. It is ironic that these new issues were raised at a time when there was a shortage of doctors. The Anglo-Boer War of 1898–1902 in South Africa had produced the need for a large number of British doctors in Africa and necessitated the employment of two Bengali doctors from India, a precedent that was not favorably regarded.

Chamberlain's committee issued its findings, often referred to as the Amalgamation Report, in January 1902. This report, which needed the approval of the Colonial Office before implementation, established ranks or grades for European officers and the annual salary of each grade, the latter determined by the size and importance of the medical department in the territories (see table 3). Gambia had no European in residence in the colony or the protectorate at the turn of the century, and the management of the medical service was left to the local government.[16] There medical officers were required to take a two-or three-month course in tropical diseases at either the London School of Tropical Medicine or at the Liverpool Medical Institute. The secretary of state, however, could use his discretion in exempting candidates from this prerequisite for appointment, if he so chose. Upon completion of the postgraduate course, medical officers received the Certificate and Diploma in Public Hygiene (DPH, requiring one year of study; but now carries industrial medicine with two years of study) or the Diploma in Tropical Medicine and Health (DTMH, requiring three months of study). With the exception of the principal medical officer, private practice was allowed, but the governor or the high commissioner could suspend the privilege, especially if the practice interfered with the efficient performance of official duties.

Under provision 2 the Chamberlain committee prohibited the employment of West African doctors as medical officers in the newly created West African Medical Staff (WAMS). The Amalgamation Report dealt a major blow to African doctors in the government service and led to extreme dissatisfaction, still vehemently discussed even today. The report reversed several decades of mutual cooperation and collegiality among European and African doctors. West African medical professionals were judged, except in rare circumstances, to be not as competent as their European counterparts, and since they did not

Table 3. *Salaries of European medical officers of various grades, Gold Coast, Southern Nigeria, and Northern Nigeria and Sierra Leone and Lagos,* 1902

	GOLD COAST, SOUTHERN NIGERIA, AND NORTHERN NIGERIA			SIERRA LEONE AND LAGOS		
	MIN.	ANNUAL INCREMENT	MAX.	MIN.	ANNUAL INCREMENT	MAX.
Principal med. off.	1,200	—	—	800	50	1,000
Dep. principal med. off.	700	25	700	—	—	—
Senior med. off.	600	20	700	600	20	700
Med. off. on first-year probation	400	20	500	400	20	500

Source: PRO, CO 872/72. Report of the Committee to Discuss Amalgamation.

hold respectable consultation status with European patients, African practices with this type of client ought not be encouraged. Provision 2 did not rule out the possibility of African doctors being employed in a hospital serving indigenous patients, but the practice should be limited to a few cases—at the discretion of the local governments. The committee acted in accordance with its imperial axiom: African and Indian doctors were to be placed on a separate roster from European doctors, must not participate in military expeditions, and under no circumstances were Africans to give orders to European officers. The exclusionary nature of this provision was the cause of continuous petitions for redress as intraprofessional conflict intensified throughout the period, prior to the start of decolonization in the 1940s.

AFRICAN DIASPORA MEDICAL STUDENTS PROTEST

At the University of Edinburgh some thirty-five medical students from West Africa, the West Indies, and Mauritius wasted little time in responding to the committee's report. They convened a meeting in early March 1902 to seek the revision of the troublesome provision 2. A letter, conciliatory in content, was sent to Professor A. R. Simpson (MD), dean of the faculty of medicine, requesting his intervention on their behalf, first through the academic senate and then to the Colonial Office. The petitioners referred to the British government role in training the first three African doctors in the nineteenth century, and recalled how West Africans thereafter began financing the medical education of their children in Great Britain, students who rendered invaluable service to medical science upon their return to their native land. Since the climate was detrimental to the health of the European doctors, African doctors worked unselfishly in providing health care service to the government and to the people. In spite of unquestionable devotion to the government, the institution had been severely criticized by the people of the Gold Coast for the government's lack of employing African doctors. The petitioners, therefore, could not quite comprehend how the Colonial Office did an about-face, since every civil post had been accessible to West Africans of British citizenship for over one hundred years. Yet the new regulations allowed any citizens of other European states with a double qualification to be eligible for membership in the West African Medical Staff, a group that was maintained by the taxes of West Africans.

The students then invoked the strongly British principle of no taxation without representation, and also stated that education rather than color should be the litmus test of one's political rights.[17]

COASTAL MEDICAL ESTABLISHMENTS

Just as the African and West Indian medical elite in England reacted to the prospect of reduced employment opportunities upon their return to West Africa, colonial authorities sought to resolve the complex problem of reconciling the reduced prospects of African doctors under the new act with the expectations that had been engendered by long years in the service. Colonial medical policy was in for a hard time. Chamberlain informed the colonies of the new regulations on February 7, 1902.[18] Sir Charles King-Harman, governor of Sierra Leone (1900–1904), responded with a reorganization proposal for his country's medical staff, one which Chamberlain accepted. The Sierra Leone medical establishment was to remain "fixed for the present," with one principal medical officer, one senior medical officer, seven medical officers, and five African medical officers. King-Harman apparently was able to secure the Sierra Leone African doctors' salaries at the pre-1901 level until later replacement by Europeans through attrition. Africans were to be prohibited from becoming medical officers but could continue to serve in lesser positions. Chamberlain reminded King-Harman that paragraph 21 of the report did not recommend the exclusion of native doctors from the government service in West Africa, and advised that it was not his intent that the five African medical officers, then in the service, should be replaced by Europeans, especially as long as suitable employment could be found for them. Chamberlain concluded with recommendations to resolve foreseeable salary problems. The principal medical officer's salary was to remain at £1,000 per annum, but provisions for medical officers who joined the service before the new act came into force were different. The new policies would be applicable to medical officers confirmed in their appointments before January 1, 1902. Those still in their probationary period as of January 1, 1902, could, following confirmation, receive £440 per annum. Medical officers with at least two and not more than three years completed as of the same date would, if recommended, be appointed from that date with salary and increments in accordance with the new regulations.[19] It is safe to assume that other governors responded in kind and made similar alterations in their medical staff salaries and appointments. However, African doctors did not lag behind in seeking redress, for the minimum salary of Sierra Leone doctors was £300 and the maximum £400, no matter how many years of service they had accrued.

African doctors in Lagos sought to bring their salaries into line with those in effect elsewhere along the coast, despite the fact that the new salary schedules were not intended to cover African medical officers. It must be remembered that African medical officers were not included in the WAMS salary clause on ranks and grades. Drs. Jenkins Lumpkin, Oguntola Sapara, Orisadipe Obasa, and W. A. Cole of the Lagos branch of the West African Medical Service first submitted a memorandum to the principal medical officer on November 10, 1903, in deference to the colonial chain of command. Their terms of service ranged from two to ten years, which, according to them, meant that their service exceeded the scheme of 1901, namely the WAMS. The doctors noted that while European medical officers in the colonies received the same salary as those of similar rank, their own scale was not comparable to that of African doctors in the Gold Coast and Sierra Leone. Whereas under the old scheme the maximum salary of Lagos doctors exceeded that of their Sierra Leone colleagues by £50 (except for that of the senior African doctor), Sierra Leone doctors under the new scheme were slated to receive £50 more. Doctors in the Gold Coast and Sierra Leone, the Lagosians decided, were now appointed on the scale of their maximum salary with the same allowances. Their petition ended not by requesting to be placed on the same scale with European doctors but "at least on the same footing as that of Native Colleagues in the other West African Colonies."[20]

The principal medical officer forwarded a reply to the Lagosians some three months later, on February 12, 1904. The questions had gone to the colonial secretary and been discussed fully, Dr. F. G. Hopkins wrote. After due deliberation, these officials could not accede to the doctor's request. Bypassing the principal medical officer on the next round, the Lagos doctors appealed directly to the secretary of state for the colonies. In a courteous letter dated March 31, 1904, that enclosed copies of previous correspondence, the doctors reviewed the salary issue and expressed concern over the fact that the maximum salary of their Sierra Leone colleagues stood at £400 and the minimum at £350. The Sierra Leone minimum was the Lagos maximum, and only two doctors had ever received that amount and only one after eight or ten years' service. So until Governor Sir William Mac-Gregor of Lagos (1899–1904), himself a doctor, had recommended a salary increase in March 1902, the Lagos doctors' maximum was much lower than that of the Sierra Leoneans. But C. H. Harley, the acting governor of Lagos for MacGregor, doubted the accuracy of the Lagos doctors' information until the principal medical office of Sierra Leone replied to him in the affirmative.[21] Ultimately, the Lagos doctors failed in their efforts to augment their own salaries. What was perhaps worse, by invoking the principal of comparable worth they caused the colonial administrators to reexamine the salary structure as it applied to West African doctors and bring down the maximum salary of the Sierra Leoneans by £50. On November 30, 1904, Governor Leslie Probyn of Sierra Leone (1904–11) received a directive from the secretary of the colonies. Henceforth, the salaries of Sierra Leone African doctors were to be set at £300 per annum; annual increments of £10 would be allowed, to a maximum of £350 per year. So now African doctors in the Gold Coast and Lagos made the same pay.[22] From that point on these doctors launched a number of different strategies aimed at the amelioration of their unequal conditions vis-à-vis the Europeans in the region, and their quest for employment in the Colonial Medical Service drained energies that might otherwise have gone into efforts to improve their group status.

Dr. William Awooner-Renner's Career and Colonial Situation

Nothing more exemplifies this state of affairs than the troubled career of William Awooner-Renner in Sierra Leone under colonial rule. Awooner-Renner (MRCS, 1880; LKQP, LM, 1880, Ireland; MD, 1881,

Brussels, with high distinction), was the brother of barrister Peter Awooner-Renner of the Gold Coast. Born in Waterloo some miles from Freetown, the brothers migrated in the 1840s with their mother to the principal city of Kwitta (Keta) in the Awuna chiefdom of the Gold Coast colony. There they lived with their successful merchant uncles who paid for their education in Europe. On the completion of their medical and legal training the Awooner-Renner brothers returned to Sierra Leone; Peter went into legal private practice, and William secured a position in the medical service.[23] Dr. Palmer Ross, the colonial surgeon, prepared an evaluation of Awooner-Renner as assistant colonial surgeon as early as 1886, four years after his initial appointment to that position. Awooner-Renner, he wrote, had performed his job in an acceptable manner, patients were satisfied following consultation, and the doctor had demonstrated a good knowledge of the medical profession. The administrative chief of the colony reported further that Awooner-Renner was beyond reproach in social and moral character. This evaluation prompted his promotion to senior assistant surgeon in 1886, and apparently this administrative appraisal went unchallenged into the dawn of the twentieth century.[24]

The available information concerning Awooner-Renner's career during this period suggests that he made invaluable contributions, especially regarding the applied use and transfer of medical technology into the colony. From 1886–1902 he filled the post of acting colonial surgeon and principal medical officer in the absence of the colonial surgeon. He was appointed to these posts following the departure of Ross, who was transferred to British Guiana as surgeon general. His promotions were evidence that he enjoyed the confidence of the governor. However, although Awooner-Renner received positive evaluations for his work, he was not awarded the position of principal medical officer. Instead, the Colonial Medical Service appointed Dr. William Thomas Prout (BM, ChM 1884, Edinburgh), an Englishman, as colonial surgeon and principal medical officer in 1895. Prout's first appointment was to Mauritius in 1885 as assistant poor law medical officer, and, before his arrival in the colony in January 1895 from service in Nigeria, he had written one article on "Frambocia or Yaws" in *Hygiene and Diseases of Warm Climates*. Governor

Cardew (1894–1900), in a confidential dispatch to the secretary of state, noted that Prout held "great qualifications in the profession and knowledge in diseases of [the] West Coast [and was] deserving of promotion."[25] The salary range for a colonial surgeon was the minimum £800 per annum for Sierra Leone and Lagos, which was raised to £1,000 in 1901, but the position did prohibit private practice. Collegiality prevailed, and Prout and Awooner-Renner worked in close cooperation. Lieutenant Colonel J. E. Cuafield commented upon the medical department in a letter of January 26, 1895: "In conclusions the Board have made pleasure in stating their satisfaction with the general order of cleanliness and discipline of the Colonial Hospitals which Dr. Renner has maintained during the period he has been in charge of the Department."[26]

On September 29, 1903, Awooner-Renner wrote to the governor requesting parity in salary with his European colleagues in the WAMS. He called attention to the fact that after nineteen years and eight months of service in the department he was being reimbursed according to a salary range established seventeen years ago. He complained that the WAMS had blocked his promotion in Sierra Leone and in other colonies. He drew attention to the lack of uniformity in employment practices by the WAMS in the Gold Coast and in Sierra Leone. He stated that Dr. D. H. R. Waldron, a West Indian with sixteen years of service, and Benjamin Quartey-Papafio were not only members of the WAMS but received the same pay as European medical officers. Awooner-Renner, however, was not asking for membership in the WAMS in Sierra Leone but, as the senior African medical officer in his majesty's service in West Africa, he held tenaciously to the belief that his salary should be the same as European medical officers in the WAMS. Awooner-Renner reminded the governor of several occasions, each lasting about six months, when he stood in while Prout was on leave. In addition to acting colonial surgeon and principal medical officer, he was simultaneously acting medical officer of health, president of the quarantine board, inspector of health and shipping, and deputy coroner of the police district. Awooner-Renner concluded by reminding the governor that Joseph Chamberlain, the secretary of state for the colonies, had commended him for his role in preparing the annual medical report of 1894.

Parity of African doctors in their appointment to the WAMS in the Gold Coast, albeit temporary, was not without salutary effects in Sierra Leone, for the medical department supported in part the application of Awooner-Renner. Prout recommended to the secretary of the colonies that the applicant be placed on the same footing with African doctors in the Gold Coast with regard to salary, in accordance with his long period of service, and that his salary be raised from £350 per annum with the presumed allowance of £50 to a maximum of £500. The governor apparently had the last word. In a letter to the secretary of state he stipulated that the doctor was to receive a raise to £400 and annual increments of £50 to a maximum £500 with yearly increments of £20. However, the maximum scale required additional years in service.[27] So this offer still left Awooner-Renner at a disadvantage with respect to his European peers.

When Prout retired from the Sierra Leone service in 1906, Awooner-Renner applied for the position for the second time since 1895. By then colonial administrators were familiar with his work, and substantial amounts of information about him were on file, including correspondence and evaluations. However, in a letter dated April 23, 1906, applying for the post, the doctor pointed to additional factors that qualified him for the position: "I have promoted the advancement of the knowledge of Tropical Medicine by my various Medical Reports published in the British Medical Journal, the Journal of Tropical Medicine and the Medical Journals of Brussels. In asking for the Post Principal Medical Officer I think I have sufficiently shown to your lordship my ability to carry out the administrative work of the Medical Department, the Sanitation of the Colony and the administration of the Quarantine Laws."[28] Awooner-Renner reminded the establishment of the fact that he had held the highest post in the past without failure or reward, and that his being a native should not bar him from the position. The doctor felt that much of the credit rewarded to Prout was in fact work done by him and had been underreported.

While Prout supported Awooner-Renner as principal medical officer for the vacant position over the English candidate—senior medical officer Thomas Hood (MRCS, LRCP)—Governor King-Harman made seniority an issue. In spite of the fact that Hood had agreed to serve under Awooner-Renner, the governor refused to grant approval for the arrangement because it would be in violation of the laws governing the functioning of the West African Medical Staff (number 678). This regulation stipulated that only the senior medical officer should serve as acting principal medical officer. Awooner-Renner had acted as principal medical officer, the governor noted, at a time when he held senior rank before the creation of the WAMS, but Hood's appointment under the new rules made him senior to the principal medical officer. How could the principal medical officer now recommend that the senior medical officer in the medical department be superseded, the governor argued? The governor's case was technically valid since Awooner-Renner was denied membership in the WAMS, in spite of his long service to the colony. But the governor's interpretation of the regulations essentially blocked Awooner-Renner's possible promotion.

The governor reviewed the reasons for the formation of the West African Medical Service, and just in case one main provision had been forgotten, he stated "that it was undesirable that European Medical Officers should be under the orders of a 'native' Medical Officer and this fact will dispose of Dr. Renner's application if it is decided that the reform is to be retrospective."[29] In place of the promotion, the governor wrote, Awooner-Renner should receive a personal allowance of £75 per annum for his long and meritorious service.

Awooner-Renner left for England in June 1906 for a leave to take a special course in gynecology. No doubt realizing the numerous retirement benefits that higher rank would bring, he applied for the position of senior medical officer in a letter from Liverpool on October 2, 1906. If approved, this position would enable him to act as the senior medical officer in the West African Medical Staff when the person already in that rank acted as principal medical officer. He reminded the secretary of state that European junior medical officers of the WAMS had superseded him to that post only because he himself was not a member.

The Colonial Office responded to the governor in Sierra Leone with regard to Awooner-Renner's request for promotion to the relative rank that he already held—namely senior medical officer—in October 1906. It appears that officials in London supported the doctor's bid. Governor Probyn, in reviewing the case with the medical department, held that the colonial medical office had already agreed to a personal grant of £75 to Awooner-Renner, mainly as compensation for the adverse effect that the WAMS was presumed to have had upon his mobility. It was customary for the senior medical officer to take charge of the Colonial Hospital, which was an extremely heavy duty. The governor lacked confidence in the proposed appointee's ability to perform the various duties of the office in a satisfactory manner and went on to accuse Awooner-Renner of malpractice in the Colonial Hospital, although its specific nature was not stated. "Just before Dr. Renner proceeded on leave, an incident took place at the hospital. Had Dr. Renner been in strong health, he would admittedly have been the blame for the accident. It was on account of his weak health that he was exonerated from blame. I merely mention the above circumstance in support of the opinion that Dr. Renner, with the best intentions in the world, would not be able to satisfactorily discharge the duties of Senior Medical Officer."[30] In the meantime, Awooner-Renner withdrew his bid for promotion to the rank of senior medical officer upon learning that the Colonial Office had sanctioned the personal grant on his behalf.

The search for Prout's replacement as principal medical officer ended on February 16, 1907, and the appointment bears ironic testimony to the high standards that the WAMS claimed to uphold. Dr. Robert Michael Forde, a graduate of the Royal University, Ireland, holder of diplomas from the Royal College of Surgeons and Physicians, and certified in the course at the London School of Tropical Medicine, became the new principal at the salary of £900. Forde had first served in the Gold Coast colony, beginning in October 1891, and apparently moved from there to Sierra Leone. Governors were required to supply the Colonial Office with evaluations of officers in the territories, and in his confidential report of January 1910 the acting governor, Henddon Smith, wrote about Forde in the following manner: "A Poor Administrator, lethargic and hardly up to the requirements of the present day Principal Medical Officer. Tactful and nice mannered. Dr. Forde has made no contribution during the past year to medical or sanitary science."[31] In spite of the personal allowance awarded to Awooner-Renner, this appointment must have been devastating to him. In addition, Forde's appointment was a factor in the acceleration of internal friction and decline in the quality of the Colonial Medical Service.

Governor's Critique of WAMS: Confidential Evaluations

At least for Sierra Leone, the medical standards of the WAMS had not improved some six years later. In 1916, commenting upon the principal medical officer's confidential reports on the officers of the WAMS, Governor R. J. Wilkinson (1916–22) forwarded the following observations to the Colonial Office: "I have added my own comments in the case of the more capable or more important officers. I wish I could have added in any single instance that an officer had some acquaintance with African languages and customs or was known to have a real sympathy with the natives or creoles. I may add that when I arrived in the Colony [Sierra Leone] I found that the Acting PMO could not tell me the number of any local anopheles [species of mosquito] or anything about its special habits. The most disheartening feature about the WAMS is this general lack of interest in the country and people."[32] While Governor Wilkinson's criticisms about the lack of cross-cultural awareness among most members of the WAMS in Sierra Leone seem justified, the WAMS also had its own problems with the salary issue of professional parity.

Members of the WAMS held longstanding grievances against the Colonial Office over the disparity in the salaries between medical men and other professionals. This morale problem might well have led not only to a lack of concern for the well-being of indigenous people but also for that of European patients throughout West Africa. An unidentified officer of the WAMS wrote to the editor of the *Lancet* complaining about pay. The medical officer, he noted, started at £400, his salary increasing in installments to £500. Following long service, a small number—at present no more than three or four—became senior medical officers at £600–700 annually. The deputy principal medical officer received £800–900, and £1,000–1,200 went to the primary medical officer. He thought that these salaries were indeed low compared to the risk the medical officers took in the tropical climate, and he went on to contrast the pay of medical officers with that of other professionals and nonprofessionals who spent less time in training.[33]

When the confidential evaluations of the WAMS are considered, not much objectivity is sacrificed in concluding that Awooner-Renner was mistreated by the service. He labored for long periods in efforts to safeguard the health of European residents and the African population in general, and, while he was president of the Quarantine Board, he formulated preventive measures against yellow fever and other infectious diseases. He planned these measures in such a manner as not to alarm merchants in adjacent territories, which could have harmed their commercial interests through quarantines.[34] In spite of his contributions in advancing medical science in the colony, Awooner-Renner suffered a new indignity upon his retirement in April 1913, when his pension was reduced from the £293 he was expecting to £270 annually. Colonial officials justified the cut by charging that Awooner-Renner's earnings from his private practice had exceeded the amount allowed under the Pension Ordinance of 1901, an accusation that called his integrity into question. "I hereby certify on my honor," Awooner-Renner apparently wrote to Governor Sir Edward Mereweather (1911–15) on July 21, 1913, that "I have received during the years 1903 to 1912 as the result of my private practice the total sum of £6,096.17.2."[35] In effect, the £6,096 averaged out to £610 per year for the period in question. His private-practice earnings followed the creation of the WAMS in 1902 and were clearly meant to compensate for income foregone when the promotions he had sought were denied. Following his retirement from the Colonial Medical Service, Awooner-Renner went into private practice full time, and in 1917 became vice mayor of Freetown.

In 1912 there were 214 medical officers in the WAMS, only 8 of whom were non-Europeans. T. Hutton-Mill, who as barrister took the colonial inquiry's case against John Farrell Easmon in 1897, went on the offensive in favor of the employment of African doctors in the Gold Coast WAMS. In October 1912 he made the following statement before the Legislative Council: "Native Medical Practitioners should be eligible for employment in our Government Service if they are qualified and efficient in as much as the Government of other West African Colonies. . . . As the revenue of the Colony out of which provision for the large expenditure under the heads of "Medical" is mainly derived from the natives, it is only fair that some of the appointments in the Department[s] should be opened to qualified natives. . . . [They] spend large sums of money in sending their sons and their relatives to England to qualify in the medical profession and it is a decided hardship that on their return to their native land they should be denied employment in the Government Service."[36] The acting governor promised to address the secretary of state on the matter, and the council moved on to other business. More African doctors were becoming available for possible government service as Hutton-Mill spoke. Two months before his appeal, August 23, 1912, Charles Elias Reindorf (MB, BS, 1910, Durham) had entered his name on the local register of the Gold coast.[37] He was the son of Rev. C. C. Reindorf, the pioneer historian of Ghana. Dr. E. Tagoe was the next available Gold Coast doctor, who became the first West African to receive the DPH (University of London) in 1924.

Dr. W. H. Langley, PMO: "Negrophobist"

The problem of employment for African doctors in Nigeria was little different from the Gold Coast situation. Nigeria had five African medical officers who were still serving in the government or who had ended their employment. They were W. A. Cole; C. J. Lumpkin, who had retired; O. P. P. Obasa who resigned; A. la Oyey who held questionable status; and O. Sapara. Dr. W. H. Langley, the principal medical officer, was asked by the secretary of state what he thought of enlarging the scope of work for African doctors in the government. In responding, Langley preferred to reply through his correspondence, a way to avoid general circulation, rather than to record in the minute paper, which was read by larger numbers including Africans. He observed: "Already I am described—very unjustly—in the Native Press as a 'Negrophobist.' . . . I may use terms and arguments which might lend colour to the accusation; therefore, although I do not fear possible untoward consequences to myself, I consider it would not be diplomatic for me, in view of the position I hold, to leave my attitude open to censorious criticism."[38] Langley's reference to "Negrophobist" implied that the Lagos press had accused him of making racist statements about Nigerians. If the number of African doctors were to be increased, Langley warned, the WAMS would have to reduce its numbers through retirement and thereby allow for the creation of a subordinate native medical staff. R. A. Savage (MB, BS, 1900, Edinburgh) a Nigerian of the Cape Coast, had registered in Nigeria on July 15, 1911, but Langley advised against his employment. "There are several reasons why I would not recommend Dr. Savage. One is that he has an English wife, who usually lives with him at Cape Coast, where, as a rule, there are few white women. In a populous centre like Lagos, her lot would be a harder one than it is now, anyhow, he, himself, is not desirable."[39] Langley never stated explicitly why he did not want Savage in Lagos but, because of Langley's alleged racist reputation, the welfare of Savage's British wife in Lagos was his least concern. British imperial behavior generally discouraged interracial relationship, particularly marriage, and Langley's rejection of Savage's appointment in Lagos might be attributed to his affinity for social distance between Africans and British women.

Presumably, Langley argued against adding more African doctors to the medical service by trying to make a case for their general incompetence. He moved next to provide a listing of unprofessional practices by African doctors. Sapara, for example, had allowed clerks to take longer sick leaves than current policy allowed, which contravened the General Order of April 12, 1912, which became operational in May. Langley presented figures to show his point. While his backing of the order caused much resentment, it saved the government hundreds of pounds per year and reduced opportunities for display of sympathies by African doctors, who were more lenient in granting sick leaves than Europeans. Langley admitted that his information about African medical officers was not acquired through personal investigation but mostly from information taken from older colleagues. A Dr. Curtis Adeniji-Jones, already dismissed from the government service, had recently diagnosed and treated a female patient for an intestinal obstruction, when the actual cause of her illness was an ectopic pregnancy. Fortunately, the patient made a quick recovery following surgical intervention by two European doctors. It appears likely, Langley surmised, that the woman could have died had his diagnosis and treatment not been corrected. The treatment dealt with the administration of different purgatives, including "croton oil! and some enemata," whereas her case was one of pregnancy within one of the small tubes between the womb and the ovaries.

Recalling other instances of mistaken diagnoses from his days of service in the Gold Coast, Langley mentioned a case in which Quartey-Papafio listed puerperal fever as the cause of death for a female patient. However, puerperal fever was a complication of childbirth, and this woman had not been pregnant in the two or three years preceding her death! In fact, a postmortem examination showed that she had died from cancer. In a second case Quartey-Papafio attributed the death of an infant to teething. Here the postmortem showed the problem to have been extensive ulceration of the large intestine and a severe liver infection.

Langley said that these and many other examples of negligence and incompetence justified a system that Dr. Savage had attacked in the Gold Coast Leader newspaper, "namely, that no authority is given for the burial of the dead unless the application is accompanied by a Death Certificate from a Government Medical Officer." This same complaint—about the death certificates—was combined with other charges against the Government Medical Service, Langley finally noted, and reverberated in the Lagos press in a flamboyant and illiterate manner. This charge was instigated by African members of the service or by those now aspiring to membership. The Lagos representatives of the Aborigines' Protection Society continued to attack the government and make matters difficult, Langley observed, and were always pressing for the employment of African doctors. For the loss of employment in the WAMS left the African doctors with hardly any option other than private practice.

Demand for medical services has always depended on what the average person thought was desirable treatment for sickness. Where people accept the efficaciouness of scientific medical treatment, their attitudes about it are in harmony with the ideology of the profession. However, for a medical renaissance to occur, a variety of factors must combine to support it, including population growth, urbanization, relative prosperity, and cross-cultural exposure. In West Africa the opposite of these conditions prevailed in the twentieth century; there was a limited demand for doctors in private practice in Africa and secure employment meant dependency on the Europeans.

Private practice did exist in the eastern and central provinces of Nigeria in such cities as Warri, Bonny, and Calabar. The mercantile community and the chiefs consulted with Western-trained practitioners, but complaints over high fees led the Colonial Office to approve a new scale of fees for both patients and colonial officers. In general, however, private practice was an uncertain undertaking, and it also tended to have lower status than public employment. Sapara reported that a popular saying among the people in the Krio language was as follows: "If you be proper, Doctor, dem Consul [governor] go give you job [Sapara reported the common assumption that if a doctor was any good the government would give him a job]."[40] Outside of Freetown, Sierra Leone, where people understood the value of scientific medicine and the model for sanitary reform in the region, private practitioners had to compete with traditional healers. Because people were accustomed to compensating the traditional healers with foodstuffs, animals, or handiworks, the private practitioner initially felt obliged to offer his medicines without the expectations of cash payments, as a way of gaining the confidence of his patients. Payment in kind, however, did not help to recover his own expenses in purchasing the medicines or the cost of his medical education. In spite of this alternative of payment in kind, African doctors continued their protest against the WAMS.

Dr. Mayfield Boyle and Criticism of WAMS (1909)

One of the most incisive and scathing criticisms of the WAMS came from a Sierra Leone physician who trained and worked in the United States. Mayfield Boyle was born of Krio parentage with Nova Scotian origin in 1878. He attended public schools in Freetown at a time when there was already a tradition of African achievement in medicine and when the local press was active (see figure 7). Besides the Sierra Leone Weekly News, another important publication of the time was the Negro, edited by Edward Wilmot Blyden (1832–1912), the important Sierra Leone Pan-Africanist, educator, and historian. Boyle was undoubtedly influenced by Blyden's cultural nationalism in his own worldview and in his subsequent choice of a profession.

Boyle arrived in the United States in the 1890s and enrolled at Alabama A. and M. College in Normal, which he attended from 1896–98. It is not inconceivable that Boyle was influenced to come to the United States by Blyden. Indeed, during his lifetime Blyden had made eight trips to America and visited several historically black colleges and universities in the South, his last tour taking place in 1895. Perhaps Southern educators requested his help in recruiting African students to attend their colleges. Africans studying abroad often did so with missionary financial support and were expected to return to Africa upon completion of their education to serve in the ministry. Boyle apparently received some missionary funding, for in 1898 he entered Howard University, Washington, D.C., to study theology. Two years later, and without explanation, he transferred to the medical school. In 1902 he received his MD, earning the distinction of being Howard University's first African to graduate from the College of Medicine in the twentieth century. Subsequently, he was licensed to practice surgery in Maryland (1903), Pennsylvania (1906), and the District of Columbia (1909). Although Boyle was interested in returning to West Africa, he never did; medical degree certifications

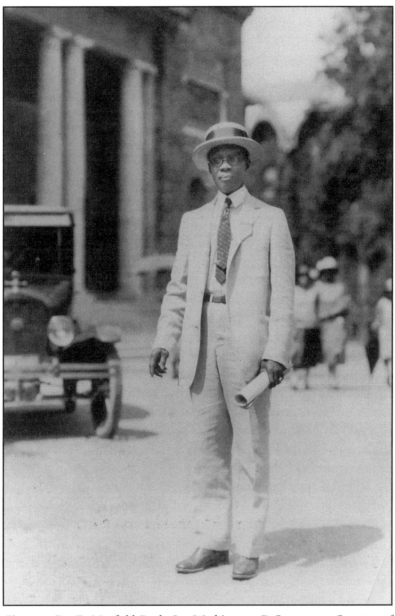

Figure 7. Dr. E. Mayfield Boyle Sr., Washington, D.C., c. 1902. Courtesy of Leone B. Thompson.

from the United States were not acceptable for licensing or medical practice in British West Africa. This factor alone in colonial policy played a major role in his decision not to return.[41]

Rev. J. R. Frederick, the West Indian pastor of the Wesleyan Methodist Church in Freetown that Boyle had attended as a youth, presented Boyle's application for employment to the principal medical officer on March 3, 1909. The apparent intent was to have Boyle registered as a practitioner under missionary authority rather than through the WAMS; this was a common practice and was about to receive legal recognition under the proposed Medical Practitioners Ordinance of 1908, which had not yet passed. Dr. R. H. Keenan, a senior medical officer of the WAMS, took responsibility for the routine process involved in Boyle's application, and in an interview with Frederick said, "it [was] near impossible to say [whether Boyle was to be employed or not] until the ord. was actually passed or approved and what its terms would be & whether they would be such as to enable Dr. Boyle to be registered."[42]

Meanwhile, Boyle's application received further scrutiny that brought him into a direct confrontation with the British Medical Council. This regulatory body drew up professional regulations that stipulated a physician must have received the medical diploma from a recognized institution in a British possession in order to register as a practitioner in British West Africa. The regulations included a list of the acceptable certifying institutions outside of the United Kingdom.[43] Unfortunately for Boyle, Howard University was not on the list, nor was Boyle apparently apprised about the restricted list of degree-granting institutions recognized by the Colonial Office.

The issue, however, of retaining the 1901 exclusionist rule of West Africans and Indians from the WAMS was referred again to a departmental committee of that body in 1908 for review and was sustained.[44] The decision apparently did not become known in Sierra Leone for some time because it was not until October 1909 that Albert Easmon forwarded a copy of the committee's report to the editor of the *Sierra Leone Weekly News* for reproduction. Shortly thereafter, the editor printed portions of the document. Based on a consensus of

British colonial medical officers who had served in West Africa and who had access to the report, paragraph 53 upheld the continued exclusion of West African and Indian physicians from the WAMS.

The writers of the report agreed that African physicians might be employed in certain isolated instances, such as in hospitals providing health care to mostly Africans. In these situations the local governments could make the final decision. But the report dealt a monumental blow to the possibility of significant professional interaction between European and African medical authorities in the reiteration of the exclusionist policy. This policy effectively reduced the number of qualified African doctors serving the coastal elites and curtailed the extension of scientific public health services to the underprivileged urban and rural African populations. This policy statement also represented a victory for pseudoscientific racism in an era of changing power relations, and it provoked alarm among the West African elite both at home and abroad.

Boyle received a copy of the edition of the *Sierra Leone Weekly News* containing the committee's report and was infuriated with its contents. In a lengthy letter to the Colonial Office, Boyle excoriated the committee for its undisguised racist attitudes and its profound ignorance of the accomplishments of Africans and diasporic blacks in medicine. Boyle's abridged letter is as follows:

No. 73

Dr. E. Mayfield Boyle to Colonial Office.
(Received 4 January, 1910)
1310 G Street, N.E., Washington, D.C., U.S.A.,
17 December, 1909

Sir,
Extract of the report of the "Departmental Committee on West African Medical Staff," which your Majesty commanded to be presented to both houses of Parliament on July, 1909, have reached me, thro' a West African Journal. . . .
Never have West Africans been so wantonly insulted as when the

Departmental Committee . . . alleged the inferiority of West African Native Doctors to European Doctors, stating further that "it is in general inadvisable to employ natives in West Africa as Medical Officers in the Government Services." This statement, which, in its expatiation, soon takes the form of a contention, rooted upon racial apathy, is sufficient to reveal even the most disinterested reader some of the real causes of the recommendations and insinuations of that Committee. We hold that while we are British subjects we are Africans and certainly ought in Africa, if nowhere else, enjoy life, liberty, and the pursuit of happiness without the encroachment of Europeans. . . .

West African Scientific Doctors are the reflectors of medical schools in Great Britain and Ireland. Their education was obtained not only at great costs but at the feet of the masters of those very Europeans recommended to supersede West Africans in West Africa. Unless the processes of training of West Africans abroad differ from those of Europeans—Englishmen in particular—or unless the Departmental Committee is prepared to show by some new process of reasoning or evidences of scientific research that the "sable livery" of African is indicative of inferiority, Your Majesty will, in the face of the declarations of the schools which have conferred upon West Africans the degrees of proficiency to pursue their professional calling, admit that the report is but a culmination of an infernal scheme of selfish aggrandizement long fomenting in the circles of European negrophobists. . . .

Civilization is full of instances of the negro's capability to do and to achieve and even the Departmental Committee may read and learn.

There has recently been returned to Haiti a negro who studied medicine in Paris, where he was subsequently elected to membership of a University Hospital Staff, a position which he held for several years before resigning to return to his native country. In one of the largest medical institutions of Boston, Mass., U.S.A., is a Liberian Neurologist who, with all of the race prejudice so rampant in the United States, has been prevailed upon by his white conferees to remain in this country. Dr. Daniel Williams, of

Chicago, a negro, was the first man on record to operate on the human heart. His diagnosis was blood clot over the viscus. Dr. Wheatland, of New Port, Rhode Island, also a negro, is a specialist in electro-therapy and a man of national repute. It is noteworthy that Dr. Wheatland studied in a medical school (Harvard) whose faculty is composed of white and coloured. It is needless to multiply references in this country, in Canada, British West Indies, South America, Australia, and other places where negro professional men rank high above the ordinary; but it can not be denied, however, that in its submergence of these facts the Departmental Committee has victimized no less a personage than the Secretary of State for the Colonies. . . . If negroes elsewhere can master the art of sciences of medicine, why should they not in West Africa?

Civilized West Africans have always proudly recognized their allegiance to Great Britain. . . . But there is a limit to the human endurance. . . . As British subjects we demand in return for our loyalty no less than the privilege of equal opportunity of British subjects elsewhere, especially in our own fatherland. . . . [W]e suggest a professional examination for all candidates of British West African Medical Appointments, whether they be Africans or Englishmen, whether they studied in Great Britain or elsewhere. . . . Increase in salary, promotion and even the tenure of office may be made imperatively contingent upon evidences of original research work done by the incumbent or upon his being able to show qualifications of advanced work as provided by schools and examining boards of the United Kingdom. . . . "The mind"—not the colour of the skin or racial characteristics—"is the standard of a man."[45]

Boyle ended his letter with a proclamation of the late sovereign, Queen Victoria, requiring equal justice to all subjects, without regard to race or creed. His letter clearly had a belated impact. Some years later, in reviewing what they were beginning to regard as unjust medical policy, officials of the Colonial Office made reference to Boyle's letter.

The Boyle letter requires additional commentary on several issues. It shows not only his awareness of and keen interest in policies affecting the medical profession in his homeland, but it also provides useful insight into the social and medical history of Africa and the diaspora. In spite of the fact that Boyle had been away from Africa since the 1880s, his knowledge about the West African community also indicates the high level of linkages and the flow of information between blacks in Africa and the United States. It would be incorrect for readers to conclude from Boyle's strong language that he harbored racist sentiments. In Adelaide Cromwell's social assessment of nineteenth-century Freetown, where Boyle grew up,

> Color as a distinguishing characteristic does not appear to have been overtly important in Creole society of Sierra Leone at that time. Position seems to have been based exclusively on origin, money and education or occupation. And as persons of any shade could have the requisite amount of each of these and through intermarriage or miscegenation many colors were found in the same immediate family, there was, in fact, no separate mulatto status—a position accorded one in some countries [for example, the United States, Jamaica, or Brazil] merely by virtue of the color of one's skin. The color lines, to the extent that they existed, or were acknowledged, were between English and African. To be Creole did not mean to be mulatto. Of course to be mulatto probably did mean one was Creole, but not necessarily elite Creole.[46]

Hence, color was not a prerequisite for advancement in Sierra Leone society, although ethnicity would continue to be a factor. Boyle's long residence in the United States coincided with the most racist period in U.S. history and may have sensitized his attitudes about race. With regard to ideology, Boyle manifests the cultural nationalism of Blyden, who shared a deep reverence for African culture and values and rejected in part the Western cultural movement. For writings of this genre stressed a hierarchy of races with the Negro in a category near the bottom. Blyden began to adhere to most of these ideas in the 1870s, the decade of Boyle's birth, and believed that "each race was equal but distinct."[47] Hence, Boyle inherited a fixed notion about race—a notion influenced no doubt by the Darwinian theory of the "survival of the fittest."

Meanwhile, Boyle continued to pursue excellence in medicine. For example, in 1904 he attended lectures in clinical medicine at Johns Hopkins Medical School given by the world-renowned clinician Sir William Osler. In further postgraduate work he studied diseases of the heart, clinical laboratory diagnostic methods at Harvard University Medical School in the summer of 1921, and completed additional courses at Harvard in 1922 and 1924. In 1923 Boyle began to study diagnostic radiology with Dr. Max Kahn and Dr. Joseph C. Bloodgood at Johns Hopkins, but Boyle had to actually enter the facility through the back door because of racial policies that even this eminent Baltimore institution had developed. When one realizes that Dr. Wilhelm Conrad Röntgen (a German physicist, 1845–1923) did not discover the X-ray until 1895,[48] Boyle must indeed rank as one of the black pioneer practitioners in the use of radiology. While associated with Bellevue Hospital in New York City, he completed further courses in radiology under Dr. Charles Gottlieb, X-ray specialist of Beth Israel and Lincoln hospitals, and in the fall of 1927 he completed courses in radiology methodology and interpretation under Professor Alexandra Marcus at the College of the City of New York. Boyle also found time to present papers at medical conferences and published his findings in the *Journal of the National Medical Association,* the journal of the parallel professional association to the American Medical Association.[49]

Boyle eventually settled permanently in the United States, and while the exact time is not known, it appears that he returned only once to Sierra Leone. Our focus on Boyle's life shows that he was a consummate medical professional in America, but also deterred by the policies that disadvantaged Africans. He made accommodations with some facets of the system of social stratification within the African American community in ways that his role model Blyden, the cultural nationalist, might not have approved. Two sons and two granddaughters went on to become Howard University alumni (see figure 8). Mayfield Boyle died at Provident Hospital, in late 1936 at the

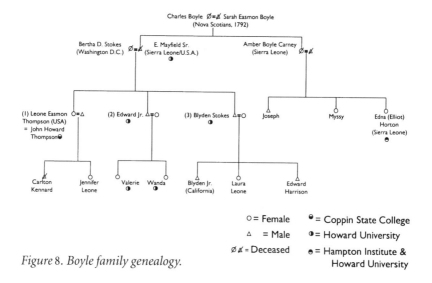

Figure 8. Boyle family genealogy.

○ = Female   ◉ = Coppin State College
△ = Male   ◑ = Howard University
∅ ⊗ = Deceased   ⊖ = Hampton Institute &
                        Howard University

Colonial Dissent: "E.C.D."

There is no doubt that medical science in Anglophone West Africa advanced under colonialism. But there is also no denying that the exclusionary nature of the WAMS and the corporate patronage system inflicted considerable suffering on African doctors both at home and abroad. Evidence of dissent among the English in West Africa came from a political officer in northern Nigeria, who worked mainly among the Hausa and the Fulani. On November 25, 1926, he signed a letter to the editor of West Africa with the initials E.C.D., reporting the existence of 18 million people in the region with just 6 doctors for the official European and "Native Staff." He proclaimed that under colonialism clerks, carpenters, schoolmasters, tax gatherers, policemen, and "dressers"—under a doctor's supervision—were trained, but he wondered why the encouragement to train doctors was not sustained. The English showed little interest in the health of the general population and seemed to have been most worried that African doctors might gain authority over English subjects, a concern that apparently was a result of their narrow focus. They seemed not to have been interested in broad public health campaigns in the countryside but simply in tidying up around their own colonial stations. The English, therefore, differed in their approach to training Africans in medicine than the French. If the French observed that some African students might not qualify in the doctorate of medicine, the option prevailed whereby their partial training could be used for a lower grade as medical assistants, whose medical certification was only valid in government service and under supervision. This was why the French system was the most marvelous medical system in West Africa, according to E.C.D. In this way the French staffed the Francophone region and brought medical service to the most remote villages. E.C.D. argued further in favor of an African Medical Service staffed by Africans who would engage the people in preventative medicine. The people would be taught and trained to engage in the most important measure: how to maintain pure water, which would banish or make less harmful hookworm, guinea worm, typhus, dysentery, and numerous other bowel complaints. He wrote: "Who can teach them the need for this better than a trained doctor, one of their own race, speaking their own language, as never a European can do—knowing their weakness, their superstitions, but knowing how to appeal to these?"[50] Finally, E.C.D. warned the establishment not to place fully qualified African doctors on a lower branch of service and "Let them not cast a reproach in this to be the British. Let their pride in their noble profession be unsullied by thoughts of ungenerous treatment." Imperial authorities paid little attention to this writer at the time, but his dissatisfaction with the WAMS was no doubt indicative of a break in colonial attitudes about the utilization of Africans in the Colonial Medical Service.

Governor Sir Frederick Gordon Guggisberg and the Training of African Doctors in the Gold Coast

While the objective of training African doctors in Sierra Leone was a nineteenth-century idea, this initiative surfaced again in the twentieth century. This time, however, the policy initiative of training Africans for medicine locally fell to the Gold Coast under the leadership of Governor Sir Frederick Gordon Guggisberg (1919–27). Guggisberg held firm to the need to provide Africans with premed through residency training locally as doctors, with clinical experience in the setting of West Africa rather than sending them to Europe. Indeed, he reported that upon the return of these students it was found (to the anger of many) that only 50 percent were properly qualified, including even some European doctors.

The French medical school at Dakar and its success in the training of African medical assistants for Francophone West Africa had become well known to British colonial officials. This school served as the model for the British who wanted to establish a similar medical school for the internal training of African doctors. Indeed, on August 30, 1921, at the initiation of Winston Churchill—then secretary of the colonies[51]—Guggisberg inquired into the possibility of establishing a medical college where Africans could be trained as medical assistants in several countries in Africa. In 1921 he sent Dr. J. M. O'Brien, a British health official, to visit the French medical school at Dakar and received an interesting report from him, but before medical assistants could complete their training, Guggisberg had already advocated the need for qualified African doctors in the Gold Coast Public Health Service.[52] On October 9, 1923, Guggisberg opened the Gold Coast Hospital at Korle Bu in Accra. In addition, between 1919 and 1923 his administration built eight more hospitals and numerous dispensaries at various places in the colony, among the Ashanti at Kumasi and farther afield in the northern territories. Since these institutions would give Africans more access to health care, this represented a shift in the thinking on the part of English colonial officials in the Gold Coast. Guggisberg was a visionary and reformer who really deserves credit for these policy shifts. His long-term objective was to develop a complete system of medical training, beginning with the secondary school at Achimota and progressing to the intended medical school at Korle Bu. He wanted as many hospitals as possible in which African doctors could complete their training. Just one year earlier, the governor had appointed Drs. A. F. Renner-Dove, G. T. Hammond, and

E. Tagoe to the medical service, while rejecting protests of the local European community in the Gold Coast.[53] Apparently, European men resented going to an African doctor and especially having him examine female family members. For example, Dunkwa was a mining and timber community housing a sizable number of Europeans; only one doctor was posted at a time to the town. Considerable dissension was expressed over Tagoe's posting in 1927, but the governor was adamant.

Governor Guggisberg, while sometimes the recipient of criticism, also received praise for his efforts to reverse the old policy that dampened the parent's spirit and diminished the aspirations of their children about entering the medical profession. Critics proposed that the government popularize medicine in the country and allow young doctors trained in Europe to be employed in the public service and use government facilities rather than enter private practice, since the latter required a greater outlay of personal funds. This was unlike entering the legal profession, one critic held, which was flooded with young Africans because colonial regulations had not yet extended to their profession. One outspoken African talked about how he at first chose mining engineering as a profession, switched next to medicine, and then abandoned it for the legal profession—all because of the risks of public service for Africans and low salaries a doctor could expect if he was not allowed to accept private patients.[54]

While Guggisberg's policies had the support and respect from the African elite, the government's progress in the employment of African doctors in public service was not fast enough. Hence, African reaction went unabated and criticism came from one of the Gold Coast's most renowned citizens. J. Casely-Hayford spoke before the Legislative Council in 1924 about the absence of African physicians in the Gold Coast hospital:

> I was certainly struck with the arrangements which in every way were perfect. I saw African nurses . . . European nurses, and I saw the arrangements and the accommodations for the European Medical Officers, but I was particularly struck not to find a single African Medical man attached to the Hospital to help in the

healing of his own countrymen in his own country. . . . [W]hen we first joined this [Legislative] Council . . . General [W. H.] Grey . . . went to the extent of describing the . . . [WAMS] as a kind of a medical trade union [author's emphasis]. He may or may not be right, but I think the idea was that the service should be opened to all and that Africans should have free access to this Service.[55]

African reaction to the lack of African doctors employed in the government public service were not without merit for the future against such a medical trade union. In 1927 Achimota graduated its first pupils, among whom were Dr. Charles Odamten Easmon, Kwame Nkrumah, and some 118 others. Most pupils of this group would become the vanguard for change in the struggle for professionalism and self-determination in the new African states.

In October 1930 the Gold Coast colonial government atoned for its shameful history of discrimination against African doctors by offering what appeared to be the first government scholarships for the study of medicine abroad since the 1850s. Five candidates submitted applications for the scholarships following the first posted notices. Similar scholarships began to be offered to African students from other colonies. The Gold Coast, however, was unusual; thanks to Guggisberg, its progress was mainly due to his leadership and progressive African and British supporters.[56]

The following chapter explores the multifaceted career of another physician whose actions sometimes did not endear him to the British middle class, especially his efforts to reform the medical trade union in the colonial era of intraprofessional conflict.

CHAPTER SIX

M. C. F. Easmon: Protectorate Clinician-Scholar

*D*r. MaCormack Charles Farrell Easmon, who was born on April 11, 1890, in Accra, Gold Coast, was nurtured in a region at a time of transition from informal to formal empire. During his eighty-two years (1890–1972), he served the Colonial Medical Service as a clinician, as an anthropologist on the social structures of indigenous societies, as a historian who made seminal contributions after World War I, and as president of the Sierra Leone Arts and Crafts Society founded in 1960.[1] Easmon's longevity and stable health allowed for more diverse occupational pursuits in the twentieth century than his nineteenth-century predecessors ever enjoyed, most of whom died young. Known as "Charlie" by relatives and friends and later as "M.C.F." in government medical circles, Easmon was a paternal descendant of the second Nova Scotian generation of the Easmon medical family; he was just seven years old when the Gold Coast government ordered his father, John Farrell Easmon—chief medical officer—to vacate the government quarters after sixteen years of service. By either choice or force, the Easmon family, severely sick from malaria and suffering from anguish, crossed a lagoon in a canoe seeking accommodation with a friend shortly after Easmon's ouster as CMO in 1897.[2]

Charlie was ten years old at the time of the sudden death of his father at age forty-four on June 9, 1900, which sent shock waves reverberating throughout Creoledom in West Africa. Charlie would carry these memories of his father's problems with the government into his adult life, and he may have some harbored ill will against the British middle class in his professional struggles.

He was a descendant of a complex maternal line, one requiring a book in itself if properly told. Charlie's maternal great-great-grandmother was a Hausa trader, Betsy Carew, and his great-great-grandfather was Thomas Carew, a Bambara butcher. Betsy and Thomas had a daughter named Hannah. Then came the Spilsbury line, and Charlie's entry here stemmed from Joseph Green Spilsbury, his great-great-grandfather, the son of a Maroon mother and Dr. George Spilsbury, a onetime colonial surgeon, who himself was the son of "a well-known London patient medicine maker."[3] Hannah Carew married Joseph Green Spilsbury, and they had three children, Anne, Thomas, and Henry. At the time of Joseph's death in 1853 he was among the nineteen biggest land and residential owners in Freetown. His wealth brought the Spilsburys and subsequent generations settler status and financial security in the burgeoning Creole society. Anne Spilsbury, Joseph's daughter, married William Smith, Jr., son of a Yorkshireman and Fanti mother in the Gold Coast. Anne and William had seven children, his second set of children, and the youngest of the Smith daughters, Annette Kathleen, or Nettie, was the mother of Charlie. The young Easmon's immediate paternal relative was Albert Whiggs Easmon, his father's brother, a practicing physician and gynecologist (see figure 9). He then shared a host of maternal relatives in Freetown, including Dr. William Awooner-Renner, an uncle, and another uncle, Francis Smith, the former puisne judge of the Gold Coast. Two other uncles, the late Drs. Robert Smith and Joseph Smith, had died in the nineteenth century.[4]

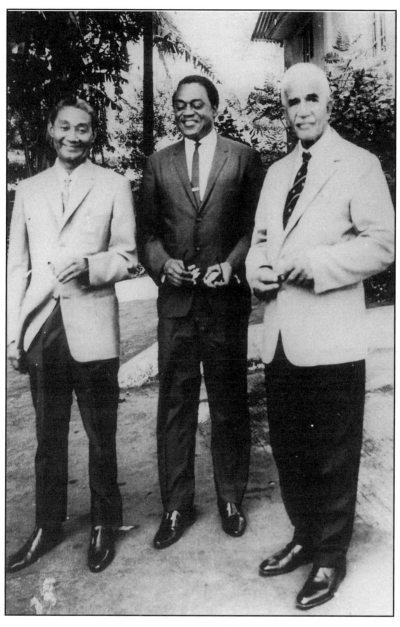

Figure 9. Drs. Raymond Sarif Easmon (left), Charles Odamten Easmon (center), and M. C. F. Easmon, Sierra Leone, c. 1968.

Mrs. Adelaide Smith Casely-Hayford (1868–1960) was the sister of Anne Kathleen Smith Easmon (1870–1951), Charlie's mother. Researcher Adelaide Cromwell illustrates the complex interlocking kinship linkages between outstanding Creole families—the Smiths, the Spilsburys, the Hebrons, the Awooner-Renners, Coleridge-Taylors, the Lumpkins, the Wrights, the Hunters, the Randalls, and the Casely-Hayfords—in Sierra Leone, Gambia, the Gold Coast, and Nigeria. Anne Kathleen, now widowed with two children, Charlie and Kathleen, needed help, and the Smith sisters did not hesitate in coming to the aid of their sister under the indefatigable leadership of Adelaide.

Aftermath of the Easmon Episode

The Easmon family moved from Accra to Freetown, Sierra Leone, sometime in 1900, where the young Easmon enrolled at Miss Smith's school and later at the grammar school. Their stay in Freetown was brief while the family made plans for moving to England. With regard to this objective, Adelaide Cromwell reported:

> The Easmon family lived on such a [high] standard that there was hardly any money left. We [the sisters to Kathleen, Adelaide, and Emma] immediately offered her [Kathleen] a home which she accepted, but of course, conditions were different and she wanted to give the children better educational advantages. This coupled with my poor state of health made us decide to return to England. So after closing the school and selling bits of housing furniture, together with all our lares and penates, there was still need for money to cover five passages: mine, Nettie's [Kathleen], the two children's and Emma's.[5]

Adelaide seized the initiative and wrote requesting free passage for the children to Sir Alfred Lewis Jones, the founder of the Elder Dempster Shipping Line, who readily agreed with "a grace I have never forgotten," said Adelaide.

The Easmons in England: Medical Training

The Easmon family and the Smith sisters arrived in England from
Freetown sometime in 1901 and took up residence in Shepherd's
Bush, at 5 Melrose Terrace. They lived in close proximity to Collert
Court, the preparatory school for St. Paul's in West Kensington,
where the young M. C. F. Easmon was enrolled from October 1901
through April 1903 and where he received two form prizes before
moving on to Epson College. This institution was a special private
school with strong connections to the medical profession, and it offered special concessions to the children of doctors. Here Easmon had
a Council Exhibition Scholarship of £30 per year and a St. Mary's
Hospital Scholarship of £145. At Epson he won two form prizes in history and divinity and played on the rugby team.

Medical training was the next part of his education. He was admitted to the University of London, St. Mary's Hospital Medical
School, and took the first examinations in June 1906 and 1907 for the
MB and BS. He passed the second examination in anatomy with distinction in July 1909 and the finals for the MB and BS in May 1912. In
the same year he qualified in England with the MRCS and in London
with the LRCP. His name now appeared on the British Medical Register, enabling him to practice in England, the Commonwealth, and
Africa. He was just 22 years old, with prizes in anatomy, histology,
psychological medicine, and practical surgery, and with certificates in
anatomy, physiology, organic chemistry, medicine, surgery, forensic
medicine, and hygiene. He received appointments as prosector in
anatomy to St. Mary's Hospital Medical School in 1909; prosector in
anatomy to the examining board of the Royal College of Surgeons
and the Royal College of Physicians in 1910; clinical assistant with
charge of the wards to the ophthalmic department of St. Mary's Hospital in 1910–11; and house surgeon to the Huntingdon County Hospital in 1912. At the "London School of Tropical Medicine (University
of London) [he] attended the 41st Session January–March 1913 and
gained the Certificate on the examination at the end of the Course
with 73% of the total marks."[6]

Easmon had indeed performed in medical training on a level comparable to that of his famous father and had upheld the scholarly

tradition of the Smith and Easmon medical families. Upon the completion of his training-level appointments in England, employment of a more permanent nature became a necessity. Perhaps aware of upcoming efforts to intervene in the decisionmaking process of the Colonial Office, the *Lancet* warned: "Attempts to influence the Secretary of State's selection through members of Parliament or other persons who are not personally well acquainted with the applicant are useless and will be regarded as indicating that the applicant does not consider his qualifications sufficiently good to justify his appointment on his own merits."[7] The *Lancet's* reference may have been to the Anti-Slavery Aborigines' Protection Society (ASAPS). This organization, headed by Rev. Sir John Hobbis Harris, was the chief lobbying agent for African medical men in the Colonial Office and Parliament in 1912.

The ASAPS had become a lobbying force for African medical professionals since the foundation of the WAMS in 1901. It had originated in about the first quarter of the nineteenth century in England to protest the cruelties exacted on indigenous Africans in suppressing slavery and other forms of inequities. By the late 1880s it had gradually changed to become an example in West Africa of groups that placed more emphasis on African control, a transition from the FéKuw (Fanti National Political Society) in the Cape Coast to the Gold Coast Aborigines' Rights Protection Society. The abolition of slavery, the growth of an African Westernized elite from their traditional African descendants, and issues involving land tenure under the British were all reasons for the organization's changing focus of protest. The organization leaders included J. Mensah Sarbah, J. Casely-Hayford, J. E. K. Aggrey, Rev. S. R. B. Attoh Ahuma, J. W. Sey, T. F. E. Jones, George Hughes, E. J. P. Brown, Dr. B. W. Quartey-Papafio, and D. Sackey QuarcooPome. It sent deputations to England, people who challenged ordinances of colonial administration and thereby formed the antecedents for modern African administration.[8]

M.C.F. EASMON AND THE COLOR BAR
Easmon completed an application for employment for the first time in London in about the first week in October 1912, through Rev. Sir

John Hobbis Harris of the ASAPS. Easmon was very much aware of the color bar in the Colonial Medical Service, but he was willing to test his newly acquired certification against a departmental committee of Parliament regulating the WAMS, which held in 1909 that "native doctors are incompetent and that their professional capabilities are not on par with those of Europeans." Easmon wanted desperately to challenge this position with his credentials and in submitting them observed: "These facts go to show, I think that my professional capabilities are on a par with those of any European about to enter the Service." The Colonial Office's response to Easmon on October 10, 1912 was immediate: "Sir, I am desired by Mr. Harcourt to inform you that your application for Colonial Medical employment will remain on record; but he fears there is practically no prospect of his being able to offer you an appointment in the West African Medical Staff."[9] This rejection of Easmon's application prompted the ASAPS to conduct research on the employment status of African doctors in West Africa.

African Physicians in the Colonial Medical Service, 1913

In early 1913 Rev. J. T. Roberts, secretary of the local auxiliary of the ASAPS in Sierra Leone, requested from Dr. Michael Lewis Jarrett (Sherbro) a survey on the admission of qualified "Native Medical Men who have undergone training, examination, and registered in the United Kingdom of Great Britain and Ireland, into the West African Medical Staff for service in British West African Colonies."[10] On February 20, 1913, Jarrett wrote a lengthy report on the number of African doctors admitted into government service since the 1860s and on the changing government policy toward their employment. The report was returned to Roberts and it included the numbers of African doctors by territory: Sierra Leone, nine; Gambia, one; Gold Coast, five, and Lagos, eight. The report noted several observations: "the service has been practically closed against the employment of Natives by that [Lagos] Government"; that the majority of these medical men were in the Colonial Medical Service at the inauguration of the WAMS in 1901 but were placed on a separate roster because of the color bar—that is, none could be admitted to the West African Medical Service except those who were of unmixed European parentage; and their designation as local medical officers carried the stigma of their not being trained in Britain. Instead, this procedure made it appear as if their qualifications were obtained in the colonies where no medical schools existed, so they were not considered bona fide doctors or medical professionals.

The irony of these restrictions was that the mercantile firms had retained the services of African doctors, and even governors of the colonies had consulted them for treatment, as the report indicated. Dr. Awooner-Renner attended the wife of Governor Sir Frederic Cardew (1894–1900) in Sierra Leone. It was well known that John Farrell Easmon was the personal physician to Governor Sir Brandford Griffith (1885–95), Lady Griffith, and their family in the Gold Coast. G. C. Denton, while acting governor in 1889, had Dr. Randall attend to his wife in Nigeria, and other high-ranking officials had not regretted placing their relatives in the hands of African doctors from time to time. Further, it was difficult for European doctors to treat special disease cases of the local people without a third person because they did not know the language, nor were they trusted as well, as the report noted:

> Besides the uneducated Native has a dread for the white man. He sees in him a person whose colour is different from his own, and consequently he cannot entirely claim his sympathy. . . . The white man is therefore unappreciated to him; while on the other hand, he sees his brother, whom as a little boy he knows and sees, grow up in his midst; he knows of his successes in the Elementary and Secondary schools and College [Fourah Bay College, Sierra Leone] of his Colony; he could remember the year, or mark certain occurrences in that year when that young man left home for England to study medicine; he hears of his successes there, and now he has returned fully qualified. . . . To himself he says I could place all my troubles before this man rather than any other.[11]

Under Jarrett's leadership, African doctors had made their case once more to the Colonial Office for employment in the WAMS and illustrated how the issue of color retarded the growth of medical infra-structure in the colonies.

Jarrett's committee expressed appreciation to Rev. Sir John Hobbis Harris for stating the limitations set for African doctors in the Colonial Medical Service in his book *Dawn in Darkest Africa*. In chapter 5 of his book, entitled "Educated Native," Harris supported the African doctors in their professional struggles:

> Has the doctor [African] failed? Again where? Not in the English and Scotch hospitals, for he has frequently carried a higher degree than he finds among his European colleagues when he returns to the coast. That he is excluded from Government service proves nothing, except perhaps prejudice. It may be asked why in the Gold Coast colony the African medical man has no place in Government service. We are told in reply, because white men, and more particularly their wives, would refuse to receive treatment at the hands of coloured medical men. This argument fails entirely when we remember that the majority of the hospital patients are not white, but coloured, and at present can only receive treatment from white doctors. . . .
>
> . . . [A]lmost every "coaster" knows how one of these heroic women [European] was . . . [on] the last bed of sickness; the distracted husband had tried everything, had implored the white doctor to try something—it hardly mattered what—to give back health to the sufferer. Suddenly a thought occurred to him! The native doctor [African physician], fully qualified, was sent for and visited the patient, and then in consultation with his white colleague, other treatment was tried. Slowly the sick one fought her way back to life and health, and to this day the husband remembers to whom he owes the restoration of one who to him was everything—and this is no isolated case.[12]

In spite of Harris's strong criticism of the Colonial Medical Service, his revelations about the quality and utility of the African doctor went unheeded in official circles.

Since the inception of the corporate patronage system of colonial health care, times had not changed for African doctors with regard to opportunity in West Africa. However, African doctors now had the Jarrett Report and Harris's book to support their ongoing claims for employment in the government service before Parliament, and Harris remained very active in corresponding to its departmental committee. Bright Davies, a Sierra Leonean and the most eminent journalist in West Africa, joined in discussing in the African press the issue of public appointments in the government.[13]

Easmon's Second Application: Sierra Leone

M. C. F. Easmon submitted a second application on May 22, 1913, for employment in the WAMS, addressed to the private secretary of the secretary of state, Colonial Office, London. His application was for an opening in Sierra Leone. Easmon had received high praise in recommendations from Wilfred Harris (MD, FRCP) and Leslie Paton (MB, FRCS) of St. Mary's Hospital in 1912. Dean Broadbent described Easmon's clinical skills as "careful and skillful in diagnosis, showing marked promise for the future. I can with confidence recommend him as a most eligible candidate for the West African Medical Staff."[14]

William Awooner-Renner was retiring in 1913 after more than twenty-nine years of service. He had worked as assistant colonial surgeon from 1882 to 1913, as acting PMO, justice of the peace, and deputy coroner of the police district. In spite of his outstanding service to the colony, membership in the WAMS was closed to him, but he was allowed to remain on the same salary standard after 1902 as before this date. Designated as a medical officer without portfolio in 1901, he was compensated at £400–500, with £20 annual increments; in 1911 his salary was set at £500 in the £600–700 scale, with an annual raise set at £25; it was set again at £654 as for the senior medical officer— who received £800–1,000—with £50 annual increments; and estimated at £944 as for the principal medical officer in the WAMS. In 1910 Awooner-Renner was moved to the King-Harman Maternity Ward of the Colonial Hospital.[15] So Easmon arrived in Freetown seeking Awooner-Renner's clinical position in the Colonial Hospital and appointment as a medical officer in the WAMS, which would place him on the same salary rating with European doctors.

The government did consider the Easmon appointment. In the interview an official handed Easmon a copy of the WAMS regulations and noted in his notes that Easmon considered himself eligible even after reading paragraph 23, which held that all candidates must be of European descent. Rejection followed and produced further questions from Members of Parliament and the African press. Dr. William Thomas Prout, principal medical officer in Sierra Leone from 1895 to 1906, opposed the Easmon appointment in the colony from the beginning, and his letters on the employment of Easmon influenced others. One official noted that "he [Easmon] had a bad father [Dr. John Farrell Easmon, with whom Prout had served with in the Gold Coast], and 2 bad uncles" (Dr. Robert Smith, Sierra Leone years of service 1865–87; and Dr. Joseph Spilsbury Smith, in the Gold Coast service 1886–94). But a high-ranking official, whose initials appear to be that of the governor, decided to "run the risk and admit Dr. Easmon to succeed Dr. Renner—in light of Dr. Prout's warning," and noting in the end "I think we have a good case for making the experiment—recognizing that it is an experiment ['experiment' here be might be in reference to whether Easmon could make an adjustment in his behavior to one of inequality as required by the NMO status; if not then the officials ran the risk of possible embarrassment in the future similar to the Easmon episode of 1897]."[16] On May 28, 1913, Edward Mereweather, governor of Sierra Leone (1911–15), appointed Easmon to the Native Medical Staff (NMS) at the standard salary rate of £300, with a raise of £10 per year to £350, and with further increase after five years of service. The maximum salary was £400 after this period. In spite of the fact that Easmon's qualification was higher than the average candidate, the governor noted, in no way was he to assume Awooner-Renner's position in the Colonial Hospital. This position was to go to a member of the WAMS, and Easmon, as were the postings of Drs. W. A. O. Taylor and William Frederick Campbell of the NMS, was to be employed according to the needs for his services in the colony or in the protectorate (see map 4).[17]

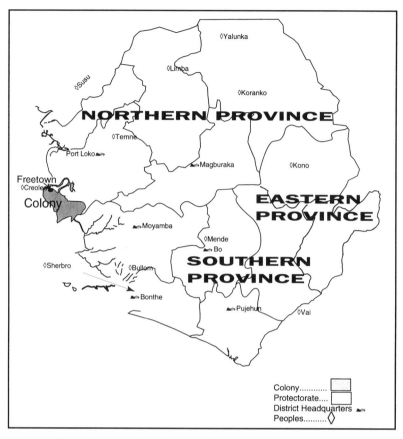

Map 4. Sierra Leone cultural and administrative areas, nineteenth and twentieth centuries.

Easmon was subsequently posted to Moyamba in the protectorate, while a number of other African doctors registered by the government in Freetown after 1910 remained in private practice, such as Albert Whiggs Easmon, Michael Lewis Jarrett, Herbert Christian Bankole-Bright, Thomas Clarkson Maxwell, and Ishmael Charles Pratt.[18] In the government service, however, Taylor and Campbell came under severe criticism by the acting principal medical officer, Dr. J. W. Collett, who noted that these officers were perfect examples of natives not suited for appointments to responsible positions, for they needed European supervision at all times in order to make them

170

maintain a reliable work ethic. Campbell had allowed a patient suffering from smallpox to be placed in the same room with patients suffering from chicken pox and, in Collett's words, while he overlooked incompetence on the part of European doctors, such carelessness was routine and had to be rectified. Hence, African physicians were not without malpractice allegations, and the authorities did not allow them to go unnoticed throughout West Africa.[19]

Easmon to Cameroon

The outbreak of World War I in 1914 would obscure such concerns because the Allied effort required West African participation to end Germany's colonization of Togo and the Cameroons. German troops numbered 7,000 in 1912 in Germany's African colonies as a whole (Togo, Cameroons, Southwest Africa or now Namibia, and Tanganyika or now Tanzania), as compared to 12,000 in British West Africa, East Africa, and Northern Rhodesia (now Zambia), or compared to 14,000 troops in the Portuguese colonies, or 18,000 in the Belgian territories. Nigeria was the most significant Allied base against Germany with the largest contingent of 4,000 Africans and 350 British officers.[20] Easmon was among them for orientation, but was posted to service in the Allied cause to the Cameroons from November 13, 1914, to July 29, 1915, with fourteen other officers of the WAMS from Sierra Leone, and granted a temporary commission as a lieutenant.[21] Togo fell quickly to Allied forces, and by 1916 the Cameroons war ended. The Allied forces had suffered some 1,000 casualties.

The war bonus issue erupted after the secretary of state for the colonies announced the beginnings of payments on January 1, 1917, to all members of the "native staff of clerks," which included clerks, general employees, the police force, prison wardens, marine staff, skilled artisans, and (in the medical departments) only nurses, dressers, lunatic asylum attendants, sanitary inspectors, and carpenters at the Lagos Hospital—all at varying rates. From what was probably a uniform document for Sierra Leone, the war bonus regulation for Nigeria stipulated eligibility requirements: "Natives in the employment of the Government of the [numerous] classes referred to . . . who have retired from the Nigerian Civil Service with or without pension since that date, or who have been transferred or dismissed from the . . . Service since that date, are entitled to claim [of] War Bonus for the period since 1st January, 1917, up to date of termination of service under the Government of Nigeria." African doctors, who were not included in the classes to be paid, yet who claimed eligibility, resented the prefixed "native" category. Since they were members of the dominant profession, they then objected to being linked to the general classes of African staff members. This was the pretext for much of the debate that followed. In 1915, to further heighten the conflict, the secretary of state had assigned the European medical officers to a higher scale of salary. The justification was twofold: inhospitable climate, and the need to maintain two residential establishments—one in England and the other in West Africa. It was logical, therefore, that even the war bonus to European medical officers would be higher than for eligible Africans. If paid, the bonus for payment to members of the native staff would be 12.5 percent of their salaries, or £44; the Europeans would get 33 percent of their salaries, or £120.[22]

This position, however, did not resolve the matter and African doctors responded with various memoranda. Hence, the debate became centered around three separate items that the African doctors essentially linked in order to hopefully gain the upper hand: the war bonus, the higher salary scale, and the duty allowance. Returning to Moyamba in 1917, Easmon interpreted the duty allowance of 1915 for members of the WAMS as a war bonus, arguing that the sum was not part of their original contract agreement, and on July 9, 1917, he applied for the same allowance to the governor through the PMO. He justified his claim by noting that he also was subject to increased living costs because of the fact that he, like Europeans in the WAMS, was not a native of Sierra Leone. The colonial authorities agreed to this point but noted that he was a native of West Africa. They reminded Easmon of his initial contract agreement of 1913, which included only annual increments and not duty allowance, noting further that he had attained his maximum salary standard in order to qualify for consideration. The governor informed Easmon that no war bonus would be forthcoming, since the duty allowance being given to the European medical officers was unrelated to the war.[23] Gambia had no African practitioner in the service,[24] and the Gold Coast had yet to hire an African doctor for its health service.[25] Hence, the war bonus issue was not raised in these colonies.

But for Nigeria it was a different matter. Drs. Oguntola Sapara, Kubolaje Faderin, Akidiya Ladapo Oluwole, and W. A. Cole petitioned the government for war bonus relief in December 1918 because of the high cost of living brought by the conflict. The native clerks, they claimed, should not be the only ones eligible for war-bonus payments, especially since one Nigerian senior or officer first class, who held the post of provincial commissioner and was recognized as a member of the European staff, was approved for and received war-bonus payments. Acting Governor A. C. Boyle denied their petition and kept them locked into their original contracts, as did the Sierra Leone government with Easmon.[26] But for Easmon there was no slackening in his struggle with the government, for race and colonialism appeared to control the dynamics of intraprofessional conflict.

Members of the WAMS of Sierra Leone who had served with the Allied forces in the Cameroons received special accolades from the British government, but Easmon's concerns had not been addressed so he submitted a petition to the secretary of state.[27] He noted that the WAMS listing of staff of medical officers from Sierra Leone who served in the Cameroons with him had a "C" after their names, but his was the only one not so designated. Most of the medical officers concurred with Easmon's contention about his name not having a "C" next to it, and since the NMOs were apparently without a staff list, Easmon opined about how he was going to receive credit. This honor was significant to him because it would shed light on his record of service in the Cameroons when it came time for promotion. Dr. H. Tweedy, the principal medical officer, finally responded to Easmon's letter of inquiry to the secretary of state and informed him that the secretary of state forwarded no communication on the issue of his recognition.

Easmon, however, found another strategy to improve his standing.

Colonial officials not indigenous to Sierra Leone could take a competence examination in the language indigenous to their assigned district and receive a salary bonus. Since Mende was the spoken language
at Bo and Moyamba, Easmon sought to be examined in Mende on the
grounds that "even though classed as a native Medical Officer I am
partly of European descent [the MaCormacks of Northern Ireland
and the Smiths of Yorkshire, England] and was neither born or educated in this Colony, nor was I domiciled here prior to obtaining my
present position in the Government Service."[28] Still a boy when his
family left the Gold Coast, Easmon's knowledge of and fluency in the
various native languages, including the Twi spoken in his native
country, was probably very limited. The executive council permitted
Easmon to take the exam, allowing the application for a separate allowance on the European scale as a special case. On February 9, 1918,
the director of education in Freetown administered a localized examination in Mende for a preliminary understanding of the language,
known as the lower standard, and Easmon scored 94.3 percent of the
marks awarded. His success allowed Easmon to receive a gratuity of
£25 for the language examination and an upgrade of his service
record.

Easmon had now resided in Sierra Leone for nearly six years and he
continued his absorption of colony and protectorate cultures by
learning both the Krio and Mende languages. Language skills were
even more essential for communication across ethnic and socioeconomic boundaries as Sierra Leone became the staging post for an unprecedented disease exchange affecting not only West Africa but also
the whole world.

Medical historians described the influenza pandemic of 1918–19 as
the most catastrophic outbreak of infectious diseases in world history. David Patterson and Gerald Pyle assess this pandemic as the
worst biological disaster since the bubonic plague of the fourteenth
century, and it struck almost every colony and community in sub-
Saharan Africa. Recently revised conservative estimates show some
30 million died worldwide and some 1.25 million died in Africa
proper, but it is more likely that 1.7–2 million people died there.[29] In
Sierra Leone perhaps 3 percent died in September 1918 alone; in the

Gold Coast some 100,000 died; and in southern Nigeria an estimated 3 percent of the inhabitants—some 250,000—perished, including 27 European officials.[30]

Influenza was not unknown to the older generation of colonial medical officers and African practitioners of the 1890s. The pandemic of 1889–93 had reached West Africa in 1891, but it was over by the time Easmon and others of his generation began to practice medicine. Influenza is caused by one of two main viruses—influenza A and influenza B—that are transmitted from person to person through the respiratory system. Deaths can also occur from pneumonia resulting from secondary bacterial infection of lungs weakened by the influenza. Numerous cultures and strains of the bacteria were erroneously isolated and identified as carrying agents of the disease before its viral etiology became known in 1933, but antibiotics capable of controlling secondary infections did not become available until about 1945. Chemotherapy for influenza does not exist even at this time, and effective vaccines were not developed until the 1950s. Since the viruses are genetically unpredictable, new vaccines must be developed constantly to deal with the variations. Patterson reports further: "The pandemic of 1918–19 was caused by the sudden creation, by mutation or perhaps by genetic recombination with a swine influenza virus, of a particularly virulent strain against which people had no previous exposure, hence no immunity."[31]

Certainly, the Sierra Leone medical establishment and population were totally unprepared for the epidemic. The medical staff consisted of three administrative medical officers, two senior medical officers, one sanitary officer, the medical officer of health, eighteen medical officers (a number later reduced to fifteen), and four NMOs. The PMO apparently attempted to recruit local African doctors in private practice to assist in the crisis but some were unwilling to assist the colonial medical establishment because of its discriminatory practices.[32] The herbalist doctors were the other resource that administered to the population as a whole. Meantime, physicians could do little but prescribe the rest with symptomatic treatment and record traces of the epidemic.

Freetown sits on a promontory and overlooks the harbor at the mouth of the Sierra Leone River. The disease first broke out in sub-Saharan Africa in Freetown on August 22, 1918. It is said that a ship from England acted as a carrier of the disease, and from Freetown the disease spread to the rest of West Africa, moving overland to Francophone northern neighbors from Dakar.

The disease affected over 60 percent of the population in Freetown with an estimated 20,000 cases.[33] Ada Hebron Awooner-Renner (1900–1992; see figure 10)—who married William Awooner-Renner, and who was the daughter of a barrister, Abe Spencer Hebron, and his wife Jane—remembered vividly the impact of the epidemic:

> I was eighteen years of age during the influenza epidemic of 1918. From the second-story balcony of our house—[the merchant prince Syble Boyle's mansion, built around 1850]—on Trelawney Street, I could see the hearse carrying a dead body for burial with one man in front pulling it and with two men behind pushing it. No one went out, and the doctors stayed in their homes. Medicines were rare. My mother gave us only quinine and lemon, mixed with eucalyptus seeds to take. People were very sick—so much so that they could not muster the strength to bury their dead. A mass grave was dug at Ascuncion Cemetery for the burial of a lot of people who died from this epidemic.[34]

Dr. Raymond Sarif Easmon, who was only five years old at the time, also remembered the daily funeral processions passing along his street. Albert Whiggs Easmon, his father, was the leading gynecologist in Freetown with an extensive private practice, and was about the only physician who did not contract influenza during the 1918–19 epidemic. Raymond Easmon observed further that "Father had literally to doctor the whole city." No doubt the strain and pressures on him were too great, too protracted for one suffering from hypertension. Shortly after the epidemic he had a stroke. For two years he was bedridden, the right side of his body paralyzed with hemiplegia (paralysis of only one half of the body). He died on Saturday, May 26, 1921, at the age of fifty-six.[35] Albert's death left only M. C. F. Easmon representing the Easmon medical men.

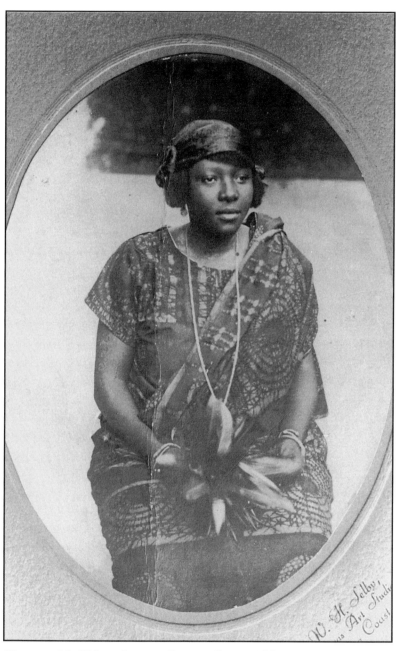

Figure 10. *Ada Hebron Awooner-Renner, Ghana, Gold Coast, c.* 1927. *Courtesy of Walter A. Renner.*

On October 30, 1918, M. C. F. Easmon submitted a report, dated October 26, 1918, on the influenza epidemic at Moyamba (the district headquarters and circuit court) and connecting towns in Ponietta district of the protectorate. This report stated that the epidemic gradually diffused along the railway line that passed from Freetown through Songo Town, Mabang, Bradford, Rotifunk and subdistrict, Boia, Moyamba, Levuma, Mano, and the Yonni chiefdom, and by September 2 the disease spread beyond the railway line to Fakais and other towns. Easmon further noted that persons associated with the messenger system and the railway contracted the viral infection first and spread it to the prisoners, wardens, and a majority of the Syrians doing business in the interior. While the older people and children seemed to have missed the contagion, the majority of cases were adult males between sixteen and forty. More men than women became ill, but about an equal number of men and women died—indicating that the smaller number of women who fell ill were much sicker than the men. The high number of cases all over Sierra Leone entailed high social and economic cost. If there were no complications, a typical bout with the disease might last ten days to two weeks. The caseloads increased exponentially, and they placed heavy burdens on the colonial medical establishment in the twenty-four outpatient facilities in medical districts of the colony. The Creoles and government officials had lower mortality than did the indigenous people because of better nutrition and stronger health before the outbreak of flu. Easmon concluded by stating that the total number of deaths was 767 in the principal towns in Ponietta district and the two chiefdoms.[36] In spite of that fact the population numbers were not known, the Temnes in the north and the Mendes and Sherbros in the south suffered numerous deaths.

The Easmon report of 1918 showed the extent of the disease in the region, but he did not report whether he himself contracted the infection, although he probably did. His success demonstrated that Creole medical officers could work in the protectorate among the indigenous people without European supervision, contradicting a myth of long standing. In Freetown the PMO recognized this factor and praised the Easmon report.

Easmon and a Hostile Reception

In the protectorate, however, Easmon's continuing demand to ranking equal to the WAMS often met a hostile reception from the British middle class. Doctors were required to make monthly tours of the towns and communities in their districts, where accommodations varied. In November 1918 Easmon made a monthly visit to Makene and wired to the officer in charge of the West African Frontier Force (WAFF) concerning his arrival. Easmon was apparently accustomed to using one of the four officers' houses. The officer in charge at Makene ordered two soldiers to accompany Easmon to the soldiers' houses, accommodation which he refused to accept. Easmon reminded the officer in charge of the type of accommodations usually available to him on tour, namely, the officers' houses. Easmon reported that the officer "at once lost his temper, raised his voice saying that he was in charge of the barracks and had decided where I [Easmon] was to stay and if I did not like it, I could go elsewhere. His manner was most offensive."[37]

Easmon made an about-face and returned to the quarters provided—the house used by the officers' servants. This house was "without proper doors or windows, [and] mere holes in the wall," was still occupied by the servants upon Easmon's arrival, the bedclothes of one were still in evidence, and the wives of the mess cooks occupied the kitchen. In 1916, Easmon remembered, the pharmacist had used the building, while Easmon stayed either in the officers' rest house or in the medical officers' house. Captain Clements was the officer in charge up until August 1918, and the new officer in charge did not know Easmon, but complied at least by having the building swept clean in Easmon's presence. In his complaint to the PMO in Freetown, Easmon stressed that the accommodations in the officer's "boys'" house lowered the prestige of the medical officer and the image of the medical department. He concluded, "I therefore beg to apply that this question of the M.O.'s quarters in Makene barracks be at once more put on a satisfactory footing and the O/C informed so as to avoid any further unpleasantness in the future."[38] Letters were exchanged between colony and protectorate officials. Captain N. E. Wrightwich of the WAFF held that Easmon was not entitled to occupy European quarters because he belonged to a subordinate department (NMO). The captain ended with further rebuttals to Easmon's complaint. In early December 1918 the PMO told the officer in charge of the WAFF that he would be most grateful if the officer would allow Easmon to occupy the bungalow desired.

Interior Medical Infrastructure

Hence, political action was not without rewards in a generally difficult rural environment that featured poor communication except along the railways, duty travel on foot from town to town or village to village over bush paths, unmade roads, and log or monkey bridges, followed by porters carrying bedding, kitchen utensils, a camp chair, and washtub. The accommodations were without electricity, portable generators, bottled gas, or refrigeration. There was no radio, and mail from abroad came only once a month. A portable gramophone might bring a respite from boredom after the day's tasks were completed.

The time was also ripe to benefit from changes in the salary structure and in the procedures for promotion. In 1920 colonial administrators introduced a new fixed uniform scale for African medical officers throughout West Africa. Junior officers had their salaries raised to £500 per year, with annual increments of £20 to a maximum of £600 per year; after the governors approval, senior officers moved to a £600 base with £25 increments up to £700. This was in contrast to the WAMS, where the lowest ranking medical officer received £660 with £30 up to £720; then £720 with £40 increments up to £800 after being confirmed; and as much as £800 with £40 increments up to £960 if a special course of study was successfully completed. Within three years the medical officer could move to £960, and later from £1,000 with £50 increments to £1,150 upon the governor's recommendation. In essence, a competent European medical officer was eligible with eleven years of service, in which three years must have been in the lower grade £660–960, for promotion to the higher grade of £1,000–1,150.

Easmon submitted his first application for promotion to a higher grade of medical officer on April 7, 1921.[39] However, he ran up against

Dr. Ernest Jenner Wright, who held the only allotted position at the higher grade of African medical officers. Though junior in grade to Easmon, he had been selected for promotion ostensibly due to an outstanding merit rating. Wright also was part English, with an African father, and who had a strong respect for English values and culture, and his ambivalence with regard to the problem of intraprofessional conflict probably earned him preferential treatment from the British middle class. On May 21, 1924, Easmon reapplied;[40] and in June 1924 officials noted that he would complete eleven years of service on July 8, 1924, and so had strong qualifications for consideration because of good recommendations and his special research in infant mortality and the sterility rate of women in the Kennema district. However, in spite of an impressive work record, Easmon had at one time come under strong criticism by a Dr. Beringer and, while none of the charges stuck, they were sufficient to prevent Easmon's advancement in the service.

Governor Slater (1922–27) next interviewed Easmon at Bo in December 1923 and, perhaps having perceived Easmon as an agitator or troublemaker, "warned him to forget his grievances and make up his mind to earn a promotion by special work."[41] Apparently, Easmon took the governor's advice to heart and expressed his sentiments in a more subtle manner to the general satisfaction of his peers and the governor, who next requested permission to include increment provisions in the estimates for 1925 for two African medical officers in the higher grade. Finally, the governor approved Easmon's bid for promotion to medical officer on January 1, 1925, after eleven years in the service, a rank he would hold until 1942. His salary was set at £625 with £25 increments to £700 because he had already spent six years in the maximum category of the lower grade (£500–600).[42]

In the course of his career Easmon manned almost every medical station in the protectorate provinces, including Moyamba, Bo, and Bonthe, and he, along with other Western doctors before him and afterward, must be given credit for advancing Western medicine among the indigenous people. Dr. Thomas Winterbottom's account of traditional medical practice in the provinces provides insight into the traditions that Easmon and other doctors later encountered. In 1794

Winterbottom, a well-trained doctor who believed in monogenesis—the belief that all human races descended from a single ancestral individual or species. While the prevailing opinion in pseudoscientific thought was otherwise, he had faith in the African capacity to develop in accord with other human species, and so he made contacts with the Temne (original inhabitants of the Sierra Leone peninsula), the Susu, Fula, Bulloms, Mandinga, and others. He observed medical practice among the herbalists to fight off witchcraft—the notion of medicine as a supernatural art and the practitioner as a witch who caused harm rather than healed in the minds of the people. Winterbottom noted that some herbalists produced amulets resembling those used in antiquity among the Jews, Greeks, and Romans to ward off diseases. He reported further on the use of herbs in a similar manner to that of mercury to produce salivation, and the confusion wrought by African herbalists in attributing a broad array of symptoms to a single cause, where in fact several separate diseases were probably involved.[43]

The healers, however, exemplified professional traits in the control of their medical resources and cultural authority. Nevertheless, their widespread practice of secrecy curtailed interpersonal association and the exchange of medical knowledge that is crucial to expand knowledge. In a recent study Steven Feierman shows that "All across Africa in the years before colonial conquest healers, and the political leaders with whom they were allied, had a much wider range of control over the social conditions of health than they had ever since."[44] While documentation is not yet extant on Easmon's testimony, he must have encountered obstacles to harmony between the two contending systems—traditional medicine and Western scientific thought—in an atmosphere marred with mutual suspicion and distrust.

Calvin Sinnette (MD) of the Howard University College of Medicine, who had clinical experience in Africa, elaborates further on the division. Modern medical practitioners were contemptuous of traditional healers, who usually protected their art through secrecy and closed treatment sessions. The two groups rarely engaged in dialogue. Western-trained scientists especially criticized the traditional practitioners for failing, except in isolated instances, to identify the active agent of disease and for frequently making claims based on unverifi-able observations rather than on statistically valid clinical trials. The absence of a degree of precision consistent with accepted Western sci-entific investigations, therefore, made it impossible to develop certain guidelines: reproducing alleged reactions or responses; predicting the effect of patient treatment with an acceptable level of certainty; stan-dardizing dosages or treatment procedures to prevent unknown toxic levels; and determining the extent of untoward side effects.[45] Sinnette, however, did not deny the significance of traditional medicine to the medical armamentarium. The degree to which Easmon made at-tempts to integrate traditional medicine with Western medicine may never be known, but he was certainly acquainted with herbalists and their healing methods.

Easmon's Clinical Publication and Practice

Easmon visited England on full-pay leave on June 15, 1922, and stayed for about seven months. Questions raised by former hospital col-leagues there compelled him to begin collecting data for a published article on the conditions and medical practice in the interior. The purpose was to interest others in the profession who might consider working in the tropics and to acquaint those already in the tropics with regions unknown to them. More was known about the larger coastal towns because of well-equipped hospitals, sanitary depart-ments, and research laboratories, and also because of the papers that were occasionally published about them. Easmon returned to Sierra Leone in December 1922 and assumed his medical duties. By 1924 Easmon had spent eleven years in the protectorate.[46] The interior of this area lacked medical infrastructure comparable to that along the coast, so Easmon was denied access not only to such facilities but also to medical innovations available to African doctors on the coast and to European doctors of the WAMS on annual leave to England. Nev-ertheless, he improved his qualifications with an MD in 1925, gained through correspondence with the University of London, and strove relentlessly for several years to obtain the FRCSE qualification (from the Royal College of Surgeons in Edinburgh), but to no avail.

The Easmon article on medical practice in the interior was published in 1925. It discussed his work at Bo, the medical station situated at the western end of the Kennema district of the central province of the Sierra Leone protectorate, during the period from September 1923 to March 1924. The article addressed such topics as the people, climate, communication, medical personnel and infrastructure, duties of the medical officer, types of cases treated, and private practice. The Kennema district was an area of 2,100 square miles with a population of 168,526 people, and the administrative headquarters featured a dispensary. The railway line connected the largest communities such as Bo, Gerihun, Blama, Kennema, and Haugha. Because the large rivers in the district were unnavigable, the medical officer worked mostly along the railway line and rarely moved far from it. Ethnic groups consisted of the Mende, Konnoh, Temne, Kissi, Lokkoh, and Sherbro, and Muslim people such as the Susa, Fula, Korankoh, and Mandingo, who were mostly agriculturalists producing palm oil and kernels and were unskilled laborers. Foreigners numbered 994 in the protectorate: Creoles 828, Syrians 113, Indians 7, Europeans 38 (5 European women), and 8 miscellaneous. Creoles supplied the mechanics, artisans, smaller traders, and government clerks. The Europeans controlled the large business firms and the senior administrative post, and some served as missionaries.

Private practice was out of the question: the majority of the indigenous people did not trust Western medicine, and foreigners were not numerous enough to support a doctor. Except for the supervisors, all government medical officers were allowed private practice, and they relieved each other from time to time at out-stations. However, the distinction between the WAMS and the NMOs remained. The government medical officer was without a rival in the district and had the last word in decisionmaking on all sanitary and medical issues. The people realized that the medical officer was in a powerful position and the only one who could command the district commissioner to cease and desist in regard to the implementation of decisions. The medical station had one dispenser in residence who was also the nurse. A sanitary inspector administered vaccinations and was assisted by sanitary assistants. Cases of serious illnesses were sent down to Freetown by train.

The first obligation of the medical officer was to take care of government officials and then the general population in attendance at the dispensary or pharmacist. Private patients were supposed to be treated last. Since British medical culture emphasized general-purpose medicine, the medical officer dealt with a wide variety of cases, including medical, surgical, gynecological, obstetric, ear, nose, throat, and eye patients. The medical officer was also in charge of each of the three sanitary districts at Bo, Blama, and Kennema, had to attend to European quarters in the town, and be ready to treat infectious cases (smallpox and chicken pox) that might arise. Meteorological observations were required daily at Bo and subjected to medical officer scrutiny. Easmon acted also as medico-legal expert of the district, and often evidence had to be given in District Commissioner's Court and the Circuit Court. In addition, the medical officer had to conduct postmortems as pathologist in the mortuary adjacent to the dispensary and had to supervise exhumations.

The dispensaries were reasonably equipped, considering their remoteness, with a stock of drugs and paraphernalia, including a portable metal operating table, instruments for minor surgery, chloroform (the only general anesthetic available), a mark and drop bottle, a Zeiss microscope with 1/12, 1/6, and 2/3 objectives, a mechanical stage and condenser, slides, cover slips, and commoner stains.

Easmon treated 2,067 new cases at the dispensary and 200 private patients during the seven-month report period. He noted that this averaged out to 80 patients per square mile for the district, while the average for the entire colony and protectorate was about 60 to the square mile. Ulcers, constipation, dyspepsia, minor injury, coughs and bronchitis, and rheumatic infections were the commonest cases. Venereal diseases—syphilis and gonorrhea—were rare but responded well in treatment to novasenobillon, stabilarsan, and bismuth salts sufarsenol. No cases of typhoid were reported in Easmon's findings, but the surgical cases were diverse and were treated under chloroform.

Easmon's private patients were mostly Creole women—there were ninety-three at Bo—who required treatment for gynecological or obstetric conditions—dysmenorrhea, amenorrhea, menorrhagia, pseudocyesis, normal and abnormal delivery, eclampsia fever, abortion, prolapse and retroversion fibroids, ovaritis and ovarian tumors, and chronic erosion of the cervix. Only a very few of these conditions were recorded among indigenous women because they would not discuss their symptoms or allow a male doctor to make the necessary pelvic examinations. This pattern of cultural behavior requires explanation; 95 percent of all women passed through the female Bundu society of secret initiation in the protectorate, where tetanus cases were high among the young, unmarried female circumcision initiates. Dr. Milton Margai (1895–1964) was the first certified doctor from the protectorate region in 1926 and the first doctor allowed to provide supervision in these rites. (By 1943 Margai became the first doctor to succeed in reducing the barriers between Western medical science and African traditional health and cultural systems through linkage. Successive training camps stressed the importance of hygiene and sterilization of medical instruments to adult women teachers of the secret initiation rites, women who had avoided Western-style treatment, and the chiefs accepted these teachings.)[47] Nevertheless, Easmon and the colonial medical system played a major role in preparing the protectorate people for the transition to come, as his publications show. Easmon had good reason to be proud of his scholarly contributions and no doubt realized their value to the government in the recruitment of doctors: "In the above account I have not been able to give any thrilling accounts of exceptional cases to be treated, but as the benefits of medical science become more and more widely known and more equipment is obtained, more and better work will be done. The foregoing particular account of eight months' work at Bo is typical of any similar period at any other district in this Colony and Protectorate and, with the changing of a few names and figures, is fair index of work in other West African Colonies."[48] Easmon finally left the protectorate for a new appointment as medical officer in Freetown in about 1926.

Colonial Office and Intraprofessional Conflict

The Colonial Office efforts in making organizational changes to unify the medical service failed to abate intraprofessional conflict—the professional disparities between African doctors and European doctors. On January 1, 1934, the new Colonial Medical Service replaced the East African Medical Service and the West African Medical Staff, with some changes in African appointments.[49] Sierra Leone now had seven African medical officers: Drs. Ernest Wright (hired July 12, 1916), M. C. F. Easmon (hired July 18, 1913), E. H. Cummings (hired July 20, 1920), E. Awooner-Renner (hired December 1, 1920), E. B. E. Hughes (hired April 1, 1924), W. F. O. Taylor (hired April 1, 1925), and Milton Margai (hired December 1, 1928), the first protectorate doctor. Gambia appointed Dr. Bright Richards (December 23, 1931) but was surpassed by the Gold Coast, with six doctors, who included Drs. Tete Mensah-Annan (hired April 7, 1920), Charles Elias Reindorf (hired January 1, 1921), Arthur Farrell Renner Dove (hired May 1, 1923), Benjamin Jonathan Odumnbaku Hoare, Gabriel Jones Dodwona Hammond (hired September 5, 1925), Edward Tagoe (hired September 1, 1926), and C. J. S. O. Taylor (hired April 23, 1930).[50] Nigeria followed with Drs. D. O. Perters (hired April 1, 1931), J. T. Femi Pearse (hired June 1, 1929), R. O. T. Cole (hired April 9, 1930), H. A. A. Doherty (hired March 1, 1932), K. Sagoe (hired July 1, 1932), A. D. Majekodunmi (hired February 1, 1933), and S. E. Onwu (hired June 19, 1933).[51]

In spite of these appointments, a number of issues remained in need of resolution in the minds of some African medical officers. On January 26, 1934, before even a month could pass under the new Colonial Medical Service, the African medical officers of Sierra Leone petitioned the government concerning their conditions of service. First they sought the removal of the word "African" in the title "African Medical Officer" because its deletion would mean the end of distinctions between European and African doctors. This practice was not used in Sierra Leone before 1902 and no comparable practice was followed in other British colonies, such as India, the West Indies, Nigeria, and the Gold Coast. Second, the African medical officers surpassed the eleven members of the WAMS in seniority, in age, in length of service, and in local experience (see table 4).

Hence, revision was in order. The word "supervision" and the category "senior officer" meant that an experienced African officer long in the service was required to work under supervision. For example, the memorandum noted that the case of a junior European medical officer placed in charge of a senior African medical officer in the Connaught Hospital surgical ward was further cause for concern, and it also mentioned other similar examples. The salary discrepancy between African and European physicians received further attention, and even the senior nursing sisters' initial salary was the same for beginning African medical officers with more extensive training. These officers were dissatisfied further with discrepancies between themselves and European officers over the issues of pensions, promotions, leave, and sick leave. The signers were M. C. F. Easmon, E. Taylor-Cummings (1890–1967), E. Awooner-Renner, E. B. E. Hughes, W. F. O. Taylor, and Milton Margai. Ernest Wright seemed to have remained outside the fray.

The officials in Sierra Leone and in the Colonial Office deduced that Easmon was the main author of the petition, since he was one of the "leading lights of African society" and had one of the largest private practices in Freetown. Easmon needed to show more gratitude to the government for allowing him to earn such a comparatively large income, colonial officials claimed, and to become the envy of Freetown African doctors in private practice.[52] A letter from Sierra Leone

Table 4. Average age and average length of service for African and European medical officers in Sierra Leone, 1934

	AVG. AGE	AVG. LENGTH OF SERVICE
African medical officers	41	12 yrs. 6 mos.
European medical officers	37	7 yrs., 3 mos.
Senior medical and hospital officers	34	—
Officers below the senior rank	—	4 yrs., 2 mos.

Source: PRO, CO 267/646.

Government House to the Colonial Office described how Easmon was the cause of a lot of unnecessary trouble. Dr. Phillip Oakley, director of the Medical and Sanitary Department—which headed the medical staff and looked after the health of the colony—proposed that Easmon's action constituted sufficient provocation to transfer him back to the protectorate at Port Loko. Since this station was generally allotted to a European medical officer, with privileges, Easmon might not have much to complain about. For on the one hand, Wright, who was recently promoted to senior African medical officer, was not a signer of the petition, and on the other hand, Awooner-Renner signed the petition and was to receive a promotion upon satisfactory completion of a certificate for attending a course on pathology in England. Wright continued in not supporting African doctors against the government, knowing that the British would support him, while Awooner-Renner stuck with his African counterparts no matter whether the British promoted him or not. Wright's behavior was the cause of much discussion in African circles. Dr. Bankole-Bright had apparently criticized him with regard to his appointment and, until matters subsided, officials thought it best to postpone the Easmon transfer to an out-station.

However, Oakley's annoyance with Easmon had not been mollified. The primary reason Easmon forwarded the petition, Oakley said, was because he was not offered the surgical ward position in the Connaught Hospital upon his return from the protectorate, and Oakley also charged Easmon with improper medical conduct: "My contention is borne out by the fact that this officer was recently in the local press for examining male and female patients together in the same room, and is therefore not qualified to be an administrator in charge of a large hospital like Connaught."[53] Furthermore, Oakley refuted each charge of the twenty-seven-page petitioners' document, and the Executive Council sanctioned his statement. So the African medical officers failed to obtain support for their list of grievances against the government.

It must be borne in mind that colonial medical departments suffered from budget constraints in the Depression years and efforts were made to recruit African medical officers at lower levels that did not entitle the recipient to benefits. The scale for medical officers was £500–525 and £600–720 in £30 increments in 1936, but the medical department wished to recruit to the new lower grade post of £400–500 in increments of £20. The intention was to appoint all future African medical officers at this scale, and to possibly place on hold the existing scale of £500–£720. In Nigeria the junior medical officers were not pensionable and were appointed at a flat rate of £400 per annum. It was possible to offer these rates and even rates as low as £200 per annum because of the large number of Nigerians studying medicine in England. Colonial officials in Sierra Leone borrowed the Nigerian model for the flat and unpensionable rate of £400 and even wanted to consider a lower rate, which may suggest that a sizable number of Sierra Leoneans were also studying in England during this time.[54]

Dr. Raymond Sarif Easmon

M. C. F. Easmon, now with twenty-three years of service, prepared to welcome his first cousin—a new medical graduate—into the profession, Raymond Sarif Easmon (MB, BS, Dunelm; DTMH, 1936, Liverpool), son of the late Albert Whiggs Easmon. Born in 1913, the year of M.C. F.'s first appointment, and now twenty-three years of age, Raymond represented the third generation of Easmon medical professionals in 1937, the year of his arrival back in Sierra Leone. Junior medical officers apparently were not completing their hospital residences in England as normally required, receiving most of their initial clinical experience in the African milieu instead. Governor Guggisberg of the Gold Coast had long advocated this approach. In Sierra Leone the director of medical and sanitary services noted the unqualified success of the junior medical officer model, which was first tried in Nigeria, and its value not only to the young doctors but to the government as well. Furthermore, the director reported on Raymond as "very promising, and from his credentials appears suitable." The young Easmon stayed in the service for two years and four months before leaving for private practice in about 1939. In 1942 M. C. F. was promoted to senior medical officer, a position he held until retirement in 1945 on pension following thirty-two years in the service.[55]

M. C. F. Easmon: Africanist and Medical Historian

In his retirement years, after 1945, M. C. F. Easmon made contributions to world scholarship beyond the realm of the clinical field. As early as 1924 he had written a book entitled *Sierra Leone Country Cloths* for the Wembley Empire Exhibition, based on his protectorate and colonial observations, and his new activity represented a continued expression of the cultural and historical interests that were manifested earlier in his publication. He became the chairman of the Sierra Leone Society and of the Monuments and Relics Commission, and founded the Sierra Leone Museum, to which he devoted many years as its full-time volunteer director. A wing of the museum was named in his honor. Easmon also served as chairman of labor boards, and as a trustee of his church, St. John's Maroon Town. In recognition of the African diaspora and the "return," he was a founding member and chairman of the Nova Scotians and Maroon Descendants Association. As a man of scholarship and charm, M. C. F. had a wide range of friends abroad and assisted many of them in queries about African history and anthropology from his recorded materials. With over sixty years of uninterrupted service to medicine and various spheres of public life, he was honored with the OBE (Order of the British Empire) in 1954, and was president of the Sierra Leone branch of the British Medical Association from 1951–53, being its representative in 1960.[56]

    M. C. F. may well be most remembered by those in African medical history for his seminal article, "Sierra Leone Doctors." This appears to be the first major study of African physicians in the twentieth century by an African. It contains eighty-nine biographical sketches of African doctors and begins before 1800 in Sierra Leone, with certifications and medical schools attended. In policy statements of 1925 and 1938, neither European nor African women medical officers were members of the Colonial Medical Service, although this policy was later reversed. However, this did not preclude Easmon from listing some six Sierra Leone African women. He chose to mention them because they had reached a particular stage in their careers in private practice, in the Colonial Medical Service, and later in independent governments: Irene Cole (MB, BS, 1944, Dunelm); Sophie Elisabeth Jenner Wright, daughter of Dr. Ernest Wright, (MRCS, LRCP, 1944; MB, BS, 1946, London); Ola Elsie Palmira During (MB, BS, 1950, Dunelm); C. Jones, the daughter of Dr. Radcliffe Jones, (MB, ChB, 1951, Edinburgh); Evelyn Caffry Cummings (MB, BS, 1951, Dunelm; medical officer, 1951); Priscilla Rosamund Kasope Nicole (LRCP and S, 1953, Ireland; medical officer, 1956); Marcella Gwynnie Ekua Davies (LCRP and S, Ireland; LAH, 1954, Combe; medical officer, 1956); and June Spain (MB, ChB, 1955, St. Andrews). Agnes Yewande Savage (MB, ChB, Edinburgh) qualified in 1929, but did not appear on Easmon's list because she was a Nigerian who practiced in the Gold Coast and the article dealt with only Sierra Leone doctors.

African gender stratification seemed to explain why so few women doctors entered medicine. Curriculum restrictions denied women access to courses in the sciences, at least in Sierra Leone. In earlier times, Dr. Ola During stated that young girls were only allowed to study mathematics for their school certificates and not science subjects such as biology, physiology, and anatomy, while the boys were allowed to study both. Concessions often had to be made for female African students by deans of European medical schools for preparatory study in science subjects before entering the first year.[57] The issue of the accessibility of a medical education for African women is one of several important questions raised by Easmon's pioneering study that merits in-depth research.

The Easmon article appears to have been the model for numerous subsequent publications. Many of the doctors who were especially active in opposing the restraints of colonialism and racism remain to be studied, such as the late Curtis Adeniji-Jones (MB, BS, 1901, Dunelm), who joined the Lagos Medical Service (1905–14), retired, went into private practice, and then became a member of the

Nigerian Legislative Council. A number of scholars benefited from the Easmon family as a whole, and the ability to show this is due to the many documents that make it possible to study their careers.

Nations and emerging nations extol their founding men and women, and Sierra Leone was no exception in this regard. Upon its independence in April 1961, Easmon was assisted by Davidson Nicol in preparing for publication *Eminent Sierra Leoneans (in the Nineteenth Century)* (1961). Beginning with the Sierra Foundation in 1792, the work focused on the lives of Creole and protectorate elites. It celebrated the virtues of nearly all the cultural groups in an attempt to integrate the peoples of Sierra Leone into nationhood, an impulse somewhat contrary to the new nation's preexisting historical and cultural realities.

Death of M. C. F. Easmon

In his midseventies, and with his health failing, M. C. F. Easmon returned to England, where he died on May 2, 1972. He was eighty-two years old.[58] M. C. F. lived some twenty-seven years after retiring, a period in which he kept active by a steady stream of significant publications and by distinguished service to his country that spanned the colonial era and independence. He was a strong family man, and members of that family had an important bearing on his professional life. He was survived by his wife, Enid Winifred Shorunkeh-Sawyerr, a daughter, Kathleen, and son Professor Charles Syrette Easmon, about whom more will be written. It is said that M. C. F.'s common-law relatives survive from his years in the protectorate at Moyamba.

The Easmon family tradition of professional careers in medicine is continued by other Easmons. First, Charles Odamten Easmon (MB, ChB, 1940, Edinburgh; DTMH, 1941, Edinburgh; FRCSE)—son of John (an accountant who died in the Jos Plateau, Nigeria) and grandson of John Farrell Easmon (1856–1900)—entered the Colonial Medical Service in the Gold Coast in 1941 as the fifth professional to emerge from the medical Easmon family. He served as a clinical assistant, although he was a qualified doctor, for his first nine months and next as junior medical office at the salary of £180 per annum. He stayed in the government service and became the first director of medical service for the government in independent Ghana in 1957. After all, Charles Odamten and Prime Minister Kwame Nkrumah were classmates at Achimota College in their formative years,[59] and they respected each other's expertise and achievements. Charles Odamten, born in 1914, died at Accra in 1994. Secondly, Charles Syrette Easmon (MB, BS, London, 1969; MRCS, LRCP, 1969, London; PhD, 1974, London; MRC Path, 1976; MD, 1981), the son of M. C. F. Easmon, teaches at St. Mary's Hospital Medical School, London. The sixth Easmon medical professional, he specializes in microbiology, and has published papers on staphylococcal and streptococcal infections, phagocytosis, and sexually transmitted diseases.[60]

David Ekundayo Boye-Johnson and the Decolonization Era

*D*r. David Ekundayo Boye-Johnson, the subject of this chapter, differs from the doctors previously discussed in a number of ways. First, he was born in the Sierra Leone protectorate and, unlike the Creoles who became doctors, Boye-Johnson had no connection by descent to the diaspora. Yet, through time he became Creole due to a cultural mechanism that will be explored. In the course of his professional training he joined in the voluntary diaspora to the United States, Canada, and Great Britain, and in the return to Sierra Leone. Secondly, unlike the Easmons and some of the other doctors who were controversial and left an abundant paper trail to facilitate the historian's work, Boye-Johnson did not do so. He was a moderate in temperament who wore the artful and cryptic mask of his ethnic duality—that is Temne-Sherbro and later Creole—and he was a consensus builder in decisionmaking. The information that is available about him, which came into the author's hands by accident, is silent on many of the issues raised in this chapter. Since he was personally caught up in the turbulence of the decolonization era as a medical officer and fortunate in encountering expanding opportunities he was able to avoid much of the intense intraprofessional conflict that had so traumatized previous generations and even some of his peers. But Boye-Johnson was compelled by the colonial situation to undergo medical training in Western Europe and in the United States before being employed in his homeland.[1] This chapter, therefore, is not just about Boye-Johnson's career; a career that must not be viewed in isolation from the experiences of other African doctors abroad. His experience was also representative of numerous other Africans seeking medical training in the West during the period of this study.

As with the doctors previously discussed, Boye-Johnson was involved in the post-1900 colonial expansion, in which African doctors were excluded from the central ranks of the government's medical service. In addition, Africans were discouraged from medical training abroad: "The objections to African doctors were they could give orders to white officers, and that the races might meet at the mess table. But there might also have been fears that it would be difficult to challenge African doctors who were able to argue with full technical authority on matters of social and economic policy, for example the health consequences of labor recruitment or of urban segregation."[2] The sixth generation of African doctors, including Boye-Johnson and others discussed here, knew the history of African medical achievements and pride in accumulating knowledge, and these influenced their desires to pursue medicine—no matter what the politics and power of the times dictated. Decolonization, however, would accelerate opportunities and lessen the professional struggle for medical mobility.

The Ward System and Creolization

The peninsula occupied by the Sierra Leone colony was twenty-five miles long and ten miles wide. In terms of its contacts with European and American cultures, the colony was very different from the interior protectorate. Communication between the two regions was difficult, and travel took place for the most part on waterways. This factor alone gave the coastal Creoles an enormous advantage over the hinterland peoples—the Temne, Susu, Mandinga, Fula, Limba, Sherbro, Mende—in education, access to training, and income (see chapter 6, map 4). The cultural distance between the two regions was reduced by two factors: the introduction of railways in the twentieth century and the longer-standing ward system.[3]

The ward system acted as a mechanism for the Creolization of the interior dwellers, enabling them to enter the ranks of the protectorate elites. Creoles, for example, often became intermediaries, or gained middleman trade status between the indigenous people and the British on the coast, following their orientation into Western culture and the accompanying privilege to exploit the hinterland on many levels of interaction. First, Creoles purchased European-imported items, including cloth and ironware, and either sold or traded them in the interior at a profit. Secondly, the indigenous people sold them palm oil, rice, kola, palm kernels, and numerous other goods to sell in Freetown. They would often employ indigenous Africans as domestic servants, cooks, and agricultural laborers, according to researcher Leo Spitzer. Through a master-servant relationship, some non-Creole children left their families and came under the trust and parental nurturing of "better-to-do Creoles for whom they performed household chores in return for the opportunity to go to school," Spitzer reports. Since this system was similar to the extended family, where everyone was treated as part of the kinship unit, it found acceptance with relative ease and usually lasted until students finished their schooling. This ward system became a common hinterland practice, and Europeans, in need of servants and assistants, participated in this form of apprenticeship. Dr. John Macaulay Wilson, of the Kafu Bullom ethnic group, was the first protectorate doctor and first doctor in Sierra Leone who was reared in this system—by Governor Zachary Macaulay in the 1790s and later by Dr. Thomas Winterbottom. Beyond this little is known about him. The late president Siaka Stevens

(1905–1988) of the Sierra Leone Republic—a Limba from Moyamba—learned Krio in the Creole household of the Smith family in
Freetown as a nine-year-old boy in about 1914. While Stevens excoriated the system, in hindsight he noted: "Although at the time I would
never have guessed that one day I would be grateful for this training, I
now see this self-discipline was an invaluable lesson. I often think that
if it had not been for this I would still be somewhere at the bottom of
the ladder."[4] The system indeed introduced Stevens to a Westernized
sense of time: "Moreover, because my playtime was so limited it became more precious to me, and I learnt to use it well, not wasting a
minute of it. My days in Kissy taught me the basis of successful living:
how to work hard and how to play hard, and, most important of all,
how to keep the two separate."[5] In the first quarter of the twentieth
century, therefore, Stevens had much in common with others who
were drawn into the ward system and in the process shed some of
their old ethnic identities.

The ward system, however, was perhaps unjustly criticized by
William Fergusson, the former West Indian governor of the Sierra
Leone colony, as early as 1842. Fergusson had observed for a long time
the arrival of the Liberated Africans into Freetown. He admired them
and sometimes supervised their assignments as apprentices to the
Creole elites. This process, however, worked to the disadvantage of
the elites' children; in relieving them from domestic and other labo-
rious chores, Fergusson concluded: "Many of the creole-born children, therefore, arrive at an adult age, not only unaccustomed to
labour, but disinclined to it, and actually incapable of working."[6]
Robert July reported that Fergusson's observation gained support as
the twentieth century dawned. A perception began to predominate
that "the Sierra Leone creoles—as descendants of the recaptives,
Nova Scotians and Maroons were by then called—somehow were ef-
fete, unequal to the rigours of building a modern civilization in
Africa."[7] This created an opportunity for the Syrians to enter the retail
trades with a competitive edge and led to the disproportionate representation of the Creoles in the professions at the expense of their providing other needed technical expertise.

Dr. David Ekundayo Boye-Johnson

David Ekundayo Boye-Johnson was born into this cultural matrix on July 11, 1912, in Rotifunk, of Temne-Sherbro parentage. He appears to have moved toward a more concealed level of Creolization than Siaka Stevens, for example, and yet he owed his professional mobility to the ward system. Scholarly literature suggests that his background was Creole. In a classic article M. C. F. Easmon listed three protectorate doctors but neglected to include Boye-Johnson. That Boye-Johnson participated in the ward system is evident by the composition of his name—which suggests a Creole identity—fitting classic upper-class Creole practices of the nineteenth and early twentieth century. It combines the Christian name David with the Yoruba Ekundayo from the Liberated Africans of western Nigeria, and the hyphenated name that was a later Creole practice and therefore the apparent reason for changing his ethnic and regional status.

The American missionary presence at Rotifunk made an indelible mark upon Boye-Johnson in his formative years, and was the decisive factor in his choice of the United States to study medicine.[8] He completed the Rotifunk Village Primary School (1917–24), the E. U. B. Albert Academy Secondary School, Freetown (1925–27), and the CMS Grammar School, Freetown (1927–29).[9] His years in Freetown enabled him to develop a web of contacts with prominent families and their children along the West African coast that would be useful for status recognition and class mobility. Through them Boye-Johnson was also exposed to dimensions of the African diaspora, especially the Maroons of Jamaica, who had a long historical presence in Freetown, and others of West Indian origin elsewhere in West Africa. Howard University had produced several Sierra Leone graduates, people who were known because of their generosity. Edna Elliot Horton (1905–94) of Freetown completed her BA degree in liberal arts at Howard University in 1933; she was reported to be the first woman university graduate in Anglophone West Africa (see figure 11).[10] These personalities and the focal role of Howard University in the diaspora were worthy topics for discussion in Freetown and no doubt Boye-Johnson heard of them.

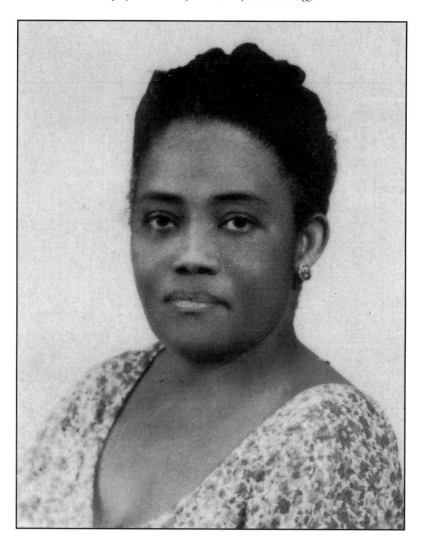

Figure 11.   *Edna Elliot Horton, Angola, c. 1956. Courtesy of Regina M. Horton.*

Colonialism introduced an institutionalized British medical culture in Anglophone West Africa. In 1902 the Colonial Office stipulated that medical graduates had to train at certain foreign institutions in order to qualify to practice in Great Britain or the Colonial
Medical Service in Africa (see appendix 1). By an Order in Council
dated March 9, 1901, the degrees of Doctor of Medicine and Surgery

of all the royal Italian universities were registrable in the Foreign List, and by the same amended order dated December 11, 1905, the degrees of Bachelor of Medicine (Igakushi) and Doctor of Medicine (Igaku Hakushi) of the Imperial University of Japan came to be registrable in the Foreign List. Hence, African doctors trained in institutions not on this approved list were prohibited from practicing in their countries of origin, a severe penalty that they were forced to accept until decolonization.

In spite of these regulations, Boye-Johnson heeded the advice of the American missionaries in Sierra Leone rather than that of his parents and friends and set off to pursue a medical education in the United States in August 1932, where he remained until October 1944. After a brief enrollment at the Hampton Institute in Virginia, Boye-Johnson transferred to Lincoln University in Pennsylvania in 1933, arriving there some two years before Kwame Nkrumah (1935–39); he graduated at the age of 24. That same year Boye-Johnson was admitted to the Howard University College of Medicine in Washington, D.C.

Howard University College of Medicine and Meharry Medical School in Nashville, Tennessee, had provided viable alternatives to Africans seeking medical training in the United States since their inception in 1868 and 1876, respectively. Both schools showed dynamic innovations in their curricula appropriate for the transfer of medical technology to Africa. Through time their African medical graduates served as representatives of the two schools influencing others to attend. (Howard University Medical School and Meharry Medical School had graduated some sixty-five African medical doctors by 1978, the school's centennial anniversary, students representing some fifteen African countries.) Boye-Johnson graduated from Howard University Medical School in 1940 at the age of thirty-one, the school's first graduate from the Sierra Leone protectorate and the third medical graduate from the region. On receipt of his degree Boye-Johnson proceeded to Provident Hospital, Chicago, in 1940 to begin a four-year internship and residency in pediatrics. His medical career, which had proceeded smoothly until that point, ran into difficulties early in 1943, prior to the completion of his residency, as surviving correspondence from the period reveals.

Tensions and frustrations began to mount in early 1943 before the completion of his residency, and a spate of extant correspondence followed. While Boye-Johnson succeeded in renewing his British passport in April 1942 without incident, when it came time a year later to renew his visa he encountered a series of frustrating bureaucratic obstacles. For example, despite a supportive recommendation from the medical director of Provident Hospital, he was required to prove to the Chicago police department that he was guilty of no felonious offenses.[11] However, Boye-Johnson found his career objective blocked on all fronts by early 1943.[12] On May 22, 1943, he applied for an immigrant visa under the British quota system through the American Consul, Windsor, Ontario, Canada, and was warned of the need to check with immigration authorities in Chicago to ascertain whether entry into Canada might be allowed.[13] The continuing series of delays on the part of the various immigration authorities were themselves sufficient cause for considerable irritation. In addition to these troubles, however, England had been sending some of its medical students to the United States since 1940 because of the war with Germany, and this factor restricted Boye-Johnson from acquiring additional training there instead of going to Canada. The fact that he was a British subject prohibited him from employment by most states in America, but he could not return to Sierra Leone to practice with an American medical certification without next studying at one of the schools on the Colonial Office approved list.

One African American doctor, who had supported Boye-Johnson's medical efforts from the time of his arrival in Chicago, came to his aid. Dr. Edward Beasley, a longtime Chicago specialist in pediatrics and contributor to the *Crisis* magazine of the NAACP, swore out an affidavit of financial support on Boye-Johnson's behalf to the state of Illinois. This guaranteed that Boye-Johnson would not become a public charge while in the United States and by itself made Boye-Johnson eligible for continued residence and a visa.[14]

With an apparent lack of satisfaction over the slow pace of the various immigration centers, Boye-Johnson wrote a long letter to the chief of the visa division at the State Department on June 29, 1943, summarizing his situation and "now begging of Department of State to invoke its powers of goodwill to all democratic peoples of the world and exert its influence on the Immigration & Nationalization Service to grant me the necessary exit and reentry permits so I may take the examination in Canada which qualification it is very important in case I cannot get an immigration visa."[15] In other words, Boye-Johnson was attempting to cover himself with alternatives of a Canadian certification in order to practice in West Africa, or to remain in the United States as a permanent resident. He ended the last of his grievances in the letter to the State Department with an emotional plea: "No matter what I do, no matter how intensive an effort I put to solve my problem I am so far, *blocked, blocked, blocked* [my emphasis]."

Boye-Johnson suffered, indeed, from extreme apprehension over a colonial policy that prevented him from returning to his own country to practice medicine. Further, he felt that the authorities in the government of the United States were obligated to assist him with obtaining an immigration visa to Canada and reentry permits. Much of the desperation expressed in this letter was soon dispelled with immigration approval for travel to Canada in 1944.

Africans and Medical Certification in Canada

Africans were not able to pursue medical training in Canada until that country met the medical certification standards of the British Medical Council. The British Medical Act of 1858 had established the Medical Register but did not make provisions for the recognition of qualifications earned outside Great Britain.[16] The Amending Act of 1886 rectified this omission, specifying the various ways in which colonial and foreign practitioners could qualify to have their names placed on the Medical Register. This meant that doctors trained in Canada who were previously debarred from employment in the colonies could now be eligible after provincial legislation complied with the Amending Act of 1886. Various colonies responded quickly to allow their medical practitioners to have reciprocity with the General Medical Council. By 1902 reciprocity was confirmed with most of the larger colonies—now referred to as the dominions—in granting medical qualifications. The Canada Medical Act of 1902 provided for the creation of a Medical Council of Canada, and in 1911 the Dominion Medical Act passed and was adopted by each of the Canadian provinces. This latter action made possible the introduction of interprovincial reciprocity with regard to medical qualifications, privileges, and application of the Amending Act of 1886. The only other requirement was that provincial legislatures had to renounce their existing right of independent registration and agree to the creation of a register for the whole Canadian dominion. Individual provinces now had a mechanism for reciprocity with other jurisdictions that met the terms of the Amending Act of 1886 and prevented a likely showdown of interprofessional struggles, that is, conflict between provincial doctors and their legislatures over the slow approval action on the Amending Act. Nova Scotia was the first to take advantage of this opportunity in 1906, and others followed: Quebec 1908 (ceased 1928), Prince Edward Island 1910, New Brunswick 1913 (ceased 1926), Ontario 1915 (ceased 1927), Saskatchewan 1915 (ceased 1926), Manitoba 1916, and Alberta 1920.

Imperial officials were becoming more sensitive about the need for improved clinical training for the tropics, and in 1941 the Office of High Commissioner for the United Kingdom at Ottawa established a school of tropical medicine at McGill University, where better clinical facilities existed than at any other empire medical school and where the summer climate was more favorable for students from the colonies.[17] This was a very important step toward meeting the medical needs of over 2 million inhabitants of the Caribbean.[18] Africans and students of African American descent, however, would have to adjust to an age-old problem that placed restrictions on medical certification even after admission.

Governor-General Sir Frederick Lugard: African Physicians and European Women

Pseudoscientific racism permeated the imperial system, and Canada was no exception. Scholars have documented racial perceptions of and behavior toward Africans and their descendants throughout the diaspora.[19] In fact, these assumptions did have a significant bearing on the ethnic composition of the black doctors' clientele in West Africa. This became a particular concern of some colonial authorities who anticipated that African medical professionals might be called upon to treat Europeans, particularly female family members, in the colonial service.

Researcher Helen Callaway has explored the lengths taken in imperial culture to maintain social distance in colonial Nigeria. Her analysis of this and of race is evident when examples show how these factors came to manifest themselves in the colonial situation.[20] In a confidential dispatch to the secretary of state in 1915, Sir Frederick (later Lord) Lugard, high commissioner of northern Nigeria (1900–1909), governor of northern and southern Nigeria (1912–14), and governor-general of (unified) Nigeria (1914–18), deliberated at length about the issue of discrimination against the "native" doctors and the distinctions between them and Africans of other professions:

> I submit that the real colour question in the case of the negro Medical Officer is accentuated in a way which is entirely peculiar to this profession [medical] and does not apply to [Africans in] law, education, and other departments. And I believe it to be reciprocal, viz., that prejudice is almost, if not quite, as great on the part of the black as on the part of the white. There are many men who, with lifelong sympathy with the negro, would yet regard it as intolerable that their wives should be attended—say, in childbirth—by a negro practitioner. *I am myself such a man* [author's emphasis]. Negroes will frankly admit to the same prejudice. It is not, as Sir H. Clifford assumes, solely due to the prejudices of the West African Medical Staff—which stand on a different plane.[21]

This unadulterated confession by the representative of the British crown in West Africa moves the dilemma of the African doctor to center stage in the ethnic professional conflict. Lugard's attitudes were shared widely enough to survive as the policy in the imperial system, maintaining the social distance between European women and African doctors and preserving structural power in the hands of the ruling race.[22] Lugard next moved to the question of color else-where in the empire.

No color bar existed in Ceylon (Sri Lanka) and India, he noted, where the medical services were open to all. The entire private prac-tice of Ceylon was in indigenous hands, people who manifested high standards in surgery and other specialties. Race was not a factor in the government service of that island, but universally did "exist in the case of negro doctors among all classes of Europeans and in all African Colonies. It also tends to show that the Cingalese [*sic*] doctor displayed the qualities which have been found wanting as a rule in the African, and could therefore claim equality with the European."[23] Speaking from personal experience, Lugard submitted that racial prejudice against the native medical officer in India did exist, in spite of the fact that a high standard of medical expertise prevailed. In re-gard to the medical service, he concluded that racial prejudice and professional restrictions based on race should be acknowledged in the Colonial Medical Service.

Dr. Peter Alphonsus Clearkin was a European medical officer who worked in Lugard's time and held the same views on race. He began service in Sierra Leone in 1914. A clever and hard-working physician, according to Governor R. J. Wilkinson's annual confidential reports on WAMS officers,[24] Clearkin left a supportive and underlying de-scription of racial biology in his memoir paper, "Ramblings and Rec-ollections of a Colonial Doctor 1913–58." He pondered with a peer the issue of whether the native mind functioned the same way as the Eu-ropean mind did. Clearkin thought that a difference between the two races did exist and resisted change. His friend replied that fourteen years had elapsed since his own arrival in the colonies, and he still did not have an answer to that question. Nevertheless, he recognized that the races were different. After nearly fifty years of working in Africa and after considerable experience with the Africans, Clearkin finally concluded that the races were distinct. In spite of the difference in language, which was no obstacle, the Indian understood and thought like the European. The inhabitants of the Caribbean spoke the En-glish language, but Clearkin had the same difficulty with their line of reasoning as he did with the Africans. Even more, he understood the thought patterns of the Cypriots, although he did not speak Greek. The Africans, he surmised, were undaunted by Western education, and so the process did not make them Europeans. Clearkin submitted further:

> There is much to be said for those old commissioners who objected to attempts being made to educate Africans and make them sham Europeans protesting that the aim of education should be to make them good Africans. Many decades will have to elapse before the African can cope with our complex civilization: it is not a matter of intelligence, they are highly intelligent, it is just that they do not think as the European does. There are few aspects of the African character on which one can be dogmatic; an African, when questioned will always give the answer which he thinks most acceptable to his questioner. They are singularly impervious to suffering in others; I have seen a whole village convulsed with laughter at one of their own suffering from severe pain after an injury. Only one who has lived and worked among Africans can understand the pleasure excited in ancient Romans by the suffering of victims in the arena. The Congo is another instance of their pleasure in inflicting pain and can be appreciated only by one who has experienced this sadistic aspect of the African character. I often wonder what is the real reaction of the African to the central fact of the Christian religion, the suffering and death of Christ.[25]

Clearkin went on to make other observations about the African character based on his European perspective and the racial scientific thought of his time. Unfortunately, his views were not unusual; they represent the kinds of attitudes that influenced European actions in Africa for a long time. West Africans encountered most of these racist notions about themselves in their travels abroad rather than in the region, and they did not take such ideas lightly. They were mindful of the need to provide an alternative view of these images in publications about African cultures and their different peoples.

By the early 1940s medical authorities at McGill were aware that racial prejudice impinged upon Chinese, Asian Indian, and African (or African-descended) professionals: "These men, the last-named especially, are not acceptable to many of the patients in hospital wards in Canada, even as students (still less as interns). They are therefore almost completely excluded by the majority of Canadian medical schools, because of the trouble their presence causes in the teaching hospitals; even McGill is unable to see its way to admitting more than four or five really dark-skinned students each year. This situation is intolerable . . . it causes tragic disappointment . . . and retards the development of the Islands as a whole."[26]

In post–World War II in Germany, Walter Awooner-Renner (see figure 12) and two Caribbean students attended the Hamburg Medical School. In 1958 they prepared for internships in obstetrics and gynecology and found it extremely difficult to find professors in teaching hospitals who would accept them. As with Canadian hospitals, patients had no empathy with black physicians and requested to be treated by someone else. These sensitivities were particularly strong in a setting like obstetrics and gynecology. This impasse was resolved when one professor of obstetrics and gynecology volunteered and offered positions for the internists with total disregard for the patient's preferences; whether any patients left mattered little to him. When it came time to examine female patients, however, the professors would skip the black students; instead, they would stand at the patient's bedside while the professor described her symptoms and discussed her diagnosis.

Awooner-Renner next told of a Nigerian medical student, Felix Igbokwe, who transferred to Hamburg from the University of Saskatchewan, where he and other black medical students had been told repeatedly—and by more than one professor—"None of you will be able to get into the clinics to treat our women." Igbokwe subsequently became chief medical officer for the University of Nsukka, Nigeria.

To a Sierra Leonean abroad, such as Boye-Johnson, Nova Scotia was attractive not only because of its status as the first Canadian province to fulfill the reciprocity agreements in 1906 but also because of its history as the former home and embarkation center of the Nova Scotian settlers to Sierra Leone in 1792. The most influential Sierra

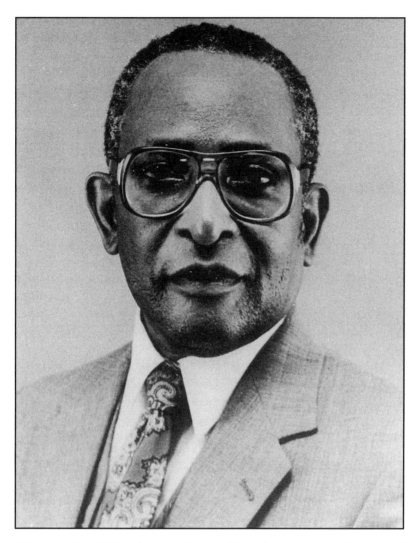

Figure 12. Dr. Walter Awooner-Renner, Sierra Leone, c. 1980. Courtesy of Walter A. Renner.

Leone doctors of the third generation (1880s–1900) had come from this settler group. Here in 1944 Boye-Johnson was awarded the Licentiate of the Medical Council of Canada (LMCC), and the Licentiate in Medicine and Surgery (LMS). He was now eligible for his name to appear on the Medical Register of Great Britain and qualified to practice in accordance with the reciprocity arrangements in the Colonial Medical Service.

Boye-Johnson returned to Sierra Leone in 1944 as medical officer in the Colonial Medical Service and held this position until 1953. Unlike Siaka Stevens who successfully sought to build a power base with the protectorate majority versus the colony, Boye-Johnson manifested the dynamic process of how new cultural expressions emerged and how ethnic groups were created from disparate ones who had lost their identity as ethnic landmarks. Cultural traits from one region surfaced in another region in the process of shifting ethnic and group identities. In Boye-Johnson's case the Krio language proper led to an ethnic overlay, that is, concealed his Temne-Sherbro origins; and in Siaka Stevens's case—a man who retreated from the colony region and returned to his former cultural base in the protectorate to build political alliances—Creole-acquired traits from participating in the ward system became partially hidden in the Sierra Leone hinterland. In contrast, Boye-Johnson continued the transition into Creoledom, at a time when other Creoles with lesser family connections to the colony were busily changing their names and allegiances to protectorate communities for political gain. This process occurred in the second half of the twentieth century as independence neared, and it was clear that the protectorate would gain political domination over the colony and its Creole population. Boye-Johnson went to the high temple of Creoledom—the Episcopal Cathedral of St. George—and married into an aristocratic Creole family—namely, the Betts, a union that would produce two speakers of the House of Representatives, two High Court judges, as well as barristers and parliamentarians. Even more, Boye-Johnson had earlier tied his aspirations to the civil service under Creole domination. In Rotifunk and Bonthe, on Sherbro Island, the American Missionary Society remained influential in Creole social circles, and Boye-Johnson, who had close ties to this missionary group in his early days, correctly understood that resuming a protectorate identity would inhibit his class mobility and status recognition. Intuition and the ward system had served him well.

But the Creole society that Boye-Johnson left in 1932 to go to the United States had changed politically by 1944. The government began to heap its largess upon the protectorate and anticolonial sentiments surfaced. By 1938–39 Krio leadership had been circumvented, and the radicalism of the 1920s and 1930s was in short supply (see chapter 8). I. T. A. Wallace-Johnson, a Sierra Leone nationalist, was jailed by the colonial officials, became sick, and was nursed back to health from a deadly disease while in prison by Dr. Raymond Sarif Easmon. Sidney Boyle (1905–)—the grandson of the famed merchant prince Syble Boyle (1850s) and Wallace-Johnson's compatriot in the proto-nationalist West African Youth League (WAYL)—was pursued by colonial authorities and left Sierra Leone in haste for England. And by the time of Boye-Johnson's return Sierra Leoneans had moved toward a strategy of gradualism in pushing for African participation in their own government.[27] While there was very little that the Creole community could do to reverse the political situation, Boye-Johnson would not be affected by these factors. His leadership strategy was geared to working within the system, no matter who was in charge. This was clearly evident as he rose through the ranks. British compliance with decolonization, however, mirrored the process of change taking place elsewhere in West Africa, reducing not only Boye-Johnson's professional struggles but others of his generation as well.

The Medical Association Movement in West Africa

The association movement was one of the harbingers of professionalism in the medical community, and an autonomous organization was crucial to success. In West Africa this movement led to many beneficial changes for African doctors in the Colonial Medical Service and in private practice. In this regard Murray Last holds that "For most of the Colonial period . . . doctors in African countries were too few to constitute a local autonomous professional association (only Sierra Leone stands out as the possible exception, outside the settler-dominated territories), and too cut off from colleagues in the metropolitan countries to be within the otherwise pervasive professional structure. Certainly in the eyes of the public, doctors in the colonial period were not recognized as members of some autonomous organisation called a 'medical profession'!"[28] This assessment, however, must be qualified.

The data support evidence to the contrary with regard to Sierra Leone's African practitioners being pioneers in associationism in West Africa. Fyfe's monumental study on Sierra Leone contains no reference to such a development. It was true that the Sierra Leone branch of the British Medical Association, an affiliate of corporate patronage, was founded in 1921 with thirty-two members and remained the only branch in the West African territory for a while. Dr. Ernest. J. Wright, an African doctor, was the honorary secretary, but the bulk of the membership—71 percent—came from the WAMS as compared with 86.7 percent in the East African Service.[29] Beyond Wright, however, the African membership must have been nominal and without autonomy because of corporate patronage that delayed the development of some professional traits (see chapter 1).

The African role in associationism, therefore, remained a minor episode. Gold Coast doctors had inherited a long history of bitter discontent with the Colonial Medical Service because they were denied employment. So they made the first attempt to break away from the British Medical Association, followed by Nigeria, Gambia, and Sierra Leone. Dr. M. A. Barnor, for example, reported that the Gold Coast Medical Practitioners' Union was established in 1933, the first medical association to be organized without European members. The Gold Coast had only a few African doctors, including association members Frederick Nanka-Bruce, C. E. Reindorf, and W. A. C. Nanka-Bruce, who were all private practitioners. At their inaugural ceremony in late 1938, Frederick Nanka-Bruce (president) outlined the reasons for organizing and how to safeguard their interest: "The element of discrimination against the African that has now found so much favour was not known in the old days and it shows how regrettably things have changed for the worse for the African practitioner, to recall that an African once held the post of principal medical officer."[30] These same doctors, however, joined the local branch of the British Medical Association in February 1953. By this time British medical officials were beginning their preparation for retirement in response to decolonization.

Nigerian doctors, however, formed the strongest associations in the colonial era. The Association of African Medical Officers was founded in June 1942, but it was at Enugu on October 30, 1942, that the doctors drafted its rules and regulations. From the time of this meeting the name was slightly changed to the Association of African Medical Officers of Nigeria. The association listed five major objectives, the last one being "to make collective representations to the Director of Medical Services and to Government matters of common interests."³¹ S. L. A. Manuwa (MD, ChB, FRCS, Edinburgh) was elected as the first chairman; E. N. O. Sodeinde (BS, MB, Dublin) as general secretary; S. O. Franklin (BS, MB, Dublin) as treasurer, and R. O. Taylor-Cole (MB, ChB, Glasgow) as auditor. The membership consisted of sixteen medical officers and one honorary member.

The factor of unequal status prompted the separate organizing efforts of the African doctors. The African group meant to convey that they manifested the traits that characterized the professions (see chapter 1). Their initiative was an important step toward medical decolonization in West Africa. On January 1, 1943, the association petitioned the Colonial Medical Service in Nigeria concerning segregation of the classified staff list of doctors, warning that the association was no longer satisfied with the practice of listing African medical officers separate from European medical officers and deemed it to be "professional ostracism or racial discrimination . . . [that conferred] in the eyes of the lay public, an inferior professional status on the officers concerned."³² Although discrimination flourished even where a separate list existed, the association noted that no other departments had separate lists where Africans held superior positions. This complaint was not peculiar to Nigeria but was voiced vehemently even in other colonies without professional associations of Africans. Through his organizing efforts, Manuwa went on to become the deputy director of medical services in 1948, and in 1951 became the first Nigerian director of Colonial Medical Services. These promotions had a profound impact elsewhere in the colonies and no doubt impressed upon other African medical officers the need to seek additional certification in order to qualify for the positions that might be created with the expected European exodus.[33]

Boye-Johnson's British Medical Diploma

In order to improve his professional status Boye-Johnson, who was working as a medical officer in the Colonial Service, went to England for study and received the Diploma in Tropical Medicine in 1949. In 1953 the school of hygiene and tropical medicine of the University of London conferred upon him the Diploma in Public Health. Boye-Johnson's dissertation for this certification was entitled "Concerning the Promotion of Public Health in the Colony and Protectorate of Sierra Leone." Portions of his study dealt with the available statistical information in Sierra Leone and he stressed the need to move beyond statistical estimates in census data by documenting the disparity between colony and protectorate statistics concerning the same matter. He further explored the major endemic diseases of Sierra Leone and problems relating to their control, along with the use and nonuse of sulfonamides and treatments in clinics, hospitals, and dispensaries. The analysis of cases covered the years 1941–50. He concluded with the observation that major obstacles to the improvement of public health were the lack of professional personnel and adequate funds. His conclusion was later echoed by colonial officials. Diseases creating a crippling economic effect had to be tackled first, he argued, and rural areas needed urgent attention as a matter of policy.[34]

Boye-Johnson completed his study leave abroad and found conditions favorable for employment not just for himself but for other Sierra Leone doctors as well. He received a promotion to senior medical officer, a position he held until 1956. He became acting assistant director of medical services from 1957–59, along with another stint as senior medical officer 1959–60. Dr. Edward Awooner-Renner was already director of medical services (DMS) in the early 1950s, the first Sierra Leonean to hold this position. In spite of the fact that the independence process was underway by 1951, the gradual nature of colonial politics in Sierra Leone meant that the nationalist struggle for independence was hardly present when compared to the Gold Coast or

Nigeria. Dr. Milton Margai, who would become the first prime minister in 1961, was a chief minister but not a full minister—merely a policy adviser to the minister of health. However, the DMS was a member of the Executive Council. In Sierra Leone, therefore, promotion and power were closely monitored by colonial authorities, even while most of the officials were planning for their departure under the changing of the guard.

Expatriate Medical Exodus and Boye-Johnson's Rise

The era of the 1950s in Anglophone West Africa was a time of political awareness. Optimism prevailed almost everywhere among Africans as the impetus for decolonization grew, and Africans abroad made plans for the return and participation in independence celebrations. Africans of most professional persuasions championed the cause of Africanization—the replacement of European personnel with Africans. Expatriates, some disheartened by the fact that their projects might not be completed, including planned roads and sanitation systems, made preparations to leave the region as the nationalist struggle threatened to dismantle colonial rule. Their pensions and the form of payment were issues of concern. For example, Governor Robert de Zouche Hall (1953–56) was uncertain at first about the reaction in Sierra Leone over the proposed special list of lump-sum payments to expatriates in order to prevent their exodus. He noted to the secretary state for the colonies, "Doctor Margai has shown its [the government's] intentions [for Her Majesty's Overseas Colonial Services, HMOCS] are acceptable,"[35] although action in the Executive Council would be delayed. The date was May 12, 1954. In fact, both Awooner-Renner and Margai slowed the Africanization process. When Awooner-Renner died in 1955, Dr. T. P. Eddy, an Englishman, assumed his position as DMS until about 1959, passing over Boye-Johnson. However, Eddy was also a member of the British Medical Association (BMA) and represented their interests in matters of salary questions at a time in which the BMA had become an anathema in Nigeria and Ghana.[36] When Eddy left his post as DMS, the position was assumed by Dr. H. M. S. Boardman, who had spent several years in the Nigerian Medical Service and hence had seniority over Boye-Johnson. With the 1961 date of independence approaching, a mass exodus of middle-class Europeans had begun, and Pakistani medical doctors were contracted to take the place of European physicians.[37] The expatriate exodus, however, had its antecedents in the 1950s as shown through vacancies in the three larger colonies (see tables 5, 6, and 7, Ghana, Nigeria, Sierra Leone, 1951–55).[38]

In spite of being passed over at an earlier time, Boye-Johnson's fortunes changed for the better with the expatriate exodus, decolonization, and the situation that developed of too few African doctors. He served as PMO (health) in the Ministry of Health in the years 1960–62, was then appointed deputy CMO in 1962, and then CMO and chief medical adviser (1963–67), as well as simultaneously being the head of the National Health Administration of Sierra Leone (1963–67). For his efforts, both professional and political, Queen Elizabeth II bestowed upon Boye-Johnson the OBE. In the international arena Boye-Johnson was licensed to practice medicine in the United States, Great Britain, Canada, and in the rest of the Commonwealth. He traveled widely—in Africa and the Middle East, to Britain, the United States (where he made at least five visits with his wife, Florie Boye-Johnson by boat), France, the USSR (observing its medical culture), and Switzerland—attending conferences and representing the government of Sierra Leone. He served on the executive board of the World Health Organization (WHO) and received USAID fellowships to study medical care in the United States and Puerto Rico, and a WHO fellowship to study public health planning in Panama, Trinidad, and Chile.

Other changes taking place in postcolonial Africa brought career benefits to large numbers of African doctors trained abroad as obstacles to employment were gradually removed; obstacles that Boye-Johnson and others of his generation had faced. Feierman correctly connects these changes to a stronger point in West Africa and African history in general. The time after World War II was one in which the social services of British colonial Africa were being transformed in fundamental ways. The British abandoned the idea that colonies ought to be self-supporting. They wanted a very different labor policy (there

Table 5. Reasons for the exodus of European medical officers from the Ministry of Health, Gold Coast, 1951–55

YEAR	NO.	RESIGNED	RETIRED	OTHER	TOTAL	%
1951	147	6	5	9	20	13.6
1952	191	10	5	14	29	15.2
1953	201	6	8	8	22	10.9
1954	217	4	7	12	23	10.6
1955	318	—	9	20	29	9.1
Totals		26	34	63	123	

Source: PRO, CO 554/1186. Minutes of Meeting of West African Directors of Medical Services, 1954–56.

Table 6. Reasons for the exodus of European medical officers from the Ministry of Health, Nigeria, 1951–54

YEAR	NO.	RESIGNED	RETIRED	OTHER	TOTAL	%
1951	546	23	8	12	43	7.9
1952	571	11	23	21	55	9.6
1953	573	15	10	23	48	8.3
1954	569	10	13	6	29	5.1
Totals		59	44	62	175	

Source: PRO, CO 554/1186. Minutes of Meeting of West African Directors of Medical Services, 1954–56.

Table 7. Reasons for the exodus of European medical officers from the Ministry of Health, Sierra Leone, 1952–54

YEAR	NO.	RESIGNED	RETIRED	OTHER	TOTAL	%
1952	75	2	2	3	7	9.3
1953	86	1	2	5	8	9.3
1954	88	4	3	5	12	13.6
Totals		7	7	13	27	

Source: PRO, CO 554/1186. Minutes of Meeting of West African Directors of Medical Services, 1954–56.

was a move in many colonies away from migrant labor), much more productivity from agriculture (to help Britain deal with the sterling crisis after the war), and a new social policy that would provide more services than the colonies had before. The Colonial Development and Welfare Acts were connected to this change. The new growth of social services meant that there was now a need for many more doctors.

By the 1950s colonial officials were faced with the shortage of medical doctors because of rising demand. Populations grew at a rate sometimes faster than economic growth. Colonial officials began to reassess the policy against the employment of foreign-trained doctors whose names did not appear on the British Medical Register. J. B. Williams, who chaired a committee to deal with this issue in the Colonial Office, wrote in the minutes of the meeting:

> I feel myself that the policy which we are adopting at present, mainly from fear of pressure from the British Medical Association, of refusing to employ foreign doctors except on terms which exclude the vast majority of them (i.e. by insisting on qualification registrable in the country) is quite indefensible in the circumstances of to-day. It is a betrayal of the interest of the Colonial peoples by deliberately withholding from them medical help which they might have; it flies straight in the face of that objective to which we all pay lip service, i.e. closer integration of the Western world, and it lays us open when the facts are fully known to the world at large (as they are bound to be sooner or later) to the most damaging kind of criticism of our whole Colonial policy. It seems to me therefore that we ought to tackle seriously the question of encouraging Colonial Government to amend their laws to admit to practise doctors with non-British qualifications.
>
> In saying this I recognise that we may find that we dare not pursue such a policy because of the power of the British Medical Association which has on more than one occasion hinted to us that they would go to extreme lengths (such as blacklisting all Colonial appointments) in order to prevent us from throwing open the colonies to foreign doctors.[39]

Another committee member also expressed uneasiness over the BMA's insistence upon a "closed shop," but while he agreed with Williams in part, he still hesitated about employing foreign doctors, expressing concern about maintaining standards and ethics. The regulations were changed to permit greater discretion in hiring for local medical officers. Directors of medical services gained the leeway through these amendments to grant a license locally to a qualified trained doctor with multiple categories of registrations. The registration of foreign doctors was facilitated, easing the way for Africans who had studied abroad to qualify for employment upon return home.[40]

The State Department and Technical Assistance Abroad

The Department of State in Washington, D.C., also played a role in promoting the acceptance of these changes in the 1950s. Through the British embassy in Washington, it raised a question over the recognition in colonial territories of medical qualifications gained in U.S. universities. During 1955–56 more than 250 students in the United States came from British colonial territories, most of them enrolled in medical and premedical courses; fewer than 20 percent came from territories where they were allowed to register as medical practitioners upon their return. Problems were bound to increase because the State Department was directly encouraging students from British territories to enroll in U.S. medical schools. It emphasized further that technical assistance was needed and welcomed in colonial territories; it was not good politics for the British to resist the U.S. efforts of providing medical expertise.[41] Technical assistance became an avowed aim of the State Department and, under the International Educational Exchange Program, the Fulbright and Smith-Mundt acts were the mechanisms used "to promote a better understanding of the United States in other countries, and to increase mutual understanding between the people of the United States and the people of other countries" in the era of Cold War competition (see chapter 8).[42]

These issues obviously caused concern to the British. Foreign students in the United States could very easily fall prey to American anti-colonial sentiments and the recently increased efforts of American blacks to broaden their civil rights might easily inspire greater political unrest in British territories. In spite of the new efforts toward the acceptance of doctors with foreign certification, Commonwealth students with hopes of working back home placed little faith in the new policy effort.[43]

The Independence Era and End of Colonial Medical Regulations

The independence movement in the African territories accelerated in the 1950s, and the British Medical Council (BMC) recognized the need to acquiesce in broadening its legislation governing the qualifications acceptable in colonial territories for registration or licensure to practice medicine. The BMC divided the colonial territories into three groups. Group A comprised twenty territories that excluded American-trained doctors from practice unless they also possessed qualifications approved by the General Medical Council. Group B consisted of six territories that accepted American-trained doctors, although three rejected U.S. qualifications obtained after January 1, 1952. Group C comprised eleven territories whose legislation permitted American-trained and foreign doctors to register and be licensed as medical practitioners. In February 1952 U.S. vice consul Robert Ross submitted to the medical department in Lagos—a cabinet-level agency—a list of U.S. medical schools whose graduates were being accepted for practice in England. This list included the Chicago Medical School, Meharry Medical College, medical schools at Howard, Harvard, Johns Hopkins, Stanford, Indiana, and Wisconsin.[44] The AMA, in conjunction with the official regional accreditation associations, supplied a list in October 1957 to the BMC of approved medical schools and internship programs, a list that was accepted. So from then on medical councils in each territory in liaison with the chief medical adviser were implementing changes that allowed for more flexibility.[45]

Ghana and Medical Autonomy

Following independence on March 6, 1957, and accompanying the change of name from the Gold Coast to Ghana, organizational changes favoring medical autonomy in the newly independent country progressed quickly. The new federal government was to deal with the Commonwealth Relations Office and no longer the Colonial Office. The BMA, whose sole purpose initially was to safeguard expatriate interest under corporate patronage, lost its authority after March 5 in Ghana. From that time the newly formed Ghana Medical Association became the sole representative body for African doctors and dentists there, and the government Medical and Dental Council would evaluate medical standards and qualifications. Dr. Kwame Nkrumah, president of the Republic of Ghana, and the first patron of the Ghana Medical Association, addressed this body at the observance of the first volume of the *Ghana Medical Journal*, on August 21, 1962.[46] (Dr. W. A. Hawe, an Englishman, was Nkrumah's physician.) The Nigerian Medical Association was founded about 1951 with 1,575 registered practitioners.[47] This procedure was repeated in Sierra Leone on November 27, 1964, the foundation date of its Medical Practitioners Union. These associations had constitutions and bylaws governing their members, and the founding members felt that it was no longer tenable to be members of the BMA, for its membership was no longer compatible with their new, independent status.[48] Boye-Johnson, who was still in the government of Sierra Leone, was not an active member of the Medical Practitioners Union, but was a member of the government's Medical and Dental Council (1963–67) and instrumental in responding to the needs of African doctors and changing registration requirements. While the struggle for medical professionalism did not end with the coming of independence, the new era reduced intraprofessional conflict and the pain endured by African doctors under colonialism in Africa and in the diaspora.

Before his death on August 10, 1978, at the age of 67 in Freetown, Boye-Johnson had lived through the foundation era of the Cold War. He witnessed its changing policy impact in West Africa, especially in Guinea and Ghana. While Sierra Leone stayed to the right of the political center and took an anticommunist stance—as did Gambia and Nigeria—Guinea and Ghana tilted to the left of the center toward Moscow, Beijing, and the Eastern bloc. Boye-Johnson's extensive foreign travels, intimate social relations with the American embassy in Freetown, communal connections in West Africa, and his long years of employment in the government health service apprised him of the East-West conflict. The general medical culture of the West had governed his medical focus and, while still in the government, he had observed the impact of socialist-trained African doctors on the medical profession in independent Africa. A new medical culture had appeared in Gambia, Ghana, Nigeria, and Sierra Leone. The infusion of Cold War ideology provided the impetus for new scholarships abroad and training to not just a new medical generation (the seventh) but other professionals as well in Africa. African medical practitioners trained in the colonial era, however, did not take kindly to the new African communist-trained doctors returning to West Africa in the independence era.

Let us turn next to this neglected generation of physicians—the communist-trained—in African medical history, and to the foreign policy initiatives from Moscow that made this development possible. The British awareness to these initiatives was heard around the world in Churchillian elegance in a speech given at Westminster College, Fulton, Missouri, on March 5, 1946, where the phrase "iron curtain" was first heard.[49]

CHAPTER EIGHT

African Physicians: From the Cold War to Perestroika

> From Stettin in the Baltic to Trieste in the Adriatic an iron cur-
> tain has descended across the continent. Behind that line lie all
> the capitals of the ancient states of Central and Eastern Europe.
> Warsaw, Berlin, Prague, Vienna, Budapest, Belgrade, Bucharest
> and Sofia.
>
> Winston Churchill, Fulton, Missouri, March 5, 1946

The British prime minister's use of the phrase "iron curtain" at
Fulton, a town of 11,000 located in the rolling countryside of central
Missouri, not only awoke the town from its American innocence but
sent global shock waves about the advance of communism in the
world. The Cold War had begun and this new order laid the ideological foundation for the competitive East-West rivalry in Africa in the
postwar period. This rivalry in West Africa introduced two medical
cultures with different objectives. The medical culture of the West
was general-purpose medicine; a single doctor was trained to treat
patients with a variety of illnesses. The medical culture of the East was
based on specialization; a single doctor was trained to deal with
one illness and had to work in a group of different specialists to treat

one patient with a variety of ailments. This type of training posed problems in Africa generally, since there were few doctors. A medical culture that did not conform to the model would be poorly tolerated. Dr. Nathaniel Akabi-Davis, a successful orthopedic specialist, discussed this development, maintaining how much diplomacy had to be exercised in handling the new, intrusive medical culture and making adjustments to the old order.[1] This explains why the African medical profession was also affected by the return of African doctors trained in Russia and the Eastern bloc. West Africans had to make accommodations with a new medical culture that required clinical adjustments, although existing studies reveal very little about this problem. This topic is the focus of this chapter, covering the colonial and postindependence eras. In order to understand the effects on African doctors in this generation (seven), one must consider first the dynamics of foreign-policy initiatives in East-West relations.

Communism had made little headway in Africa in the postwar years. The Communist International's (Comintern) purpose from 1919 to 1943 was to promote global revolution based on Marxist-Leninist philosophy, only to become a fatality of World War II,[2] while the postwar partition of Europe went unaffected. Decolonization in West Africa in the 1940s and the 1950s generally adhered to its imperial legacy of anticommunism. Stalin's death in 1953 and the subsequent fading of his cult, however, allowed a new generation of Soviet policymakers to renew initiatives in the Afro-Asian World. In 1955 the Bandung Conference in Indonesia, which was the first significant meeting of the new Asian and African leaders, perceptibly changed the Soviets' myopic view about the merits of diplomacy in the Third World. And in 1956 the Communist Party of the Soviet Union (CPSU) recognized the need to cooperate with bourgeois African leaders in the first independence movement in order to advance socialism, for some African leaders seemed interested in the communist cause. The Congo briefly under Patrice Lumumba, Guinea under Sékou Touré, Mali under Modibo Keita, and Ghana under Kwame Nkrumah, all had anti-Western policies and became the most acceptable pawns in the new communist strategies for recruitment. These countries were, therefore, vulnerable to communist penetration in the eyes of Western powers and subjected to extensive surveillance (see appendix 2).[3]

By the 1960s political leaders in some of the newly independent states were beginning to voice a modified brand of Marxist rhetoric. Soviet and Eastern bloc trade missions appeared in Africa,[4] and Soviet-African friendship societies operated as proxies for influence in and out of the Soviet embassies and consulates. Before long these developments had begun to touch the medical profession, and African students began to be recruited for medical training in Moscow, Prague, and other Eastern bloc locations.[5] Moscow decided to accelerate its initiative in Africa because of the increasing interest shown in Africans by the United States and U.S. educational institutions.

The Cold War and Sub-Saharan Africa

Moscow and Washington were relatively indifferent to sub-Saharan Africa in the immediate postwar era. Moscow concentrated on strategic centers of land power in Europe, and Washington countered with its Marshall Plan for Europe and subordinated its sub-Saharan interests to Western colonial powers in Africa, now U.S. allies. Unless there were obvious foreign-policy gains for the USSR, Stalin held that revolutions in Africa would have to await the leadership of the nascent proletariat. Soviet policy toward Africa modified after Stalin's death in 1953, becoming more accepting of the leadership of the petit bourgeois class, once regarded as the "African agents of white colonialism." Not only was the African working class embraced but also the "national bourgeoisie," because the nationalist struggles were seen as potential stepping stones to socialism. By 1956 the CPSU was in full support of these initiatives in Africa.

The new, more realistic Soviet policy found expression at the United Nations, where the Soviet delegation called for an end to the Western colonial presence in Africa. As early as 1954, N. V. Yushmanov and D. A. Ol'derogge, two leading Soviet Africanists, had edited an ethnographic survey called *Narody Afriki* (Peoples of Africa), which served as a guide for Soviet strategy in Africa as the Cold War increased the competitive momentum. Notwithstanding that this document stressed the inferiority of Africa cultures,[6] Moscow showered the newly sovereign African states with attention, both welcome and unwelcome. It extended diplomatic recognition to them but also put in place a network of agents and informants in their labor organizations, political movements, women's associations, cultural groups, youth leagues, and scholarship programs.

By 1956 the expatriate exodus had produced an acute and worsening shortage of trained personnel that had begun to be felt in London. Governor B. Harris of Gambia warned that the USSR might take advantage of the exodus to promote its own objectives in Africa. Soviet offers of technical assistance, he noted, would look very attractive: "not because of any acceptance of foreign ideologies but because of the urgent need for development and the failure of Britain to provide the staff of the highest calibre, when required[. This] is one of the most potent factors, not only in assisting territories toward self-government but in retaining their confidence in Her Majesty's Government."[7]

Indeed, the USSR subsequently negotiated protocols of cooperation in the fields of science and culture with the United Arab Republics (UAR—Egypt and Syria), Guinea, Ghana, Ethiopia, Mali, and Somalia in the years 1957–61. Other countries, including Nigeria, Togo, Liberia, Morocco, Tunis, Libya, and Senegal, did not conclude such agreements, but the USSR supported cultural and scientific relations with these countries through both state institutions and social organizations. In 1960 the USSR gave guided tours to at least 200 Africans interested in Soviet education, science, culture, health, and sports. Of the 777 African students studying in the USSR in 1960–61, 140 attended Peoples' Friendship University (renamed Patrice Lumumba University in 1961), which was established specifically for students from Asia, Africa, and Latin America. African students were also enrolled at Moscow State University, Leningrad State University, Kiev University, Central Asian University in Tashkent (also established in 1961 specifically for Asian, African, and Latin American students), and the Tashkent Agricultural Institute (see map 5). Of these students 350 came from the UAR, 76 from Ghana, 75 from the Sudan, 62 from Guinea, and 23 from Somalia; the remainder

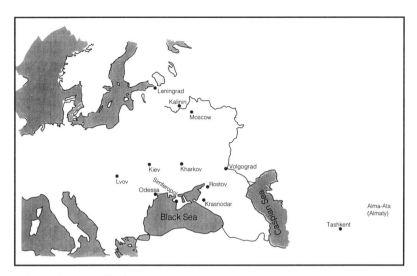

Map 5. Soviet medical centers, 1985

came from some 17 other African countries. Most of the students were enrolled in preparatory facilities or standard programs of higher Soviet education.[8]

Soviet policymakers used a plan of grouping African states as a means for selecting those suitable to their interests. For example, in West Africa, as the decade of the 1950s came to an end, Ghana and Guinea were the two main supporters of socialism in the region and received most of the attention from the USSR. This explains why African students from Sierra Leone and Nigeria do not appear in the listings of the U.S. Department of State or in the USSR compilation for 1959–60. According to Soviet observers, Sierra Leone, along with Cameroon, Chad, Dahomey (Benin), Gabon, Côte d'Ivoire, Madagascar, Niger, Senegal, Tanganyika (Tanzania), and Uganda, were too closely linked at that time to the foreign policies of the former British and French colonial powers for Eastern bloc support. Nigeria, along with Kenya, Liberia, Somalia, Togo, and Upper Volta (Burkina Faso) were assigned an intermediate, more ambiguous category because they lacked strong socialist tendencies. My own fieldwork in Sierra Leone in 1984 and 1985, however, together with the ministry of health data, confirm the presence in that country of a number of

Soviet program activities—including some in the medical field—and the *Gambia Gazette* (April 1986), and the *Nigerian Medical Directory* (1970–71) show the tentative lists of doctors trained in Soviet (four of them) and other socialist countries (sixteen). (For Ghana and Sierra Leone, with larger numbers of Soviet and Eastern bloc–trained doctors, see appendixes 3 and 4.)

Qualified Specialists

Medical training facilities in the Soviet Union and the socialist countries generally emphasized the production of highly trained specialists. Professional education was directed by the state, and the individual professions, such as medicine, had no separate autonomy. Professors were allowed to set minimum curricular standards for students, with the objective of preserving a high average level of education; specialists were created in response to societal needs. The African doctor trained in the Soviet Union, therefore, experienced a different system than that of the Western countries.[9]

The Soviet-trained African doctor was accustomed to work within a team of specialists that emphasized collective responsibility; in contrast, patient care in Great Britain and the United States emphasized individual responsibility. This meant that the Soviet medical trainee did not need general medical knowledge for degree certification. The lack of knowledge by one doctor about a specific diagnosis would be made up for by another doctor in the team. However, the Soviet style of medical training was not particularly well suited to the reality of the African situation, where there was a high ratio of patients to physicians and where the greatest need was for medical care at the basic level. Indeed, there are still not enough doctors in West Africa for group medical practice to serve patients' needs adequately, especially away from the larger cities (see tables 1 and 2). In this kind of setting a general practitioner is more valuable than a specialist.

The medical school curriculum in the Eastern bloc, under reform since 1968, leaned heavily in favor of specialization and it deemphasized the general practitioner. Medical certification required seven years of training. The first three years included the basic science courses and English for non-English-speaking students and Russian for those needing training in that language. Clinical training of various sorts was provided in the next four years. In the seventh year the student performed an internship in a sizable *oblast* or city hospital, and those intending to specialize could pursue their interests in fields such as general surgery, ENT (ear, nose, and throat), ophthalmology, urology, orthopedics, or pediatric surgery. Students were assigned to a medical service institution for the next three to five years. Valuable experience was obviously gained during the period, one that appears to be equivalent to the "house job" practical experience phase of the medical student in Great Britain. Broader training might follow for those in the therapeutics—psychiatry, neurology, or dermatology— and the same can be said for those pursuing obstetrics and gynecology, and pediatrics.[10] In Russia, however, a separate protocol had to be signed between the Soviet central government and the respective African government in order for the African medical doctor to complete the residency phase. In the absence of such protocol, if an African government decided that the shortage of doctors was too acute and so could not wait for the doctors to complete the residency, African students would return home in a questionable state of preparedness to begin their medical careers.

It was said that the first African doctors trained in the USSR had a very limited value to Africa and were barely health officers; in the USSR, perhaps, they would have been sent out to rural areas as health officers and general physicians in the Ukraine or Byelorussia (now Belarus). Professors in the socialist countries attended international seminars in Western Europe and constructed their class syllabi on the same order as in the West. According to Sierra Leone doctors who studied in the Eastern bloc, the medical requirements at the Medical Institute of Sofia, Bulgaria, and the University of Novi Sad, Yugoslavia, were similar to those operative in the Western European tradition with long years of study required. The published and oral interview data show that the medical curricula in Poland, Hungary, and Czechoslovakia had the same structure until the fall of communism in Eastern Europe.[11] In spite of the early initiative toward specialization as our study will later show, the Soviet Union has produced some great successes among African doctors, including those who have gone on to become highly respected surgeons and physicians.

Despite these problems, the Soviet-trained African doctor embodied a new challenge to the traditional dominant social status of the medical elite in Africa. Theoretically, for example, professions try to heighten their status and increase the social distance between themselves and others. Larson examines the role that the accumulation of knowledge plays in the autonomous development of special occupations. Professions with the power to evaluate their own members and the right to self-control reduce the element of external regulation. These privileges, however, can be lost if that profession's value to society diminishes or under conditions of revolutionary social change. The high status of the physician undergoes demystification where emphasis becomes centered upon preventive as opposed to curative care. Under these conditions medical specialization fits in the context of the medical team, and "the physician tends to lose at least some of his 'inherent' superiority."[12] And paramedical personnel, such as the famous barefoot doctors in China, dilute the physician's monopoly of medical knowledge.

Sierra Leone Nationals: First Group 1959

Sierra Leone nationals sought desperately to study medicine in the USSR and other Eastern bloc nations because Sierra Leone lacked a medical training infrastructure and the socialist countries gave scholarships. In spite of the fact that in the nineteenth century Sierra Leone produced professionals in large numbers in proportion to its territorial size—doctors, lawyers, civil servants, and journalists—the nation has now become a backwater with one of the highest infant mortality rates in the world. The need for a university medical training facility had been raised in the nineteenth century by one of West Africa's most famous physicians. Africanus Horton initiated the first effort aimed at eliminating the peripheral status of the West African medical profession. As chapter 3 describes, he wrote to the War Office as early as 1861 recommending the establishment of a medical school in West Africa. British officials, however, rejected his proposal outright.

Some 101 years later the medical school issue surfaced again. According to World Health Organization records, a proposal to found a Sierra Leone medical school was under active consideration in the early 1960s, but once again the initiative came to nothing. Under the U.S. Agency for International Development (USAID), the United States had been investing in health projects since 1942, and Accra, Ghana, apparently received some aid for a medical center in the early 1960s.[13] Sierra Leone almost received support at the same time but, according to my physician informant Olu-Williams (see figure 13):

> The American government was willing to help in the establishment of a medical infrastructure in about 1961, following independence, which was to be of an internationally recognized.... Unfortunately, Sir Milton Margai, the first prime minister, died in 1964, and Albert Margai, his brother and successor, did not believe that the proposal should be given high priority; the program dropped out of contention; and the funds were diverted elsewhere. Since then, the American government offered its usual aid with help from the Rockefeller Foundation to foster the medical school, but Albert, again, did not give the proposed funds priority.[14]

Sierra Leoneans studied abroad or elsewhere in Africa, for Nigeria and Ghana acquired medical training facilities in the mid-1950s, and their scientific communities rose in importance in part because of these resources. The USSR and the Eastern bloc nations not only supported Sierra Leoneans but also Gambians, Ghanaians, and Nigerians in their quest for medical training through scholarships, and these Eastern bloc–trained doctors came to outnumber the Western-trained professionals in health care delivery in government hospitals. However, the initial step in reaching the Soviet Union was not an easy one, especially for Sierra Leoneans.

The first group of Sierra Leoneans went to the USSR illegally in late 1959. Sierra Leone, which had fallen out of step with the pace of decolonization elsewhere in West Africa, was now, on the eve of independence, in the throes of a bewildered and truncated nationalist movement; that is, the coming of independence in Sierra Leone was

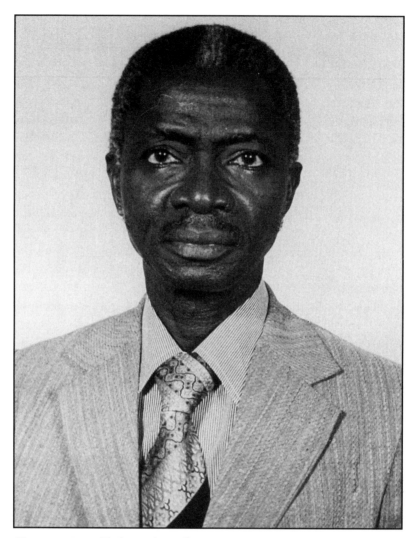

Figure 13. *Dr. Alfred E. Olu-Williams, Sierra Leone, c.* 1980s. *Courtesy of Alfred E. Olu-Williams.*

not a rupture with colonialism, for independence was more like a graduation into an elite group—a circle held together by the English language, affection for English culture, and with a strong belief that London was the center of the world. This perspective was held by citizens of the former colony and protectorate alike. Controlled by a colonial government with a strongly anticommunist orientation, Sierra Leone had no diplomatic relations with the Soviet Union. The expatriate exodus had left Sierra Leone with an acute shortage of trained personnel that was perhaps worse than any other country in the region. Several organizations with connections to Moscow were anxious to provide scholarships for students who wished to study in the USSR. These included the Afro-Asian Solidarity committees, the Sierra Leone Women's Organization, the International Union of Students based in Prague, and the Friendship Society (see appendix 2 for the communist presence in Africa and the absence by name of Sierra Leone for the period up to June 1959 but cited thereafter from July–September 1959).[15] The Afro-Asian Solidarity Committee sponsored one group who left Sierra Leone disguised as soccer players on their way to a game in Conakry, Guinea. From there the students boarded an Aeroflot plane for Moscow. Whether they would be able to practice medicine in Sierra Leone upon return never entered their minds, especially since a more sympathetic regime might be in power by that time.

Aeroflot to Moscow: Sierra Leone Students

This group included A. A. Taqui (MD), who it is said was the first student to register at Friendship University. Taqui is now an outstanding pediatrician at the Ahmadu Bello University Teaching Hospital in Zaria, Nigeria. Ivan Johnson-Taylor (MD; see figure 14) was also a member of the first group; today he is one of the most qualified surgeons in Sierra Leone. Others who trained in the USSR also returned but did not pursue medical careers.[16] It is said that most of the students in pursuit of professional development in Moscow had links with the political opposition to the Margai forces who were preparing to assume the reins of power from the colonial government.

Sierra Leone inherited a radical nationalist tradition from I. T. A. Wallace-Johnson, a journalist; Trinidadian George Padmore (formerly Malcolm Nurse), who had also studied law at Howard University; the West African Youth League (WAYL); in part from the trade unions; and from protest movements in West Africa. As early as 1930

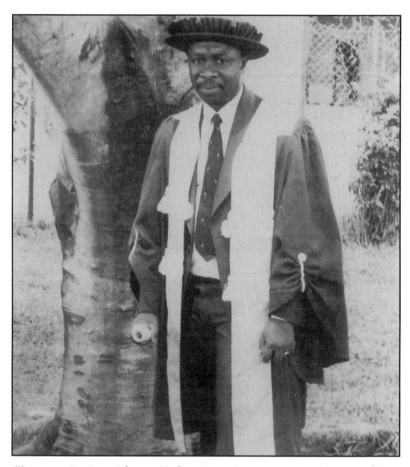

Figure 14. Dr. Ivan Johnson-Taylor, Sierra Leone, c. 1970s. Courtesy of Ivan Johnson-Taylor.

Wallace-Johnson attended the Comintern's Hamburg Conference of Negro Workers. It was an important conference, also attended by Jomo Kenyatta of Kenya, and E. F. Small of Gambia. Here it was decided that Africans should lead their revolution independently of blacks in other parts of the world. Following the conference, Wallace-Johnson, Padmore, and several others traveled to Moscow to participate in the Fifth Congress of the Red International Labor Union.[17] Wallace-Johnson also studied at Moscow's Peoples' University in the

1930s. In 1938 he founded the WAYL to promote socialist ideas and anticolonialism. While the WAYL spoke for working people in the region, its members included some Westernized social elites. It disseminated its views through the controversial *African Standard* for agitation against colonialism. Eventually, Wallace-Johnson went to jail for his political activities in Sierra Leone, a move that further fueled the opposition. Padmore, who had joined the nationalist struggle for independence in Ghana, became an official adviser in 1957 to Prime Minister Nkrumah. He and Wallace-Johnson worked closely together on issues of self-determination before the latter's death in 1964. In spite of Wallace-Johnson's and Padmore's ties to the Communist Party, both retained some independence of thought and action and tried to adapt radical principles to the specific African context in which they were working and organizing.

Under the leadership of Siaka Stevens, a trade unionist and admirer of Wallace-Johnson who eventually became Sierra Leone's first minister of mines, land, and labor, the opposition had renewed its call for a general election before independence in mid-1960. By October 17 of that year it had galvanized itself into a full-fledged political party known as the Elections Before Independence Movement (EBIM); and later it came to be called the All People's Congress (APC). The EBIM had ties to the Afro-Asian Solidarity Committee and was instrumental in organizing the first group of Sierra Leone students to go to Moscow. It would also assist the second group, but not before some of its members, including Stevens, entered Pademba Prison in Freetown for their political activities. The youth secretary, along with the entire executive committee of the APC, was detained in May 1962 and not released until three months later.[18]

By this time several youth activists who had also gone to jail with the APC leadership had become persona non grata to the government. They secretly traveled from Sierra Leone to Guinea and from there to Moscow, where several (including at least two women) pursued medical studies. Many in this group came from the former interior protectorate, as is shown by their names and ethnicity of origin in appendix 3.

Racism in the USSR:
Russian Women and the Death of a Ghanaian Student

In spite of communist rhetoric proclaiming a classless society free of racial bias, reality for the African students was quite the opposite. Gary Lee, an African American who spent four years in the Soviet Union as a reporter for the *Washington Post,* repeated a story told in Moscow by a Moscow advice columnist. This appeared in the *Washington Post* in April 1991: "The other day, a pregnant woman called up hysterically asking whether her child, fathered by an African, would come out black. Another wanted to know if the black would wash off her boy-friend's skin."[19] Russia was not without other embarrassing racist incidents that impinged on its foreign relations. The murder in 1963 of Edmond Asare-Addao, a Ghanaian medical student engaged to marry a Russian woman, focused resentment over these problems and triggered the first mass demonstrations in Red Square since the 1920s.[20]

The hostile racial climate caused many students to interrupt their studies and leave the USSR. Some Sierra Leoneans went to West Germany to complete their medical training. Several of them failed in the pursuit of medicine—due to poor performance, mental breakdown, the politics of the times, or even alcoholism. There were some outstanding practitioners who emerged from the groups that went to the USSR in the early 1960s, but more than likely the Margai regime provided no welcoming mats for those professionals who had left the country with intelligence agents on their heels. The reverse was true for professionals returning to Ghana; certainly, they were welcomed on their return to a country that maintained friendly relations with the Soviet Union and helped to arrange their studies there. The reception of Nigerian returnees is less certain, but their return was not such an important factor because of the existing medical centers in Nigeria for training and teaching. Gambian records officially show that only two doctors were trained in the East, although the actual number might be larger.

The year 1965 was a propitious year for Sierra Leoneans to study abroad because of a change in the government. The new prime min-

236

ister, attorney Albert Margai, the brother of Sir Milton Margai, and admirer of Prime Minster Nkrumah of Ghana, was the first Sierra Leone head of state to establish diplomatic relations with the USSR. On his assumption of power he almost immediately gave government approval for the first time for students to study in the Soviet Union. About fifteen scholarships were given directly by the Soviet government to study in diverse fields, with the majority in medicine. This group, it was said, was the best in terms of the quality of the training they had received in Sierra Leone before going to the USSR, and they were distributed throughout the Soviet Union in the various universities, rather than in just one institution. None of these students went to Patrice Lumumba University, which had become subject to much criticism. Nevertheless, Lumumba University continued to receive students through the channels established earlier by the APC acting in liaison with the Afro-Asian Solidarity Committee. The two units continued their cooperation and the initial groups were followed by others, the majority training in medicine.

While the Sierra Leoneans were in the USSR, their newly independent government passed statutes accelerating the decolonization process in the professions. Sierra Leone attorney Raymond Awooner-Renner recalled in 1985 that for the legal profession change did not come quickly. For example, the British Colonial Legal Practitioners Ordinance of 1960 still regulates to this day who shall be licensed in Sierra Leone. One must not only must be educated in the British legal system but be certified as a barrister in England, Northern Ireland, or the Republic of Ireland, or as an advocate in Scotland. Before December 1927 one merely had to be a student of the Inn of Court in order to be admitted as a legal practitioner in the Sierra Leone colony.[21]

The Medical Practitioners and Dental Surgeons Act of 1966 showed more flexibility than the Legal Practitioners Ordinance. The Medical and Dental Council permitted medical practitioners registered in Great Britain to be placed on the permanent register of Sierra Leone as well as those who, in the opinion of the council, held equivalent standards with Great Britain but whose certification was issued elsewhere. The council also had the authority to provide temporary registration to doctors and dentists who might later appear on the permanent register.

The Sierra Leone Medical and Dental Association (SLMDA) pushed for even more flexibility in the 1966 act, which allowed for only two categories of registration—provisional and permanent. Beginning in 1968 the SLMDA pushed for an amendment to the 1966 act in the Sierra Leone Parliament to allow for three categories of registration: (1) provisional medical officers, for those whose names had never appeared on a Medical Register; (2) temporary medical officers, for those with preregistration experience but who were non-Sierra Leoneans, allowing foreigners to practice; and (3) permanent medical officers, for those with preregistration experience with internship, or for those never previously registered. Postgraduate experience of the third category qualified one to enter independent practice. The amendment proposal was made into a bill and put through the attorney general's office but had not been ratified by 1985. Sierra Leoneans trained in the USSR and the Eastern bloc would function under what was called a "Conclusion of Cabinet," which recognized the three categories proposed by the SLMDA and allowed the physicians to register in the ministry of health.[22]

The First Generation Returns: Trouble Ahead

The first generation of doctors trained in the Soviet Union challenged the existing, Westernized medical culture of Sierra Leone in ways that ranged from their more informal habits of dress, to their orientation, to group practice. Their sense of a professional identity distinct from the Western-trained medical practitioners eventually culminated in the 1979 creation of the Sierra Leone Association of Soviet Graduates.

The reticence of medical informants in Sierra Leone and in Ghana to discuss the clinical effectiveness of the new doctors made data collection difficult. Medical informants in Sierra Leone and Ghana were uncomfortable discussing the clinical skills of the Soviet-trained doctors, but strong criticism of the Soviet system was widespread. After all, the African press did allow some of the malpractice cases to be reported to the public—even if they were officially not supposed to do so—and possibly the African practitioners trained in the West found it titillating to leak the information.

Soviet medical programs in the 1960s presented four fundamental problems for African students.

1. Medical students were not always routinely provided with clinical experience following their first four years of academic work. Students who were assertive on their own behalf might be assigned to work in a clinical setting; other graduates might return to Africa still lacking experience in practical procedures and requiring supervision.

2. Confusion over language differences, especially for specialized medical terminology, was another source of difficulty. (Keep in mind that the first year was spent in language training in both the USSR and other Eastern bloc countries; some students might even have to repeat their studies.) In an interview in Freetown in March 1985 William Roberts (MD), who was trained in the Soviet system, reported that students might have to learn the word for a single medical term in two or three languages—Russian, French, and English—in addition to their indigenous African language in order to converse with patients back home. Even then, confusion abounded. For example, the Russian word for ganglion can be used as "lymph nodes"; so if a Russian-trained doctor used "ganglion," it means "nerve bundle."[23] So one must study medical terminology in different languages in order to resolve this problem. Syndromes, for example, could be most confusing since the Soviet professors would use their author's names, with Russian spelling, whereas in English (or other Western languages) the authors might well be completely different, and their names would be spelled in the Anglicized form.

3. The third problem was that drugs were designated by different names in different countries. A physician prescribing a certain

compound by the proprietary name he had learned in medical school might not be understood by a pharmacist who knew the same compound under a completely different name. Eventually, practitioners and pharmacists were pushed into using generic names to avoid misunderstanding.

4. But perhaps the most serious problem had to do with the African doctors' preparation for the health conditions that awaited them at home. Infectious diseases that have been all but eradicated in other parts of the world still constitute a primary health problem in Africa. But Soviet medical training emphasized cardiovascular disease, malignancies, and viral infections, conditions that are common in developed countries.

Roberts described what could happen when the Soviet-trained doctor returned to a tropical setting: "My first experience was with a child [in Freetown] who came in with a convulsion. I thought it was viral meningitis. I was then told that it was cerebral malaria. I diagnosed another case as rheumatoid arthritis that was actually another form of arthritis. In developed countries such cases are rare. That is why I stress that we need research centers in Africa and that all medical training should be done in our own environment."[24]

The host countries of medical training could have reduced this diagnosis trauma by allowing their trainees the privilege of preregistration before their return. A program requiring "housemanship" or resident internship is crucial to the resolution of this problem. Based on the data in hand up to 1971, none of the Sierra Leoneans studying medicine in the USSR were allowed to preregister upon completion. So when they finished the course, medical degrees or diplomas were immediately issued and the newly trained doctors returned directly home.

West African Ministries of Health to the Rescue

The West African ministries of health made adjustments in their medical registration requirements in efforts to integrate the new doc-

tors into the practice of general medicine. Their efforts brought to an
end the last clinical vestiges of intraprofessional conflict. In Ghana a
longer term of residency was designed for the returning doctors, especially those from the USSR. Emmanuel Evans-Anfom (MB, ChB,
1944; DTMH, 1948, Edinburgh; FRCS, 1955, Edinburgh; see figure 15),
who served as chairman of the Medical and Dental Council, remembered the problems that the Ghana medical establishment faced with
the returning doctors. Ghana had apparently kept its better-certified
students in the science fields, the best students in medicine, the next
group in engineering. Those who could not qualify in Ghana took
scholarships abroad, particularly in Eastern Europe (see map 6). The
places most commonly accommodating them were Warsaw, Krakow
(Poland), Budapest (Hungary), Prague (Czechoslovakia), Novi Sad,
Belgrade (Yugoslavia), Bucharest (Romania), Sofia (Bulgaria), and
Leipzig, Karl-Marx-Stadt, and Halle (German Democratic Republic).
The entry requirements were lower in those countries than in Ghana,
where the British system was followed. The students however, faced a

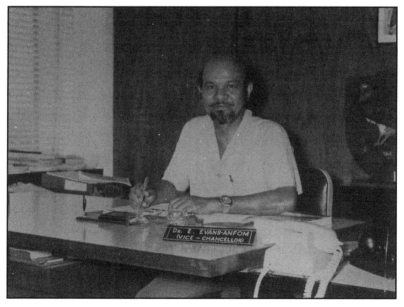

*Figure 15. Dr. Emmanuel Evans-Anfom, Ghana (Kumasi), c. 1970s. Courtesy
of Emmanuel Evans-Anfom.*

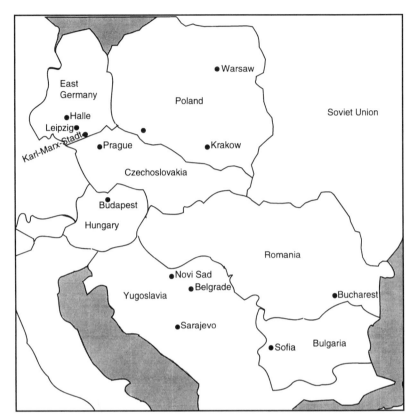

Map 6. Eastern European medical centers, 1985

number of problems, and "a lot of [sensitive] politics around [abound] when they first came back," according to Evans-Anfom.[25]

The Sierra Leone government also developed a model program to deal with what had become one of its most sensitive health professional problems. This was done in consultation with some of Sierra Leone's highly esteemed veteran doctors, such as Marcella Davies, chief medical officer of the ministry of health and the first woman appointee to that position in Anglophone West Africa; Alfred Olu-Williams, chief surgeon; Egerton Luke, medical officer and surgeon; and Nathaniel Akabi-Davis. The ministry of health established the Department of Clinical Studies in 1971. The first institution to provide medical training in Sierra Leone,[26] the department was staffed by some thirty specialists in medicine, surgery, pathology, obstetrics and gynecology, orthopedics, and ophthalmology. All these specialists were drawn from the ranks of doctors who had completed their training in Great Britain in the pre-1961 colonial era. The department was housed in a new single-story building constructed near Connaught Hospital, and formal lectures were given in an adjacent library. The new director, Robert Wellesley Cole (BS, MA, MB, MD, MS, FRCS, FRCSE)—who actually practiced in England—and his colleagues organized a schedule of morning lectures for the new doctors, followed each afternoon by clinical ward duty. Most of the participants were new doctors trained in the USSR and the Eastern bloc countries. The new policy promulgated that all doctors who had not done an internship or had not preregistered before coming to Sierra Leone had to go through the process of a rotating internship in the Department of Clinical Studies.

This meant that doctors moved in rotation in a program that required a year of residency in the Connaught Hospital and various clinics in Freetown—first with six months in medicine and six months in surgery. The requirements were later changed to a two-year program. The clinicians understood that the responsibility the new doctors faced exceeded that of their colleagues in developed countries. This was especially true for those called upon to take positions as district medical officers. In 1972 the Sierra Leone government ended the scholarship program in undergraduate medical education in the USSR. By 1976, however, some 120 Sierra Leone doctors had come through the Soviet system.[27] To be fair, the Soviet Union had little experience with medical needs of tropical Africa until the British and French exodus of the 1950s. The USSR had about three regions in its vast territory that can be designated as tropical: Uzbekistan, Tashkent, and Kazakhstan. Soviet medical educators may at first have felt their highest priority was to return newly trained doctors as quickly as possible to fill the void of professionals in African health care systems. For example, in 1959 Nigeria had just 1 physician for every 70,000 people in its population. In Ghana the ratio in 1960 was 1 for every 18,000.[28] Raymond Easmon recorded a doctor–patient ratio of less than 1 to 20,000 for the whole of Sierra Leone in 1973.[29]

European doctors who remained in Africa and the postcolonial changes that allowed American doctors to register in Africa helped to reduce the doctor–patient ratios. Even more beneficial, however, were the number of graduates coming out of African medical schools. Nigeria graduated its first medical class of thirteen out of fourteen at the University College Hospital, Ibadan, in November 1960. And Ghana graduated its first medical school class of thirty-four in 1969.

Not impervious to criticism, the USSR moderated its curriculum to fit the needs of African medical trainees through feedback received from African health officials and from professional observations in African countries about how their African trainees were functioning. With firsthand knowledge of African health needs, and aware of the image of Russian medical culture in the eyes of the West, the USSR modified its African training program and several African doctors returned to the USSR for further training.

Dr. Juma Muchi of Tanzania

Medical education reforms in the USSR, therefore, reduced the number of problems encountered by earlier students. For example, Dr. Juma Muchi of Zanzibar (Tanzania) is an example of one who benefited from these medical reforms. He left home in 1968 to study medicine at Krasnodar State Medical Institute (USSR) near the Black Sea, where he received his MD in 1975. There, he met other medical students from Gambia, Sierra Leone, Ghana, and a sizable number from Nigeria. In addition to one year of Russian, students were also required to study Latin to lay the foundation for a common medical vocabulary. While the lectures were given in Russian, students knew English equivalents through the study of Latin. Further, Russian professors often spoke three or four Western languages and could easily give students medical terms in other languages besides Russian. According to Muchi's report, medical students did five years of basic medicine, and in the sixth year, prior to the qualifying year, they pursued one year in rotation. For Muchi this phase included three months in internal medicine, three in surgery, three in obstetrics and gynecology, and three in infectious diseases—what the Russians called "diseases of the tropics." This residency was conducted with Russian patients and doctors.[30]

An analysis of the African physician in socialist Tanzania is beyond the scope of this study. However, our interview with Muchi provides comparative evidence concerning the manifestation of British medical culture in East Africa. After the Zanzibar Revolution of 1964, a shortage of doctors developed that remains to this day, as the Arabs and other foreign doctors left. Doctors from China, Cuba, Italy, Denmark, and the USSR came in to treat the acute diseases on the island. On his return from Russia in 1975, Muchi came under the supervision of Tanzanian doctors trained in Russia before the revolution. He was posted to the island of Pemba, where he worked as a general practitioner and did surgery when surgeon specialists were scarce. Since there were no British-trained African doctors in Zanzibar in 1975, Muchi was spared the kind of intraprofessional conflict endured by earlier generations on both sides of the continent. On the Tanzania mainland, however, working conditions were comparable to those in West Africa, and friction arose between Western- and Eastern-trained doctors.

In the broader scheme of medical education, the process of decolonization in Sierra Leone created new challenges to the established medical culture in health care delivery. Sierra Leone physicians trained in the socialist bloc introduced group specialization into an existing health care system dominated by general-purpose medicine. Some professional tensions still persist today as the two cultures seek accommodation, and the ultimate outcome of this process is still to be determined. The high ratio of patients to doctors was somewhat lowered by the influx of new physicians from 1967 to 1985 into all the nations of the Anglophone region. Medical specialists from the Eastern bloc continued to trickle back into the region after 1975. Even more important in the long run for development was the fact that African doctors from the socialist bloc appeared to be more sensitive to the need for reform of a decentralized system that no longer met the needs of the people. Without regard to medical culture, all physicians must be required to show evidence of their continued competency in medicine and certification in tropical diseases. Ordinary

Sierra Leoneans urgently emphasized the need to improve medical standards in the country as a whole, but few were prepared to challenge a widespread perception of mediocrity in existing medical practice.

Socialist-Trained Physicians and "New Directions"

As a group, the socialist-trained doctors have advocated specific kinds of reforms to West African medical delivery systems. First, the government should take firm control of drug distribution and regulate drug prices. This would reduce excessive profiteering between governments, influential individuals, and multinationals. This could be achieved by the establishment of government-owned pharmacies that would maintain prices below those in commercial firms. Government pharmacies would be staffed by civil servants and stocked with high-priority drugs. Eligibility requirements for those purchases would be determined by a system similar to Medicaid in the United States. Drugs, therefore, would be sold to people in possession of an identity card—people who would pay a nominal fee that was deducted automatically from their salary or income—and an individual or family members would be eligible to receive full benefits automatically as the need arose. Further, this program would be open mainly to government workers, lower-income groups, and their children. The doctors also urged, medical cultures notwithstanding, that the nursing standards in hospitals should be restored at least to the preindependence level, for medical education would suffer without proper attention to the development of nursing and the acquisition of hospital equipment.

Perestroika and Glasnost

In 1985 Charles Quist Adade reported that dramatic changes occurred in the Soviet Union that would impact on the medical profession. The reforms associated with perestroika and glasnost prompted efforts to blend the two medical cultures of the Soviet Union and sub-Saharan Africa.[31] Perestroika—or former President Mikhail Gorbachev's policy of restructuring and renovating the Soviet socialist system—was inspired by the need to replicate further the curriculum structure observed in Great Britain and Continent. This meant that Africans studying medicine in the future in the USSR would generally take the same courses used in Europe and in Africa, although these plans would take time for implementation for a variety of reasons, especially because of the fall of the USSR and communism in 1991.

By 1985, however, the Soviet Union had some 13,000 African students studying in the country and sharing the benefits of the restructuring. There were a total of more than 30,000 students from 130 Third World countries studying five- to six-year courses in about 150 specialized professions, of which about 10 percent were Africans. The Patrice Lumumba University enrolled some 35,000 students. By this same year, 1985, the Soviet Union had trained some 52,000 Third World professional specialists, and some 5,000 African engineers and other technical specialists were also trained in Soviet institutions.

Soviet educational planners began to structure degree programs to correspond to Western institutions. In the old system the first degrees, such as the Bachelor of Science and Bachelor of Arts, were combined. Several countries refused to recognize these diplomas because of this factor, and ideological indoctrination in the form of Cold War rhetoric permeated nearly every form of classroom discourse. Under the new system, however, three years of study must have been successfully completed before the students could be awarded the first degrees (BS or BA). Next, students would be awarded the Master of Science (MS) and Master of Arts (MA) certification.

The new changes, Adade noted, would impact on medical training with regard to the reduction of the much maligned specialists in West Africa. The Soviet medical authorities had become sensitized to the problems African doctors faced upon their return to their respective countries through Soviet embassies. Reports on the clinical studies previously outlined in this chapter might also have reached these authorities. Even more, Africans with Soviet MDs often returned to the Soviet Union for further training at the advice of their African supervisors. The authorities came to know more about the need to restructure their medical requirements along the standards of general-purpose medical culture, and to emphasize the use of pharmacopeia nomenclature underlined by the WHO, in which African medical doctors hold prominent posts today.

Soviet Professional Representation in Sub-Saharan Africa

African physicians trained in the Soviet Union and Eastern bloc countries have demonstrated the efforts made in meeting universal medical standards in their countries of origin. This is true for Anglophone West Africa as well as elsewhere in Africa. The doctors in our study also share this determination with other world professionals trained in the Soviet Union. By conservative estimates these include one head of state, ten cabinet ministers, fifteen directors of major enterprises, five rectors of universities or colleges, and twenty rectors and deans in numerous developing countries.

The East-West conflict within Africa laid the foundation for a mosaic laboratory of professions that still plays a significant role in development. The merits of this conflict are even more evident when objective efforts are made to evaluate the declining state of African affairs with the demise of the Cold War. This seemingly sudden occurrence has necessitated a rethinking of possible solutions for the development of medical professionalism in Africa.

Epilogue

*B*ritish colonialism imprinted the legacy of the modern medical profession in Anglophone West Africa in the nineteenth and twentieth centuries. African physicians were willing participants in this process, but its development in West Africa was quite unlike its manifestation in Great Britain, whose tripartite class structure of gentry, middle class, and workers defined rigid social tiers. British doctors for the most part remained in their class of origin in Great Britain—the middle class. Colonialism altered this class arrangement by admitting middle-class British doctors to the elite ranks of colonial society, where they consolidated their positions through a system of nonhistorical association of invented traditions, backed by imperial power and the ideology of pseudoscientific racism. As employees in the Colonial Medical Service, African physicians were marginalized under this system for over 157 years under a common theme described as intraprofessional conflict. This stronghold was broken with the emergence of the association movement and medical autonomy, two of the essential hallmarks of professionalism.

Colonialism, however, began with the introduction of a single medical culture called general-purpose medicine in the nineteenth and twentieth centuries. During the Cold War and the dawn of the independence era, African medical students were offered scholarships to the Soviet Union and Eastern bloc countries. So they returned as communist-trained medical doctors with a new medical culture—one centered on specialization—which met resistance from the existing medical culture of the West. Conflicts in medical practice followed in the manner of a new dimension of intraprofessional conflict between these two cultures. African doctors representing the Western medical culture responded to this problem with a resolution in the form of clinical programs of adjustments in development. So new doctors were integrated into the general-purpose medicine of the colonial medical generation. These adjustments were instrumental in reducing the acute shortage of doctors brought on by both the late development of medical schools in West Africa and the exodus of European doctors in the 1950s.

This study, however, holds serious implications for the social history of medicine in West Africa. First of all, the corporate patronage system that determined the role of the Colonial Medical Service in the region was a colonial tragedy for the whole population. Integrated health polices were not allowed, even though (in retrospect) they would have made for healthier populations and better relations. Diaspora medical institutions—including Howard University and Meharry—were frustrated in their attempts to improve the African situation, knowing that the doctors they trained and certified would not be allowed to practice in their country of origin in West Africa until late in the twentieth century. The limitations of colonial science also stymied any progress. Officials lacked vision in their resistance to the training and use of more African physicians and other professional classes, groups that would provide leadership for Africa. What they created in the nineteenth century—an open and generally mobile society—was gone by the 1900s and closed to African mobility: caused by pseudoscientific racism, and the fear of the British Medical Association that their jobs would disappear. Monogenesis and polygenesis thought triumphed in science, the pulpit, and in the colonial mind; sexual stereotypes arose in conjunction with these beliefs and encouraged efforts in colonial policymaking to prevent African physicians from treating European women as patients. Enlightened colonial statesmen did come forward in dissent, including Governor Guggisberg of the Gold Coast and Sir William MacGregor (MD), governor of the Lagos colony, but the era did not produce enough of them to enable change in their day. But Africans themselves could have shown more effective leadership, even under the weight of colonialism. This study shows there was the formation of an African elite in pioneering frontier medical communities, and these families continued to dominate over several generations, assuming the role of developing professionalism under unique conditions; yet, for the most part, they were previously ignored in various historical and social studies of the time and area.

I hope that my efforts here will encourage the adventurous to travel down new avenues of research. Communalism and intraprofessional conflict as a recurring and binding theme must be revived—pushed to a state of renewal, imposed on new constructs (in and outside Africa) and organizational developments, or used in the revisions of earlier ones with regard to the professions. Intraprofessional conflict in the colonial era was manifested in a particular way in the medical profession of Anglophone West Africa, yet mitigated in another way in Francophone West Africa—which pursued a policy of assimilation—and in an entirely different way in the West Indies, where few middle-class Europeans came to practice medicine. These different experiences under colonialism would be a fruitful topic of research. Future studies might prosper from looking at the African medical doctor in private practice and consulting patients coming from different classes; this might tell us about the rapidity in the spread of Western medicine among the nonelite class and its challenge to the African herbalists, or the appeal of the herbalists to the masses.

There is still a need for research on the traits of professionalism in Africa. Corporate patronage and intraprofessional conflict staggered these, allowing the least important traits to develop more fully and suppressing the more important ones, including medical autonomy and association. A history of professional ethics and corresponding litigation over malpractice in Africa (as it is done in the United States) has yet to be written. Similarly, one reads a lot about existing economic associations in independent Africa—for example, the Economic Community of West African States (ECOWAS), the South African Development Coordination Conference (SADCC), and the revival of the East African Community (ECA), or the African Alternative Framework to Structural Adjustment Programmes for Socioeconomic Recovery and Transformation (AAF-SAP)—but little is known about the professional associations that preceded these organizations: their role in decolonization, their relationship with contemporary African governments (which can be quite adversarial at times), or about African associations in the West resulting from the migration of professionals. In addition, association members in Africa either served or maintained liaisons with various institutions around the world. There is a need, therefore, to reconstruct the history of these medical institutions, private clinics, legal institutions, or whatever companies were involved in Africa in this way: their country, their founding men and women, and to show how medical institutions effected treatment and cures for their patients, especially documented cures using medicines rooted in African pharmacopeia. Even more, let us not forget that Africans trained in the former USSR and Eastern bloc countries are now represented in a wide range of professions in Africa and beyond. This present study covers only part of such a significant development and much more research is needed on this issue.

In the context of professionalism and developing institutions the social construction of a scientific public in African societies remains a neglected theme for research. Researcher Thomas Kaiser (University of Arkansas, Little Rock) shows that the emergence of modern science in the West was dependent upon this public, which was itself the product of a certain level of literacy that preceded the invention of the printing press. While a variety of factors can be credited for the expansion of scientific literacy, the printing press accelerated the creation of a reading public in science and in other fields. This scientific public did not include all persons and even all readers. National boundaries and social estates placed limitations on who might be included and excluded: for instance, those who for want of education could not articulate the language of science or the manipulations of its conventions.

The foundation of a scientific public in the early modern era did two things: (1) sustained a wider audience for the pedagogy of science; and (2) established standards for evaluating claims to knowledge. The Western tradition and the African tradition both held currents of "secret knowledge" (for example, forms of Renaissance magic, and the Poro societies of West Africa), but the formation of a scientific public—informed by books, periodicals, academia, and scientific societies—devalued these traditions through interprofessional relations and jurisdictional control. Forms of knowledge that affected the scientific public inevitably gained more favor. Disinterested parties ruled out "discoveries" not brought before the public and tested by objective inquiry, while literacy undermined traditional authority by making the acquisition of truth more democratic. Traditional institutions whose authority rested on claims of a privileged access to secret knowledge lost their stature in the judgment of an enlightened public informed by the rise of professionalism. Now the question comes as to what degree can we trace the emerging social construction of a scientific public in sub-Saharan Africa?

Such a distribution of a scientific public and culture is more numerous than one might think. Researcher Harold Marcus's (Michigan State University) study on Ethiopia, a country known throughout the course of history as Da'mat (seventh century to third century B.C.), as Axum (first century A.D.), as Zagwe (eleventh century to thirteenth century A.D.), as Solomonic (fourteenth century to sixteenth century A.D., the fourth group empire), Contraction (1540–1700, Muslim invasion and Oromo movements), and as Abyssinia (1700–1855), might provide an excellent case study in the development of a scientific public during these historical periods; it had a medieval literature in its own written language of Ge'ez, technology, and a worldview based on the Judaic and Christian heritages. Part 1, chapter 2 of this study briefly discusses one such era, the years 1464–1591, when the famed University of Sankore in the western Sudanic Songhai empire flourished. Similarly productive was the frontier coastal community of Sierra Leone, where professionalism on the

Western model emerged during the nineteenth century. More cases exist, however, and are in need of unraveling by the resourceful and productive student or scholar in sub-Saharan Africa. Since scientific public centers have been the threshold for advancement in the past, this remains so for the present and the future. These proposed studies, therefore, will be beneficial to West Africa and to Africa as a whole in providing alternatives to their problems of development, for the Cold War's termination has proved a setback for sub-Saharan Africa. The industrialized world has changed its focus and a major share of its multilateral development aid now goes to the former communist entities.

Today's scientific public centers in West Africa and in Africa in general are in a state of decline. However, efforts must be made to stabilize and to restore them to the standards that marked the independence era in 1960, and medical standards must be included. Today, most nation-states have high infant mortality rates that astound the imagination, and most of the surviving children, who constitute the future of Africa, are suffering from malnutrition. Diseases are of epidemic proportion, and the population, roughly 600 million, might be doubled in twenty-five years unless governments act with family planning programs. In any event, population increase will impose undue strains and pressures on health services; for in some countries newly trained African doctors are already being rushed into practice for either the government or as private practitioners without diplomas in tropical medicine. This results in everyone suffering: the children, the patients, the nurses, and the doctors. Complicating the crisis further is the fact that large numbers of Africans with technical expertise are out of their countries, living either in the West, the Middle East, or other African countries with better economies and living standards. This is the African brain drain, hampering West Africa's development now more than the European exodus of the 1950s. There are no easy solutions to government deficits and mounting health problems. A start could be made by the West through debt forgiveness and rescheduling of loans. This should be followed with aid to scientific and medical centers, which ought to consist of not only the redistribution and reallocation of various supplies but also provision of the most updated scientific journals and books to mitigate the existing book famine. Democratic African governments, those with officials elected by the people, need to participate: they must gain the confidence of the West and international donors by stamping out corruption and inefficiency in their governments, stopping the funneling of funds abroad, and showing African self-help initiatives of investments in small-scale development projects to the world instead. These recommendations are not new but worth reiteration and implementation. Let us not forget that scientific data has shown through DNA samples that humankind originated in the Great Rift Valley of East Africa, a development described recently by French paleontologist Yves Coppens as the "East Side Story." Hence, we all originated in Africa and are linked to its diaspora—either in prehistoric, ancient, or modern times. Now is the time for the world to show compassion to the inhabitants of that continent in order to lessen the suffering, while there is a chance for restructuring and hope is still alive.

Colonial List of Qualifying Foreign Medical Schools for the Medical Register

LICENSING BODY	DEGREE(S)	QUALIFIED FOR:
Punjab University	MD, etc.	Medicine and surgery
Ceylon Medical College	Surg.	Medicine and surgery
Dalhousie Univ.	MD, etc.	Medicine and surgery
Halifax Medical Coll.	Mast., Surg.	Medicine and surgery
Laval Univ.	MD	Medicine and surgery
Nova Scotia Provincial Medical Board	Lic. Med.; Surg.	Medicine and surgery
Univ. of Adelaide	MD, etc.	Medicine and surgery
Univ. of Calcutta	MD, etc.	Medicine and surgery
Univ. of Madras	MD, etc.	Medicine and surgery
Univ. of Malta	MD, etc.	Medicine and surgery
Univ. of Melbourne	MD, etc.	Medicine and surgery
Univ. of New Zealand	ChB; Lic. Med.	Medicine and surgery
University of Sydney	MD, etc.	Medicine and surgery

West Africa's Relations with the Soviet Bloc, July–September 1959

TYPE OF DELEGATION	COUNTRY	FROM	DATE	PERSONALITIES	NOTES
Communist-bloc and Communist international organizations' delegations to Africa					
Diplomatic	Guinea	China	June	Pai-Jen	CPR ambassador to Morocco.
	Guinea	Hungary	August	Janus Radvanvi	Ministry of Foreign Affairs "goodwill" visit.
	Ghana	USSR	September	Scherbov Gorelov	Members of diplomatic corps. Arrived in Ghana "for talks with USSR embassy."
Trade	Guinea	Hungary	August	Janus Radvanvi	See Diplomatic delegation above.
	Guinea	Bulgaria	August		
	Guinea	USSR	August		
	Ghana	USSR	July	Ivan Maslov	Of "Soviet Foreign Trade Organisation" (ten-day visit).
	South Africa	East Germany	September	Rudolf Blankenburger	Director of Foreign Trade.
	Ghana	Poland	August		See Specialist delegation below.
	Ghana	Hungary	August	Janus Radvanvi	Invited by Ghana govt. Ten scholarships in Hungary offered by delegation to Ghana.
				Dr. Alexander Prejes	
	Ghana	East Germany	September	Tibor Sebestven	
	Guinea	East Germany	August		

TYPE OF DELEGATION	COUNTRY	FROM	DATE	PERSONALITIES	NOTES
Specialist	Ghana	Poland	July	Benedykt Menel, Stanislav Siekierski, Vladimir Friling, Edmund Chudek, Alexi Maczmarek, Eugeniusz Mazanek	A further twelve expected. Industrial survey specialists invited by Industrial Corp. to survey production of electric light bulbs, radio sets, glue, lime, and iron ore mining.
	Ghana	Poland	August	S. Takuski, B. Szyhalski, J. Yabtkonski, Z. Kuszynski, A. Arendt, M. Michtowski, S. Landau	Engineers advising the Industrial Development Corporation.
	Guinea	Czech	July	Macuch, Bradacek	Doctors
	Ghana	Hungary	August	?	Two engineers invited by the Office of Electrification to study the possibility of constructing hydroelectric power stations.
	Ghana	Czech	August	Vladimir Hara, Stefan Simek	Industrial experts.
Press and radio	Guinea	East Germany	July	Karel Friedrich Reinhardt	Representative of Deutschland-sonder.
Communist international front organizations	Guinea	USSR	July/August	Orestev	Pravda correspondent in Ghana.
	Senegal	WFDY	May/June	Lo Cheik Bara	Deputy secretary.
	Guinea	WFDY	May/June	Lo Cheik Bara	General of WFDY.

(continued)

TYPE OF DELEGATION	COUNTRY	FROM	DATE	PERSONALITIES	NOTES
	Ivory Coast	WFDY	May/June	Lo Cheik Bara	Visit regarding World Youth Festival and WFDY Assembly. Claimed to have visited Ghana but may not have done so.
Academic	Ghana	WFDY	May/June	Lo Cheik Bara	
	Ghana	USSR	August	Peter Ivanovich Kupriyanov	Graduate of the Institute of Oriental Studies, Moscow. Carrying out research in social and economic fields for UNESCO.
	Liberia	USSR	?	Peter Ivanovich Kupriyanov	Reported to have spent three months in Liberia under arrangements of UNESCO.
	Guinea	USSR	?	Peter Ivanovich Kupriyanov	Paid brief visit to Conakry from Liberia.
Communist party	Guinea	USSR	September	S. R. Rashidov	For the Fifth National Congress of the Guinea Democratic party.
	Guinea	Czechoslovakia	September		
	Guinea	Bulgaria	September		
	Guinea	Romania	September		
	Guinea	East Germany	September	Professor A. Kurella (candidate-member of the SED politburo)	
Youth	Guinea	USSR	September		

Afro-Asian	Guinea	USSR China	September		Chinese and Soviet AAPSC Permanent Secretariat members visited Guinea to discuss the Second Afro-Asian Conference to be held in Conakry.

African delegations to Communist-bloc countries and Communist international front meetings

TYPE OF DELEGATION	COUNTRY	TO	DATE	PERSONALITIES	NOTES
Sport	Ethiopia	USSR	July		Football team.
	Ethiopia	Czechoslovakia	July/August		Football team.
Government	Ghana	Poland	August	William Amoro William Ntonso K. B. Ayensu A. E. A. Ofori-Atta	For the 48th Conference of Interparliament Union.
	Guinea	Hungary	July	Keita M. Famara	Official delegate.
	Liberia	USSR	July	R. Morris (deputy minister of trade and agriculture)	Invited by USSR deputy minister of foreign trade. Unofficial.
	Guinea	USSR	August	Diallo Saifoulaye	"Goodwill" visit.
	Guinea	Czechoslovakia Bulgaria	August/September	L. Diane	Attended Bulgarian state holiday celebrations.
Afro-Asian	Cameroons	USSR	June	Ernest Ouandie	
	Cameroons	East Germany	June	Ernest Ouandie	
	Cameroons	China	July	Ernest Ouandie	Invited by Chinese Committee for Afro-Asian Solidarity.

(continued)

TYPE OF DELEGATION	COUNTRY	TO	DATE	PERSONALITIES	NOTES
	Kenya	China	July	James Ochwata	Invited by Chinese Committee for Afro-Asian Solidarity.
	Ghana	USSR	September	Martin Appiah Dankwa Ohene Adu K. K. Apladu S. O. Kobbina	For the Conference of Afro-Asian Cooperative Movements, Tashkent.
Cultural	Liberia	USSR	August	Director of Information Office and others.	For film festival.
	Cameroons	China	June	Benjamin Matip	Guest of Chinese Writers' Union.
	Cameroons	North Vietnam	August	Benjamin Matip	
	Guinea	USSR	August		For film festival.
Women	Guinea	China	August	Marian M. Camara	Invited by China Women's Federation.
Trade union	East Africa	China	July	James Ochwata	Described as "former secretary general of the East Africa Trade Union" for May Day celebrations.
	Ghana	East Germany	May	E. Ohene-Yeboah	For May Day celebrations.
	Guinea	Bulgaria	August	Camara Oumar Din Dia Mamadou	Invited by Bulgarian T.U.
	Nigeria	East Germany	September	M. Imoudu (ANTUF)	African T.U. meeting allegedly attended by more than two hundred representatives from eighteen African countries. Only Imoudu named.

TYPE OF DELEGATION	COUNTRY	TO	DATE	PERSONALITIES	NOTES
Religious	Nigeria	USSR	September	M. Imoudu	Went on from above conference.
	Kenya	USSR	July	James Ochwata	On invitation of Moscow Patriarchate. Ochwata described as "head of Coptic Church of Kenya, Uganda, and Tanganyika." Said to be " performing duties of Bishop of his Church, who has been gaoled."
Youth	Guinea	East Germany	August		Nine college students, for three weeks, under cultural agreement.
	Senegal	China	August	N'diaye Aroumane	Delegation of the Youth Movement of Progressive Union of Senegal.
	South Africa	China	August	Herby Pillay	Member of the Executive Committee of the Youth Action Committee of South Africa. Invited by the All-China Youth Federation.
	Sierra Leone	China	August	Victor Pratt	Chairman of the Fourah Bay University Student Council. Invited by the All-China Youth Federation.
	South Africa	USSR	September	Gaby Toure	Representative of the Youth Action Committee of South Africa; attended International Students Seminar on Higher Education in the USSR.

TYPE OF DELEGATION	COUNTRY	TO	DATE	PERSONALITIES	NOTES
	Nigeria	USSR	August		Went on from the Youth Festival, Vienna.
	Mauritius	USSR	August		Went on from the Youth Festival, Vienna.
	Kenya	USSR	August	Nathan Odembeza	Went on from the Youth Fesitval, Vienna.
	Senegal	USSR	August	Yussef Diop	Went on from the Youth Festival, Vienna.
	Guinea	USSR	August		Went on from the Youth Festival, Vienna.
	Mauretania	USSR	August	Ahmed Baba	Went on from the Youth Festival, Vienna.
	General Union of West African Students	USSR	August	Orlu Gubu Emil	Went on from the Youth Festival, Vienna.
	Cameroons	USSR	August	Aloys Marie Ndjog	Went on from the Youth Festival, Vienna.
	Guinea	Czechoslovakia	August		Went on from the Youth Festival, Vienna.
	Ghana	Czechoslovakia	August		Went on from the Youth Festival, Vienna.
	Guinea	East Germany	August		Went on from the Youth Festival, Vienna.

TYPE OF DELEGATION	COUNTRY	TO	DATE	PERSONALITIES	NOTES
	Ghana	East Germany	August		Went on from the Youth Festival, Vienna.
	Ghana	Hungary	August		Went on from the Youth Festival, Vienna.
	Ghana	Poland	August		Went on from the Youth Festival, Vienna.
	Unspecified	Bulgaria	August		Went on from the Youth Festival, Vienna.
Economic	Mali Federation (Soudan)	Czechoslovakia	September	Dr. Hamacire N'Doure (minister of trade)?	Official.
	Guinea	Czechoslovakia	July	Keita N'Famara	Official delegate.
	Guinea	Hungary	July	Keita N'Famara	Official delegate.
	Ghana	China	September	P. K. Quaidoo	Official delegate.
	South Africa	East Germany	September		Official delegate.
	Ghana	East Germany	September	A. J. Dwuona Hammond	Official delegate.
Nationalist	Uganda	China	July	Kiwanuka	
	Cameroons	USSR	August	Isaac Tchoumba Nikanor Njiawue	UPC refugees.
Miscellaneous	Ghana	Czechoslovakia	September		For an International Seminar for Cooperative Members of Economically underdeveloped countries.
	Ghana	East Germany	September/October	G. E. Ampomah D. K. Amankwa	Meeting of the Association of German Cooperative Societies.

(continued)

TYPE OF DELEGATION	COUNTRY	TO	DATE	PERSONALITIES	NOTES
	Guinea	USSR	August	Camara Daoud	Delegation from the Guinea Democratic party invited by the Supreme Soviet.
	Ethiopia	Czechoslovakia	August	Haile Mariam (secretary general of the Ministry of Pensions)	International seminar on social security.
International organizations					
Youth Festival, Vienna	Madagascar		July	Akereben Jolide	
	Togo		July	Michel Ayih	President of the Togo Festival Committee.
	Belgian Congo		July		
	Ivory Coast		July		
	Uganda		July		
	Ghana (from the United Kingdom)		July	Desmond Tey Mrs. Tey Djane Miss Amoo Amerodje	Forty-member delagation from the Cultural Society in the United Kingdom.
	Mali Federation (Soudan)		July		
	Kenya		July	Nathan Adembeza?	From London.
	Senegal		July	Kane Ali Bocar Yussef Diop	Chairman of the African Youth Council.

(continued)

TYPE OF DELEGATION	COUNTRY	TO	DATE	PERSONALITIES	NOTES
	Guinea		July	Tibou Tounkara	Delegation of thirty-eight. Tounkara is vice-president of the African Youth Council.
	Cameroons		July	Aloys-Marie Ndjog	
	Maurentania		July	Ahmed Baba	
World Peace Council	Cameroons		August	Nikano Njiawue	World Conference Against Nuclear Weapons.
	Ghana		August	E. C. Quaye	World Conference Against Nuclear Weapons.
World Federation of Democratic Youth	Senegal		August		WFDY Assembly, Prague.
	Togo		August		WFDY Assembly, Prague.
	Ivory Coast		August		WFDY Assembly, Prague.
	French West Africa		August		WFDY Assembly, Prague.
	Cameroons		August		WFDY Assembly, Prague.
	Guinea		August	Aloys-Marie Ndjog	WFDY Assembly, Prague.
	African Youth Council		August	Tounkara	WFDY Assembly, Prague.
International Union of Students	Unspecified		August		IUS Secretariat Meeting, Budapest.
World Federation of Trade Unions	Guinea		September		WFTU course for Africans, Budapest.
	Senegal		September	Seydou Diallo	
	Cameroons		September		
	Congo		September		
	Madagascar		September		

TYPE OF DELEGATION	COUNTRY	TO	DATE	PERSONALITIES	NOTES
International Union of Journalists	Ghana		June	Bernard Dorkenoo (Ghanaian journalist then based in Guinea)	International Meeting of Foreign Editors, Prague.
	Guinea		June	Sy Abdoulaye	
Communist International Teachers Organisation	French Africa (unspecified)		July		Administrative Committee meeting, Sofia.
China's National Day	Nigeria	China	September	M. Imoudu	
	Senegal	China	September	A. Diagne	Representing the IUS.
	Senegal	China	September	Alioune Badara Payes	Representing the WFDY.
	Moyen Congo	China	September	Matsika Aime	Representing the WFDY.
	Ghana	China	September	Grace Ayensu	Representing the WIDF.
	Guinea	China	September	Barry Diawadou (minister of education)	
	Mauretania	China	September	Ba Abdul Aziz (secretary general of the National Union of Mauretania)	

Ghanaian Physicians Trained in the USSR and the Eastern Bloc, 1984

NAME	QUALIFICATIONS	DATE OF QUALIFICATION
Abraham, Agnes Augustina	MD, Univ. Kiev	1967
Abude, Fritz Ernest	MD, Univ. Hungary	1970
Acquah, Bernard	MD, Univ. Moscow	1971
Acquah, Joseph Abonko	MD, Univ. Moscow	1972
	MB, ChB, Univ. G.	
Acquaah, Robert Kelly	MD, Univ. Volgograd	1972
Adade, Andrew Adu	MD, Charles Univ., Prague	1973
Adam, Issah	MD, Kalinin Med. Inst.	1972
Adamo, Robert Christopher	MD, Univ. Kharkov	1971
Addo, Edward Adotey	MD, Kharkov Med. Inst.	1972
Adibo, Moses Erasmus Komla	MD, Univ. Belgrade	1973
	DPH, Univ. Otago, New Zealand	1970
Adjei, Kwaku Christian	MD, Univ. Bucharest	1972
Adjei, Samuel Osei	MB, BS, Univ. Sarajevo	1972
Adom-Gabusu, Aikins Kofi	BRACH, Kharkov	1969
Adu-Ameyaw, Frederick	MD, Kiev State Medical Inst.	1968

(continued)

NAME	QUALIFICATIONS	DATE OF QUALIFICATION
Afari, Edwin Andrews	MD, Univ. Odessa	1967
	DPH, Univ. Liverpool	1974
	DIH, Royal College of Physicians	1975
	DTM&H., Royal College of Physicians	1976
	MSC, OCCMED, Univ. London	1975
Agadzi, Victor Kofi	MD, Peoples Friendship Univ., Moscow	1966
	DPH, Makerere Univ., Uganda	1972
	DTCD, Univ. Wales	1973
Agyekum, Owusu	MD, Leningrad Military Medical Academy	1972
Agyekum, Adu Kofi	MD, Odessa Med. Inst.	1969
Ahenkora, Dennis Kwasi	Diploma, Inst. of Med., Bucharest	1972
Akomaa-Boadu, Stephen	MD, State Med. Inst., Odessa	1972
Akwaboa-Nkansah, Charles	MD, Lvov Med. Inst.	1969
Akyea, Daniel Kwaku	MD, Warsaw Medical Academy	1970
Amable, John Kwaku	MD, First Leningrad Med. Inst.	1972
Amissah, Albert Baiden	MD, Peoples Friendship Univ.	1966
Amoyaw, Francis	MD, Charles Univ.	1969
Amponsah, Samuel Rexford	MD, Univ. Lvov	1971
Amponsem, Joseph Kwaku	MD, 1st Med. Inst., Leningrad	1972
Amuah, Joseph Christophorus	Arztliche Prufung, Univ. Kiel	1971
Anderson, Kwesi Octavius	MD, Univ. Lvov	1968
Anipare, William Erasmus	MD, Warsaw Med. Academy	1969
Annang, Christopher Okpoti	Diploma, Likar a Academia Medye ag., Poland	1974
Annani, Max Anum	MD, Kalinin State Med. Inst.	1969
Annor-Adjei, Dan Nicholas	MD, 2nd Med. Inst., Moscow	1972
Antwi, John Francis	MD, Univ. Lvov	1969
Appiah, Adolph	MD, Kharkov Med. Inst.	1970
Appiah, Andrew Kwame	Arztliche Prufung, Univ. Munich	1968
Armah, George Joseph A.	MD, Univ. Warsaw Medical Acad.	1974
Arthur, Isaq Mohammed	MD, Univ. Odessa	1971
Arthur, Joseph Alexander	MD, Kalinin State Med.	1968
Arthur, Victor Botchey	MD, Univ. Stravropol	1972
Aryee, Kingsford Isaac	Arztliche Prufung, Univ. Mainz	1970
	Anerkenning als Mals-Nasen-Ohrenazt, Univ. Mainz	1975
Asamoa, Emmanuel Eddie	MD, Univ. Belgrade	1971
Asamoah-Adu Alexander	MD, Univ. Szeged	1970

(continued)

NAME	QUALIFICATIONS	DATE OF QUALIFICATION
Asanakpo, Nancy Johnson	MD, Patrice Lumumba Univ., Moscow	1967
Asare, Felicia Kyerewaa	MD, Univ. Moscow	1968
Asare, Joseph Bediako	Lekarz Medycyny Cracow Med. Inst.	1971
Asare, Yaw Agyeman	Arztliche Prufung, Univ. Kiel	1971
Asare-Adjepong, Samuel	MD, Univ. Moscow	1973
Asare-Brown, Dora	MD, USSR	1972
Ashitei, Christopher Amaa	MD, USSR	1972
Asiedu, Alex	MD, Rostov State Med. Inst.	1969
Asiedu, Augustina	MD, Univ. Rostov	1968
Assani, Bernice Dwrotimi	MD, Univ. Kiev	1968
Atando, Seth Wellington	MD, Univ. Moscow	1965
Attobrah, Fred Boateng	MD, Univ. Odessa	1970
Atutonu, Nelson Kofi Kakraba	MD, Warsaw Med. Acad.	1964
Austin, Samuel Abel	MD, Lvov State Med. Inst.	1972
Avumatsodo, Emmanuel K.	MD, Univ. Skopje	1980
Ayettey, Joseph Mensah	MD, Univ. Lvov	1971
Ayirebi-Acquah, Ebenezer	MD, Odessa State Med. Inst.	1968
Azu, Paul Mate	MD, Univ. Lvov	1968
Badu, Obed Kwasi	MD, Kharkov Med. Inst.	1970
Baffoe, Bonnie Segfried L.	Arztliche Prufung, Univ. Heidelburg	1961
Bani Bensu, Amos Kwasi	Arztliche Prufung, Univ. Leipzig	1970
Bankas, Daniel Owusu	Stomatology Odessa Med. Inst.	1979
Bansa, Walter Kwame	MD, Karl-Marx Univ., Leipzig	1970
Bawiah, Lawrence Kofi	MD, Univ. Poland	1970
Benneh, Stephen	Arztliche Prufung, Univ. Gottingen	1973
Bensah, David Churchill	MD, Kharkov Med. Inst.	1968
Bentil, William Ninsin	MB, BS, Univ. Patna	1960
	MS, Univ. Patna	1964
Bentsi, Cecilia	MD, Odessa, USSR	1967
Bentsi, Isaac Kofi	MD, Univ. Odessa	1967
Biney, Albert Kobina	MD, Univ. Moscow	1971
Boaten, Barbara	MD, Univ. Cracow	1971
Boateng, Ernest Amoah	MD, Warsaw Med. Acad.	1970
Boateng, Samuel	Staatexam Approbation, Univ. Kiel	1971
Bonso-Bruce Mrs.	MD, Univ. Moscow	1967
Brakohiapa, William Ofori	Staatsexamen, Leipzig Univ.	1966
	MD, Giessen Univ.	1971
	Facharzt fur Radiologie, Giessen Univ.	1973

NAME	QUALIFICATIONS	DATE OF QUALIFICATION
Brantuo, Daniel	MD, Kharkov Med. Inst.	1970
Brew, Bon Kwaku	MD, Univ. Kharkov	1969
Bugri, Samuel Zanya	MD, Univ. Sarajeve, Poland	1974
Caiquo, Joseph Kyemenu	MD, Tashkent State Med. Inst.	1968
	DPH, Univ. Sydney	1977
Caiquo, Tsease Kyemenu	MD, Univ. Kharkov	1967
Crentsil, John Michael	MD, Kharkov Med. Inst.	1969
Croffie, Elizabeth Ama	MD, Univ. Kharkov	1969
Cubagee, Deborah Brigitte	MD, Sged Med. School	1970
	DPH. Univ. Toronto	1976
Dadsi, Kobina Gyasi	MD, Med. Academy of Warsaw	1972
Dakor, Francis Teye	Approbation Als Arzt, Univ. Leipzig	1972
Darkoh, Godfried Seth	MD, Univ. Leipzig	1969
Darkor, Francis Teye	MD, Karl Marx Univ.	1972
Darku, Joe W.	MD, Military Med. Acad., Leningrad	1970
Dodoo, Joseph Amanor	MD, Univ. Lvov	1967
Ewusi-Mensah, Kwawi	MD, Univ. Zagrab	1971
Fordjour, Joseph Kwadwo	MD, Lvov Med. Inst.	1968
Forkuoh, Benjamin Kwaku	MD, Charles Univ.	1971
	Specialist Cert. in Gyn. and Obst., Charles Univ.	1975
Fredua-Agyeman, Alex O. K.	MD, Charles Univ.	1970
Fredua-Agyeman, Agnes	MD, Charles Univ.	1970
Fummey, Olabisi Vida	MD, Belgrade University	1972
	Diploma in Paediatrics, Belgrade Univ.	1974
Gordon, Seth	MD, Odessa Med. Inst.	1970
Grant, Alexander Sapara	Lekarza Medecyny (MD), Med. Acad., Cracow	1973
Gudugbe, David Yao	MD, Charles Univ.	1973
Hammond-Aryee, Clement	MD, Kalinin Med. Inst.	1968
Hayfron, William Wilfred	MD, Univ. Szeged	1971
Heming, Theophilus	MD, Univ. Lvov	1968
Hoidbrook, Alexander	MD, Krasnodor Med. Inst.	1969
Hutton-Mills, Fairbanks	MD, Univ. Hungary	1970
Hylton, Alfred Solomon	MD, Univ. Lvov	1969
Kassim, Mohammed Sulley	Diploma, Academia Medyczm Warszawie	1969
Kissi, S. A. Y.	MD, Rostov Med. Inst.	1979
Kissi, Darling A.	MD, Rostov Med. Inst.	1969

(continued)

NAME	QUALIFICATIONS	DATE OF QUALIFICATION
Kom, Francis Wogbe	MD, Charles Univ.	1970
Koranteng, Gladys	MD, 1st Moscow Inst.	1968
Koranteng, Reynolds Gyekye	Medicinae Doktoris, Charles Univ.	1972
Koranteng, Seth	MD, Univ. Moscow	1967
Kuffuor, Emmanuel Osei	MD, Univ. Hungary	1970
Kukah, Patrick Kwadwo	Diploma Ledarza, Med. Acad., Wroclaw, Poland	1979
Kwashie, Adwoa Asiedua	MD, Univ. Budapest	1980
Lamptey, Isaac	MD, Univ. Novi Sad	1971
Lamptey, Maria	MD, Univ. Novi Sad	1979
Mallet, Donald Emmanuel	Arztliche Prufung, Univ. Tubingen	1968
Maxwell, Arthur Thomas	MD, Univ. Moscow	1977
Mbroh, Samuel Kojo Essuon	MD, Univ. Moscow	1972
Mensa-Achaempong, Philip	MD, Faculty of Medicine, Bucharest	1972
Mensah, Joseph Duncanson	MD, Univ. Odessa	1971
Mensah, Samuel A. Q.	MD, Univ. Zagreb	1975
Mensah, Sylvester Agyemang	Arztliche Prufung	1968
Myers-Lamptey, Jonathan	MD, Szeged Medical School, Hungary	1970
	Specialist Cert. in Obst. and Gyn, Szeged Med. School	1975
Narh, Edward Atter	MD, Univ. Lvov	1967
Narh, Joseph Tei	MD, Univ. Prague	1969
Nee-Whang, Christian	MD, Univ. Warsaw	1969
Nettey-Roberts, Victor	MD, Charles Univ.	1973
Newman, Isaac	Medicinae Doctoris, Charles Univ.	1975
Nkruman, Mathew	MD, Univ. Kalinin	1959
Nordor, Christian	MD, Univ. Kalinin	1969
Ntim, Alfred Yaw	MD, Univ. Kharkov	1969
Nunoo, Phillip Kwesi	MD, Univ. Lvov	1967
Ochere, Daniel Yaw	MD, Lvov Med. Inst.	1972
Ocran, Anna	MD, Univ. Budapest	1980
Ocran, Ben Kissi	MD, Univ. Kuban	1970
Ocran, Kwamena	MD, Univ. Prague	1964
Odame, Godwill	MD, Univ. Kharkov	1969
Odame-Agyekum, Kofi	MD, Univ. Prague	1968
Oduro-Koranteng, Kwaku	MD, State Med. Inst., Volgograd	1971
Okumi, Peter Harry Kofi	MD, State Med. Inst., Odessa	1967
Okwabi, Thomas Nii Amah	MD, Rostov State Med. Inst., USSR	1972

(continued) 275

NAME	QUALIFICATIONS	DATE OF QUALIFICATION
Okyne, Albert Richardson	MD, Cracow Med. Acad.	1972
Onwumere-Yeboah, Nnena	Arztliche Prufung, Tubingen Univ.	1970
Osei, E. A.	MD, Karl Marx Univ.	1971
Osei-Bonsu, Emmanuel	MD, Univ. Lvov	1969
Osei-Bonsu, James	MD, Univ. Lvov	1968
Osei-Boadu, Emmanuel	MD, Univ. Lvov	1969
Oti, William Wilberforce	MD, Cracow Med. Acad.	1971
Quaofio, Charles Nyarku	MD, Parlov Med. Inst.	1980
Quartey, Mark K. A.	MD, Patrice Lumumba Univ.	1980
Quartey, Moses Nii Kwatelai	MD, 1st Leningrad Parlov Med. Inst.	1973
Quaye, Samuel Armah	MD, Crimean State Med. Inst.	1972
Quist, Patrick Kobla	MD, Univ. Szeged	1971
Renner, Adwoa Adoma	MD, Univ. Volgograd	1971
Renner, Nylon Kojo	MD, Univ. Volgograd	1971
	Certificate in Surgery (West Germany)	1979
Sakyi-Bekoe, Kofi	MD, Odessa State Med. Inst.	1967
Sekyi-Aidoo, Kofi	MD, Lvov State Med. Inst.	1971
Seneadze, Theophilus Nami	Lekar, Warsaw	1966
Siaw, Godfried Kofi	MD, Kharkov Med. Inst.	1969
Solomon, William Tawiah	Diploma, Lakarza, Warsaw	1970
Sunnu, Galina	MD, Lvov Medical Inst.	1970
Tamakloe, Nyaho	MD, Charles Univ.	1972
Tawiah, Robinson Addo	MD, Univ. Belgrade	1968
	Cert. of Obst. and Gyn., Belgrade	1969
Tenkorang, Yaw Kani	MD, Kalinin State Med. Inst.	
Tete-Lartey, Eric Asare	MD, Odessa State Med. Inst.	1967
Tetteh, Joseph Frankie	MD, Univ. Moscow	1970
Tettey, Erasmus Kofi	MD, Med. Univ. Budapest	1971
Thomas, Arthur Maxwell	MD, Univ. Moscow	1971
Tieku, Pater Addai Kwaku	MD, Univ. JE Parkyne BRNO, Czech.	1968
	Diploma, Gyn./Obst., Charles Univ.	1974
Valentin, Tete Jean	MD, Charles Univ.	1966
Walton, Stella Esi	MD, Univ. Szeged	1966
Wellington, Godwin	MD, Univ. Szeged	1972
Wilson, S. E.	MD, USSR	1970
Wiredu, Samuel Oduro	MD, Kharkov Med. Inst.	1969
Woode, Albert	MD, Univ. Kharkov	1970
Yemoh, Ebenezer Nsia	MD, State Med. Inst., Kharkov	1971
Yorke, Andrews K.	Diploma in Medicine Charles Univ.	1975

(continued)

NAME	QUALIFICATIONS	DATE OF QUALIFICATION
Supplementary list, standing register		
Armah, George Joseph	MD, Univ. Warsaw	1974
Awua, Siaw B. Nelson	MD, Patrice Lumumba Univ.	1981
Brakohiapa, Victor	MD, Patrice Lumumba Univ.	1980
Hansen, Geoffrey Mensah	MD, Charles Univ.	1972
Rodgers, Samuel Kwabla	MD, Univ. Skopje	1980
Sobotie, Ukula Edemma	MD, Kharkov Med. Inst.	1974
Provisional register		
Abantanga, Francis A.	MD, Kharkov Med. Inst.	1982
Adadevoh, Susu Bridgit	MD, Warsaw Med. Inst.	1982
Addo, Mark Colley	MD, Univ. Bucharest	1981
Ahedor, Michael Brightert	MD, Minsk Med. Inst.	1982
Amoako-Atta, Kwabena	Diploma, Univ. Bucharest	1981
Amoakwa-Adu, Sammy Amoako	MD, Kalinin Med. Inst.	1982
Ankumah, Richard K.	MD, 1st Pavlov Med. Inst.	1982
Antwi, Ernest Kofi	MD, Univ. Moscow	1981
Asante, Baah	MD, Univ. Moscow	1981
Coleman, Albert Mark E.	Diploma, Univ. Bucharest	1982
Dadzie, Sampson Kow	MD, Odessa Med. Inst.	1981
Dua, Agyeman Otchere Tettey	MD, Lvov Med. Inst.	1982
Martin, Rolland Sowa	MD, Kalinin Med. Inst.	1981
Mensah, Wonkyi Thomas	MD, 1st Pavlov Med. Inst.	1981
Okantey, Emmanuel Nii	Diploma, Univ. Bucharest	1981
Quansah, Robert Ekow	MD, Crimea Med. Inst.	1982
Sabeng, Kofi Barnabas	MD, Lvov Med. Inst.	1982
Sampson, Kow Dadzie	MD, Odessa Med. Inst.	1981
Sevi-Tengey, Joseph Nomla	MD, Peoples Friendship Univ.	1981
Tawiah, Emmanuel Harry	MD, Volgograd Med. Inst.	1982
Wryter, Alexander	MD, Patrice Lumumba Univ.	1982
Yawson, Margaret Rosette	MD, Kharkov Med. Inst.	1982

Sierra Leone Doctors Trained in Soviet and Eastern-Bloc Universities, 1984 and 1967–76

Number of Doctors from Soviet and Eastern-Bloc Universities, 1984

UNIVERSITY	NO.
Odessa State Medical Institute, USSR	18
Volgograd State Medical Institute, USSR	3
1st Leningrad State Medical Institute, USSR	18
Leningrad State Paediatric Medical Institute, USSR	4
1st Moscow State Medical Institute, USSR	5
Krasnodar State Medical Institute, USSR	3
Kiev State Medical Institute, USSR	10
Simferopol State Medical Institute, USSR	3
Kharkov State Medical Institute, USSR	11
Tashkent State Medical Institute, USSR	1
Peoples Friendship University, Moscow, USSR	10
Lvov State Medical Institute, USSR	4
Charles University of Prague, Czechoslovakia	1
Kuban State Medical Institute, USSR	4

(*continued*)

UNIVERSITY	NO.
Kalinin State Medical/Dental Institute, USSR	2
Rostov State Medical Institute, USSR	4
Patrice Lumumba Friendship University, USSR	2
Bucharest University Faculty of G. Medicine, Romania	2
International Friendship University, USSR	2
St. Mary's Hospital Medical School, England	1
Friendship University, USSR	1
Selesiam Medical Acad-katowice, Poland	1
Lekarr Medical Academy, Poland	1
Medical Institute of Sofia, Bulgaria	2
Medical Institute Plovdiv, Bulgaria	2
Zagreb University, Yugoslavia	2
Karl Marx University, East Germany	1
University of Vienna, Austria	1
University of Movi Sad, Yugoslavia	1
2nd Moscow State Medical Institute	1

List of Working Doctors, 1969–72

NAME	OCCUPATION
Septimus George	PHO, Cline Town
Ivan Johnston-Taylor	Surgeon
Bunda Kamara	Chest Clinic Lakka Hospital
A. A. Taqi	Paediatrician, Ahmadu Bello University Hospital, Zaria, Nigeria
D. W. O. B. Roberts	Research Pathologist, World Health Organization
M. O. Taylor-Lewis	Private Practice Physician/Psychiatrist
Lottie Whitefield	

Interns in Soviet and Eastern-Bloc Universities, September 1971–August 1973

NAME	LOCATION
Kdris Bangura	1st Leningrad State Medical Institute
J. C. T. Cole	1st Leningrad State Medical Institute
A. S. Conteh	1st Leningrad State Medical Institute
S. W. George	Kiev State Medical Institute
M. A. S. Jalloh	1st Moscow State Medical Institute
S. S. Jalloh	1st Leningrad State Medical Institute
E. A. Jarfoi	Krasnodar State Medical Institute
E. A. Juxon-Smith	1st Leningrad State Medical Institute
T. J. Juxon-Smith	1st Leningrad State Medical Institute
P. B. Kamara	Odessa State Medical Institute
N. H. B. Lawson	1st Leningrad State Medical Institute
A. J. Macfoy	1st Leningrad State Medical Institute
A. R. L. Massaquoi	1st Leningrad State Medical Institute
D. S. Saisay	Peoples Friendship University
K. J. Sasay	Simferopol State Medical Institute

Interns in Soviet and Eastern-Bloc Universities, September 1972–August 1974

NAME	LOCATION
F. U. Lansena-Wonneh	Simferopol State Medical Institute
M. B. Koroma	Kiev State Medical Institute
J. I. Sesay	Tashkent State Medical Institute
E. S. Grant	Krasnodar State Medical Institute
T. S. Dumbuya	Simferopol State Medical Institute
S. I. Kamara	Odessa State Medical Institute
M. S. K. Abdulai	1st Leningrad State Medical Institute
Noah Conteh	Kharkov State Medical Institute
J. H. Simbo	1st Leningrad State Medical Institute
M. M. Sankoh	Volgograd State Medical Institute
A. L. Rogers	1st Leningrad State Medical Institute
E. A. Nahim	Kharkov State Medical Institute
C. W. Kamara	Kharkov State Medical Institute
M. B. Zubairu	1st Leningrad State Medical Institute
B. M. Kanneh	Kharkov State Medical Institute
S. O. Koroma	Odessa State Medical Institute
M. Lengor	1st Leningrad State Medical Institute
J. F. Whitfield	Leningrad State Paediatric Medical Institute
J. C. O. Whitfield	Leningrad State Paediatric Medical Institute
T. M. Williams	1st Leningrad Medical Institute
E. B. A. Sankoh	Belosian Medical Acad-Katowave
A. K. Kajue	Lekaria Medical Acad.
H. O. W. Fraser	Peoples Friendship University
H. D. Kamara	Leningrad State Paediatric Medical Institute
S. J. Wai	Kharkov State Medical Institute
P. A. Lebbie	1st Leningrad State Medical Institute
S. E. Beooles	Kiev State Medical Institute

Interns in Soviet and Eastern-Bloc Universities, September 1973–August 1975

NAME	LOCATION
W. T. Baldeh	Kiev State Medical Institute
Idris Bangara	1st Leningrad State Medical Institute
A. O. Bangura	Kiev State Medical Institute
N. E. Beury	Odessa Medical State Institute
J. A. Bona	University of Vienna
N. Broaderick	Kalinins State Medical/Dental Institute
F. Caesay	Moscow State Medical/Dental Institute
A. A. Cessay	Kiev State Medical Institute
A. K. Cham	Kiev State Medical Institute
V. O. C. Cole	Peoples Friendship University Moscow
S. Y. Daramy	Odessa Medical Institute
P. V. Dougan	Friendship University
M. E. H. Dumbuya	Lvov State Medical Institute
E. W. Faux-During	Kharkov State Medical Institute
A. B. Gaye	Peoples Friendship University Moscow
O. O. Gborie	State Medical Institute, Sofia
S. E. B. Gborie	Medical Institute, Sofia
M. F. Gbow	St. Mary's Hospital Medical School
A. T. Harding	Odessa State Medical Institute
D. E. Harding	Kubam Medical Institute
T. I. Harding	Odessa State Medical Institute
D. S. M. Jah	Kharkov State Medical Institute
Abou-Bakarr Kamara	1st Leningrad Medical Institute
P. M. Kamara	Odessa Medical State University
S. K. Kamara	International Friendship University
F. C. S. Kann	Rostov On-Dan State Medical Institute
A. B. Kargbo	Peoples Friendship University
B. Kargbo	Rostov State Medical School
M. M. Kargbo	Kharkov State University
A. S. Kebbie	Lvov State Medical Institute
G. J. Komba-Kono	Kharkov State Medical Institute
D. Mac-Boimah	Lvov State Medical Institute
J. C. Macfoy	Odessa State Medical Institute
M. A. Mansaray	Charles University of Prague
A. B. Mason	Moscow Medical Institute
H. B. Mathia	Krasnodar State Medical Institute

(*continued*)

283

NAME	LOCATION
T. S. Mbriwa	Kiev State Medical Institute
Phrancis Momoh	Kiev State Medical Institute
C. H. E. Morgan	Volgograd State Medical Institute
E. E. Morgan	Leningrad State Medical Paediatric Institute
C. J. Neale	Moscow State Medical Institute
J. A. Ngagba	Leningrad Medical Paediatric Institute
I. S. Palmer	Rostov State Medical Institute
S. A. Pratt	Patrice Lumumba Peoples Friendship University
R. C. Quinn	Odessa State Medical Institute
S. J. Rogers	Volgograd State Medical Institute
R. M. Sankoh	Lvov State Medical Institute
A. B. K. Sesay	Odessa State Medical Institute
A. P. Sesay	Peoples Friendship University Moscow
W. E. Sherriff	University of Novi Sad
Jengo Stevens	Karl Marx University-Leipzig
A. A. Taqi	Peoples Friendship University
H. R. Thuray	Kuban State Medical Institute
J. B. Touray	Kalinin State Medical/Dental Institute
M. D. Turay	Zagreb University
D. R. Williams	Bucharest University Faculty of G. Medicine
A. R. Wurie	Zagreb Medical School

Interns in Soviet and Eastern-Bloc Universities, August 1975–1976

NAME	LOCATION
J. A. Babadi	Medical Institute Plovdiv
J. S. Babadi	Medical Institute Plovdiv
J. K. George	USSR, 1978
H. Hariri	Rostov State Medical Institute
A. O. Jah	Medical Faculty Bucharest
A. Kai Kai	Lvov State Medical Institute
M. M. Milton	Patrice Lumumba Friendship University
F. B. Moigule	2nd Moscow Medical Institute
B. E. Parker	International Friendship University
A. B. Paul-Bangura	Peoples Friendship University
P. A. T. Roberts	Peoples Friendship University
S. M. Saccoh Fourah Bay College	Sofia, Bulgaria: MD, DTH, 1984; MO, BSc, Honors,
B. R. Temple	Odessa Medical Institute
D. R. Thomas	Odessa Medical Institute
A. A. Zubairu	Kuban State Medical Institute

Notes

INTRODUCTION

1. Sinnette, personal correspondence; and Hartwig, Patterson, eds., *Disease in African History,* 3–21.
2. Stone, "Prosopography," 46–79.
3. "The Declaration of Alma-Ata."

CHAPTER ONE: AFRICAN PHYSICIANS IN TIME PERSPECTIVE

1. Sinnette, personal correspondence; and see Patton, "Howard University and Meharry Medical Schools," 109–23. On the importance of the profession and abstract knowledge see the indispensable study, Abbott, *The System of Professions,* 8–9, 102–3.
2. Pickering, "Medicine and Education," 69–78.
3. Melson and Wolpe, "Modernization and the Politics of Communalism," 1112–14.
4. Berridge, "Health and Medicine," 180; Reader, *Professional Men,* 45–48, 50–68; and Brown, "British Army Surgeons Commissioned 1840–1909," 411–31.
5. Larson, *The Rise of Professionalism,* 107–8.

6. Abbott, *The System of Professions*, 87–90.
7. Last and Chavunduka, eds., *The Professionalisation of African Medicine*, 8.
8. Abbott, *The System of Professions*, 87.
9. Patterson, "River Blindness in Northern Ghana, 1900–1950," 88–117.
10. Ephson, "Herbs in Pharmacy," 1605–7.
11. Adeloye, *African Pioneers of Modern Medicine*, 13.
12. Toungara, "The Apotheosis of Côte d'Ivoire's Nana Houphouët-Boigny," 23–54. And see De Craemer and Fox, *The Emerging Physician*.
13. Abbott, *The System of Professions*, 201–2.
14. Public Record Office (hereinafter PRO), CO 879/99, Memorandum as to the employment of native medical officers in West Africa, 1908.
15. Johnson, *Professions and Power*, 46.
16. Johnson, "Imperialism and the Professions," 285.
17. Patterson, "Disease and Medicine in African History," 141–48.
18. T. S. Gale, "Official Medical Policy in British West Africa 1870–1930," 107.
19. PRO, CO 554/11, Native medical officers; Ballhatchet, *Race, Sex, and Class under the Raj*; Bolt, *Victorian Attitudes Toward Race*, 1–28, 109–56; Callaway, "Purity and Exotica in Legitimating the Empire," 1–38; and Chaudhuri and Strobel, eds., *Western Women and Imperialism*.
20. For German doctors in Africa, see Gann and Duignan, *The Rulers of German Africa*, 179–80, 204–5, 208.
21. Vaucel, "Le Service de Santé des Troupes de Marine et la Médecine Tropicale Française," 229.
22. Suret-Canale, *Afrique Noire L'Ere Coloniale 1900–1945*, 420–21.
23. Nicol, interviewed February 6, 1985; and commentary on Nicol. Walter Awooner-Renner, interviewed February 11, 1985, in Freetown. See also "Qualifying Degrees and Diplomas," 537–42.
24. Hobson, "Medical Education in Europe," 815–33; and Cooper, "Education for the Health Professions in the Soviet Union," 412–18.
25. Adeloye, "Nigerian Pioneer Doctors and Early West African Politics," 18.
26. During, interviewed in Freetown.
27. Tettey, "Medical Practitioners of African Descent in Colonial Ghana," 143; and NAG, *Ghana Gazette*, January 18, 1958, 74–79.
28. Brown, "British Army Surgeons Commissioned 1840–1909 with West Indian/West African Service," 411–31.
29. Beck, "The British Medical Council and British Medical Education in the Nineteenth Century," 150–52.
30. Fendall, "A History of the Yaba School of Medicine, Nigeria," 118–23; National Archives Ibadan (hereinafter NAI), CSO 26 File no. 16631, 2:246, "Medical Students"; and NAI, CSO 26 File no. 43212/S.19, "The Award of Scholarships, 1947/48."
31. "Editorial: Final M.B., B.S. (London) in Special Relationship," 2.

32. Schram, *A History of the Nigerian Health Services,* 280–86.
33. PRO, CO 554/2097; and PRO, CO 554/638.
34. Schram, *A History of the Nigerian Health Services,* 283; De Craemer and Fox, *The Emerging Physician,* 3.; Legum, *Congo Disaster,* 44, 65; and Slade, *The Belgian Congo.*
35. National Archives, Ghana (hereinafter NAG), Adm. 5/1/217.
36. *Proposal for a College of Medicine and Allied Health Services.* For the 1962 report, see *Report of the Commission Appointed to Advise on the Possibility of Establishing a Medical Faculty at Fourah Bay College;* and Alfonso Mejia, Helena Pizurki, and Erica Royston, *Physician and Nurse Migration.*
37. Adeloye, *Dr. E. Latunde Odeku.*
38. Cheverton, "The District Medical Office," 142.
39. Barnor (MB), interviewed in Accra.
40. Olu-Williams, interviewed in Freetown; and SLPA, *Sierra Leone Gazette,* 858–60.
41. Agbabiaka, "Doctors' Associations Banned," 437.
42. Waddy, "A District Medical Office in North-West Ghana," 164.
43. Waddy (MD), interviewed in Winchester, England. See also Waddy, "The Present State of Public Health in the African Soudan," 95–115.
44. Waddy, "Arabian Literature and Sleeping Sickness in Northern Nigeria," 283; and Khaldun, *Histoire des Berbers,* 114–16.

CHAPTER TWO: THE MEDICAL PROFESSION IN AFRICA
FROM ANCIENT TIMES TO 1800

1. Dols, Medieval Islamic Medicine, 36–41.
2. Sigerist, A History of Medicine, 321–25; Finch, "The African Background of Medical Science," 9; and Newsome, "Black Contributions to the Early History of Western Medicine," 27–39.
3. Osler, The Evolution of Modern Medicine, 10; Sigerist, *The Great Doctors,* 21–28; and Estes, *The Medical Skills of Ancient Egypt,* 1–26, 114.
4. Sigerist, *A History of Medicine,* 226–27, 297, 302.
5. Ibid., 325.
6. Rawlinson, *The History of Herodotus,* 117–18.
7. Finch, "The African Background of Medical Science," 9.
8. Sigerist, *The Great Doctors,* 22.
9. Heilbroner, *The Future as History,* 18–21.
10. Sutton, "The Aquatic Civilization of Middle Africa," 527–46.
11. Leiser, "Medical Education in Islamic Lands," 52.
12. Galdston, "Trade Routes and Medicine," 342–58.
13. McCall, *Africa in Time Perspective,* 33–34.
14. Dols, *Medieval Islamic Medicine,* 3–27.
15. Africanus, *The History and Description of Africa,* 825–42.

16. Inan, "Al-Jami al-Azhar wa Rihlat al-Alf Sana," 56–57; Lumpkin and Zitzler, "Cairo-Science Academy of the Middle Ages," 25–38; and Junaidu, *The Relevance of the University to Our Society,* 7–10.
17. Saad, *Social History of Timbuktu,* 21, 74, 269.
18. Dols, *Medieval Islamic Medicine,* 41.
19. Alteras, "The Roles of Spanish Jewish Physicians," 43–51; and Patai, *The Vanished Worlds of Jewry,* 1–14.
20. Africanus, *The History and Description of Africa,* 1005.
21. Hirschberg, "The Problem of the Judaized Berbers," 336.
22. Cissoko, "Famines et Epidémies à Timboutou et dans la Boucle du Niger," 806–21.
23. Jackson, *An Account of Timbuktu,* 33–34.
24. Henige, *Colonial Governors from the Fifteenth Century to the Present,* 171–72.

CHAPTER THREE: THE SIERRA LEONE NEXUS
1. Wyse, "Searchlight on the Krio of Sierra Leone," 2–10.
2. Kilson, *Political Change in a West African State,* 76.
3. Ibid., 68–69.
4. Fyfe, *A History of Sierra Leone;* and "The Formation of a West African Intellectual Community," 10–12.
5. T. S. Gale, "Official Medical Policy in British West Africa 1870–1930," 33–34.
6. M. C. F. Easmon, "Sierra Leone Doctors," 81–96.
7. Curtin, "The White Man's Grave," 94–95.
8. Ibid., 97.
9. Beck, "The British Medical Council," 150–52.
10. Chitnis, "Medical Education in Edinburgh, 1790–1826," 173–85.
11. PRO, CO 267/40; and Peterkin, Johnston, and Drew, eds., *Commissioned Officers in the Medical Services of the British Army 1660–1960,* 249.
12. PRO, CO 267/57.
13. PRO, CO 267/59.
14. Sierra Leone Public Archives (hereinafter SLPA), Liberated African Department, 15, Letter Book.
15. SLPA, St. George Cathedral, Freetown, Sierra Leone, notes.
16. SLPA, Requisitions of medicines, materials, and instruments, for the use of the Liberated Africans in Sierra Leone for 12 months.
17. University of Birmingham, Main Library, CAI/017.
18. Ibid., CAI/05–6.
19. PRO, CO 267/159.
20. SLPA, Governor's Council Minutes, March 29, 1841.
21. Fyfe, *A History of Sierra Leone,* 178, 211.
22. PRO, CO 267/164.

23. SLPA, Governor's Council Minutes Book; PRO, CO 267/66 (1841); and PRO, CO 267/84 (1844).
24. Fyfe, *A History of Sierra Leone,* 229; and July, *The Origins of Modern African Thought,* 132–36.
25. PRO, CO 267/187.
26. SLPA, Governor's dispatches to the secretary of state, November 26, 1845; PRO, CO 267/189.
27. PRO, CO 267/189.
28. SLPA, Governor's Council Minutes, December 20, 1845; PRO, CO 267/189; and PRO, CO 267/196, William Fergusson, Jr., on board the barque *Funchal.*
29. PRO, CO 267/196, William Fergusson, Jr., letter on behalf of mother; Fyfe, *A History of Sierra Leone,* 216, 260–61; PRO, CO 267/196, William Fergusson, Jr., on board the barque *Funchal.*
30. PRO, WO 43/869.
31. Mbaeyi, *British Military and Naval Forces in West African History,* 107–8; and PRO, WO 43/869.
32. PRO, WO 43/869; and Fyfe, *Africanus Horton,* 29.
33. PRO, WO 43/869.
34. PRO, WO 43/869.
35. Roland Oliver, *The Missionary Factor in East Africa,* 64.
36. Fyfe, *Africanus Horton,* 23–28.
37. Ibid., 32–36; and Adeloye, *Nigerian Pioneers of Modern Medicine,* 2.
38. Boahen, "Politics of Ghana, 1800–1874," 213, 217.
39. Fyfe, *Africanus Horton,* 42.
40. Horton, *West African Countries and Peoples,* 44–45.
41. University of Birmingham Main Library, CAI/0117/1–23.
42. Ibid., CAI/0117/7, Charles Callaghan.
43. Ibid., CAI/0117/7, James Africanus B. Horton.
44. Ibid., CAI/0117/7, Governor Rich Pine.
45. Adeloye, *Nigerian Pioneers of Modern Medicine,* 6.
46. T. S. Gale, "Official Medical Policy in British West Africa 1870–1930," 23–26.
47. Adeloye, *Nigerian Pioneers of Modern Medicine,* 37–38.
48. Ayandele, *African Historical Studies,* 170.
49. Adeloye, *Nigerian Pioneers of Modern Medicine,* 28, 51–52, 53–60.
50. Bullough, "The Causes of the Scottish Medical Renaissance," 13–14, 18–20.
51. Ibid., 13.
52. Ibid., 25.

CHAPTER FOUR: THE EASMON EPISODE

1. Dumett, "The Campaign Against Malaria," 191–95; and Patterson, *Health in Colonial Ghana,* 13–14. For the history of racial discrimination in colonial administration, see Patterson, "Disease and Medicine in African History,"

147; and for the changing concepts about race in British thought, see Stepan, *The Idea of Race in Science.*

2. Jenkins, "In Pursuit of the African Past," 114–29.
3. Asmis, "Law and Policy Relating to the Natives of the Gold Coast and Nigeria," 18–19, 29, 136–64; Kimble, *A Political History of Ghana,* 9–10; and Henige, *Colonial Governors from the Fifteenth Century to the Present,* 174.
4. Jones-Quartey, "Sierra Leone's Role in the Development of Ghana, 1820–1930," 75–76.
5. Hunter, *Road to Freedom,* 13–14.
6. Nicol, "Brazil, Canada, Nova Scotia, and the Guinea Coast," 17.
7. Brown, "British Army Surgeons Commissioned 1840–1909," 421.
8. M. C. F. Easmon, "A Nova Scotian Family," 57–59.
9. Mann, *Marrying Well,* 82, 98–100.
10. SLPA, Letters to the Gold Coast 1874–87.
11. Fyfe, *A History of Sierra Leone,* 423.
12. T. S. Gale, "Official Medical Policy in British West Africa 1870–1930," 15–16. See John Farrell Easmon, "Notes of a Case of Blackwater Fever with Remarks," 277–80. Easmon noted that the fever was called by French writers *Fièvre Bilieuse Mélanurique* or *Hématurique,* 277.
13. PRO, CO 96/224, Record of service of Dr. J. F. Easmon. See also PRO, CO 96/164, Dr. J. D. McCarthy on Easmon.
14. PRO, CO 879/31.
15. T. S. Gale, "Official Medical Policy in British West Africa 1870–1930," 16.
16. *Manson's Tropical Diseases* had not done so in its seventh edition, published in 1921.
17. SLPA, Minute Paper M151/1917 (October).
18. PRO, CO 96/164, Appointment of Dr. Easmon.
19. Patterson, "Health in Urban Ghana," 251–68; Curtin, "Medical Knowledge and Urban Planning in Tropical Africa," 594–613; and Cell, "Anglo-Indian Medical Theory and the Origins of Segregation in West Africa," 307–35.
20. PRO, CO 92/224.
21. Dumett, "John Sarbah the Elder," 659.
22. SLPA, Governor's confidential dispatches to the secretary of state 1882–88; and Spitzer, *The Creoles of Sierra Leone,* 53.
23. PRO, CO 96/224, Dr. J. F. Easmon applies for appointment.
24. PRO, CO 96/296, Confidential dispatch 1897.
25. PRO, CO 96/296, Dr. Easmon to the colonial secretary.
26. PRO, CO 96/296, Dr. Easmon's reply to charge of carrying on private medical practice.
27. PRO, CO 92/296; at £15,621 (c. $82,010.25—1 Guinea to £1, 1 Shilling to $5.25) in 1896, the Gold Coast Colony Medical Department's budget was

larger than Lagos colony's £8,034 (c. $43,596) in the same year and Sierra Leone's £8,047 (c. $42,246.75) in 1898.

28. PRO, CO 96/244.

29. NAG, *Gold Coast Civil List*; and Jenkins, "Gold Coasters Overseas, 1880–1919," 44–45. On Gold Coast education see Nketia, "Program in Gold Coast Education," 1–9.

30. PRO, CO 96/247; and NAG, Adm. 11/1107.

31. PRO, CO 96/269.

32. PRO, CO 96/266, Medical Service request; and PRO, CO 96/196, *The Gold Coast Independent.*

33. PRO, CO 96/296, *The Gold Coast Independent.*

34. PRO, CO 96/286.

35. M. C. F. Easmon, "A Nova Scotian Family," 59–60.

36. PRO, CO 96/297, Dr. J. F. Easmon.

37. PRO, CO 96/297, Governor Maxwell to Honourable J. Chamberlain, about Easmon.

38. PRO, CO 96/307, Dr. J. F. Easmon, charges against him.

39. Raymond Awooner-Renner (BL, London; MA, Boston; DIL, Harvard; DIL, The Hague), interviewed in Freetown; and Walter Awooner-Renner, interviewed in Freetown.

40. NAG, Adm. 12/1/15.

41. M. C. F. Easmon, "A Nova Scotian Family," 60.

42. Kimble, *A Political History of Ghana*, 98.

43. Feierman, personal correspondence.

CHAPTER FIVE: COLONIAL MEDICAL UNION AND AFRICAN REACTION

1. Denzer, "Abolition and Reform in West Africa," 81–82.

2. Kimble, *A Political History of Ghana*, 224–49.

3. Fyfe, *A History of Sierra Leone*, 464–65.

4. PRO, CO 96/296, Medical Service request.

5. PRO, CO 879/99, British Medical Association.

6. Manson-Bahr, *History of the School of Tropical Medicine In London;* and Shepherd, *A History of the Liverpool Medical Institute.*

7. *The London School of Tropical Medicine*, 10–28; and Nkwam, "British Medical and Health Policies in West Africa c. 1920–60," 125–32.

8. PRO, CO 879/99, Enclosure no. 1, preliminary report.

9. Dumett, "The Campaign Against Malaria," 195.

10. Curtin et al, *African History*, 446.

11. Larson, *The Rise of Professionalism*, xvi–xvii.

12. PRO, CO 872/72. For the response see PRO, CO 879/99.

13. PRO, CO 279/112.
14. Bodleian Library, Rhodes House, Oxford (hereinafter BLO), MSS. British Empire S22, vol. G248, West African medical men.
15. Johnson, "Imperialism and the Professions," 288.
16. PRO, CO 872/72; and T. S. Gale, "Segregation in British West Africa," 495–507.
17. PRO, CO 96/402.
18. SLPA, Minute Paper Confidential 10/1902.
19. SLPA, Minute Paper Confidential 73/1902.
20. SLPA, Minute Paper Confidential 85/1904.
21. Ibid.
22. SLPA, Minute Paper Confidential 141/1904.
23. NAG, Adm. 11/1107.
24. SLPA, Governor's confidential dispatches to the secretary of state, 56/1906.
25. SLPA, Annual Confidential Report, 1901.
26. SLPA, Minute Paper Confidential 56/1906.
27. SLPA, Minute Paper 4250/1903, Application from Dr. Renner.
28. SLPA, Minute Paper Confidential 56/1906.
29. Ibid.
30. SLPA, Minute Paper Confidential 150/1906, Dr. Renner.
31. SLPA, Governor's confidential dispatches, 1910.
32. SLPA, Governor's confidential dispatches, 1916.
33. SLPA Minute Paper 985/1907. See also SLPA, *Annual Medical and Sanitary Report*, 1912.
34. PRO, CO 879/105.
35. SLPA, Retirement of Dr. W. Awooner-Renner, medical. From PMO #887, April 25, 1913.
36. PRO, CO 98/19.
37. NAG, *Ghana Gazette*, List of medical practitioners.
38. PRO, CO 554/11, Memo by Dr. Langley.
39. Ibid.
40. BLO, MSS. British Empire S22, vol. G248. O. Sapara, "Colonial Medical Appointments in the West African Colonies."
41. Patton, "E. Mayfield Boyle," 52–53.
42. SLPA, Minute Paper 1132/1909, The Medical Practitioners Ordinance; and Horton, interviewed in Freetown.
43. SLPA, Minute Paper 4100/1909.
44. PRO, CO 554/82/4179/4212.
45. Ibid.
46. Cromwell, *An African Victorian Feminist*, 39.
47. Lynch, *Edward Wilmot Blyden*, 54, 60–83.
48. Dibner, *Wilhelm Conrad Röntgen and the Discovery of X-Rays*.
49. Leone Boyle Easmon Thompson, interview in Rockville, Md.

50. E.C.D., "Native v. European Doctors," 137.
51. Nkwam, "British Medical and Health Policies in West Africa c. 1920–60," 30, 29–34, which includes a citation of PRO, CO 554/78/4067.
52. NAG, Adm. 14/2/11; and NAG, Adm. 5/4/268.
53. *Korle Bu Hospital 1923–1973*, 4, 10–14.
54. NAG, Adm. 14/2/10; and NAG, Adm. 12/5/143.
55. NAG, Adm. 14/2/10.
56. NAG, Adm. 11/1577, Gold Coast colony, government scholarships.

CHAPTER SIX: M. C. F. EASMON

1. Abayomi Cole, "Obituary of Dr. MaCormack Charles Farrell Easmon," 19–27.
2. PRO, CO 96/307, Dr. J. F. Easmon.
3. Cromwell, *An African Victorian Feminist*, 29–36; and Casely-Hayford, *Memoirs and Poems*.
4. BLO, MSS. British Empire S22, vol. G248, M. C. F. Easmon to Rev. J. H. Harris.
5. Cromwell, *An African Victorian Feminist*, 57.
6. PRO, CO 267/549, Native medical officer.
7. BLO, Reprint from *Lancet*, September 7, 1912.
8. Kimble, *A Political History of Ghana*, 150, 330–80.
9. BLO, MSS. British Empire S22, vol. G248, R. H. Griffin to Dr. M. C. F. Easmon.
10. BLO, MSS. British Empire S22, vol. G248, M. L. Jarrett Report.
11. Ibid.
12. Harris, *Dawn in Darkest Africa*, 110–12.
13. BLO, "African Medical Practitioners," *Nigerian Chronicle*, 1912.
14. PRO, CO 267/549, Dr. John F. H. Broadbent.
15. M. C. F. Easmon, "Sierra Leone Doctors," 85–86; and SLPA, Minute Paper Rf. 1048 756/10, Medical Department.
16. PRO, CO 267/550.
17. PRO, CO 267/549, Governor Edward Mereweather.
18. PRO, CO 554/11, List of native medical practitioners.
19. PRO, CO 554/11, Native medical officers.
20. Gann and Duignan, *The Rulers of German Africa*, 216–17; and Rudin, *Germans in the Cameroons*.
21. SLPA, Minute Paper M93/1917.
22. PRO, CO 583/74.
23. SLPA, Minute Paper M93/17; and SLPA, Minute Paper M101/1917.
24. Gailey, *A History of the Gambia*, 175.

25. *Gold Coast Civil Service List;* Agboideka, "Sir Gordon Guggisberg's Contribution," 52–64; and T. S. Gale, "Sir Gordon Guggisberg and His African Critics," 271–74.

26. PRO, CO 583/74.

27. SLPA, Minute Paper M93/1917.

28. SLPA, Minute Paper M46/1917, Application of Dr. M. C. F. Easmon.

29. Patterson and Pyle, "The Diffusion of Influenza in Sub-Saharan Africa During the 1918–19 Pandemic," 1299–1307; and Patterson and Pyle, "The Geography and Mortality of the 1918 Influenza Pandemic," 4–21.

30. T. S. Gale, "Official Medical Policy in British West Africa 1870–1930," 389; and Patterson, "The Influenza Epidemic of 1918–19 in the Gold Coast," 485–502.

31. Patterson, "The Influenza Epidemic of 1918–19 in the Gold Coast," 487.

32. SLPA, Minute Paper M90/1919; and SLPA, M131/1918.

33. SLPA, Minute Paper CS236/1918; and SLPA, Minute Paper M88/1918.

34. Ada Awooner-Renner, interviewed in Freetown.

35. Raymond Easmon, letter to Charles Tettey.

36. SLPA, Minute Paper M174/1918.

37. SLPA, Minute Paper M179/1918, Dr. Easmon's complaint of unusual, uncivil reception.

38. Ibid.

39. PRO, CO 267/604, From the principal medical officer.

40. PRO, CO 267/604, From the medical officer, Bo.

41. PRO, CO 267/604, Governor A. R. Slater.

42. *Civil Service List,* Sierra Leone.

43. Winterbottom, *An Account of the Native Africans,* xiv, xxviii–xxix, 251–72.

44. Feierman, "Popular Control over the Institutions of Health," 205–6.

45. Sinnette, personal correspondence.

46. M. C. F. Easmon, "Conditions of Medical Work in a West African Bush Station," 128–31.

47. Deanna Thomas, "Sir Milton Margai," 64–79.

48. M. C. F. Easmon, "Conditions of Medical Work in a West African Bush Station," 131; and M. C. F. Easmon, "Helminthiasis in the Sierra Leone Protectorate," 305–7.

49. PRO, CO 267/646, African medical officers, petition. See also Nkwam, "British Medical and Health Policies in West Africa c. 1920–60," 146–52.

50. *Gold Coast Civil Service List,* 1922, 1925, 1926, 1927, 1928, 1929.

51. PRO, CO 267/646, From the African medical officers.

52. PRO, CO 267/646, Arnold Hudson.

53. PRO, CO 267/646, From the director of medical services.

54. SLPA, CSOM 56/36.

55. Raymond Easmon, interviewed in Freetown.

56. "M. C. F. Easmon," Obituary, *British Medical Journal*, 29.
57. During, interviewed in Freetown.
58. "M. C. F. Easmon," Obituary, *The Times* (London), May 9, 1972. The *Lancet* did not carry an obituary.
59. Charles Odamten Easmon, interviewed in Accra.
60. *The Medical Directory*, 881.

CHAPTER SEVEN: DAVID EKUNDAYO BOYE-JOHNSON

1. I owe my special thanks to the late Mrs. Florie Boye-Johnson (died April 1985), the widow of David Ekundayo Boye-Johnson, for she generously entrusted me with his personal papers on July 26, 1983, Freetown.
2. Feierman, "Struggles for Control," 121.
3. Spitzer, *The Creoles of Sierra Leone*, 70–71, 80–81.
4. Stevens, *What Life Has Taught Me*, 39.
5. Ibid.
6. July, *The Origins of Modern African Thought*, 136.
7. Ibid.
8. Boye-Johnson, personal correspondence to the chief of the visa division.
9. Boye-Johnson, curriculum vitae.
10. Horton, interviewed in Freetown; and Wilkinson, ed., *Directory of Graduates Howard University, 1870–1963*, 118.
11. Boye-Johnson, declaration of identification, Chicago.
12. Wilburn, visa division, Department of State; and Commissioner of Police, Chicago Police Department.
13. Belovsky, American consul, Windsor, Ontario, Canada.
14. Beasley, affidavit of financial sponsorship.
15. Boye-Johnson, personal correspondence to the chief of the visa division, Department of State.
16. PRO, CO 877/9/2, Canadian medical qualifications.
17. PRO, CO 859/63/4, Draft memorandum on the proposal.
18. PRO, CO 859/63/4, Memorandum on proposed diploma course.
19. Curtin, *The Image of Africa*, 46–47; Stepan, *The Idea of Race in Science*; and Bolt, *The Anti-Slavery Movement and Reconstruction*, 141–70.
20. Callaway, *Gender, Culture and Empire*, 48–51.
21. PRO, CO 879/116, Nigeria, the Governor-General to the Secretary of State.
22. For comparative practice in India, where Lugard also served before coming to Nigeria, see Ballhatchet, *Race, Sex, and Class under the Raj*, 96–122; and Callaway, "Purity and Exotica in Legitimating the Empire," 1–38.
23. PRO, CO 879/116.
24. SLPA, Governor's confidential dispatches, December 18, 1916.
25. BLO, MSS. British Empire R. 4.
26. PRO, CO 859/63/4, Memorandum on proposed diploma course.

27. Wyse, *H. C. Bankole-Bright,* 32–86, 97–104, 116–19, 136; and Spitzer, *The Creoles of Sierra Leone,* 180–216.

28. Last, "The Professionalisation of African Medicine," 10; and Barnor, "A History of Medical Societies in Ghana," 4–7.

29. "The Association and Medical Practice in the Colonies," 1–20.

30. Nkwam, "British Medical and Health Policies in West Africa c. 1920–60," cites *West Africa,* January 14, 1939, 11.

31. NAI, 4797, October 30, 1942.

32. NAI, 4797, July 12, 1949, correspondence.On BMA branches in each West African colony, see NAI, 4797 10.7.42.

33. PRO, CO 1017/399; PRO, CO 1017/400; PRO, CO 1017/404; PRO, CO HMOCS; PRO, CO 554/1000; PRO, CO 1017/369, Confidential, future of the Colonial Service; and PRO, CO 1017/369, HMOCS possible developments.

34. Boye-Johnson, "Concerning the Promotion of Public Health in the Colony."

35. PRO, CO 1017/369 (Secret) to the secretary of state, Overseas Civil Service.

36. PRO, CO 554/1186, West African directors.

37. Olu-Williams, interviewed in Freetown.

38. PRO, CO 554/1186. Minutes of Meetings of West African Directors of Medical Services.

39. PRO, CO 877/32/4.

40. *The Laws of the Colony and Protectorate of Sierra Leone, 1946,* vol. 2; *Laws of Sierra Leone 1960;* and *Legislation of Sierra Leone 1965.* For the Gold Coast see PRO, CO 877/322/4; and NAG, *Ghana Gazette,* List of medical practitioners, 1958. For Gambia and Nigeria see PRO, CO 859/1270; and PRO, CO 877/32/4.

41. PRO, CO 859/1271, Dr. H. P. S. Gillette.

42. PRO, CO 859/1271, British colonial medical students in North America.

43. Ibid.; and PRO, CO 876/248.

44. NAI, E112.

45. PRO, CO 859/1271, Legislation and categories.

46. Barnor, "A History of Medical Societies in Ghana," 4–7; NAG, *Ghana Medical Association,* 1–23.

47. Mabayoje, "The Nigerian Medical Association," 14–19.

48. "The Medical Practitioners Union," *Sierra Leone Constitution,* November 27, 1964, 1–8.

49. *Fulton Daily Sun-Gazette.* And see Yakobson, "Russia and Africa," 453–87.

CHAPTER EIGHT: AFRICAN PHYSICIANS

1. Akabi-Davis, interviewed in Freetown.

2. Blakely, *Russia and the Negro,* 74.

3. PRO, DO 35/9306.
4. Gann, "The Soviet Union and Sub-Sahara Africa," 15–18; and Bissell, "The Brezhnev Doctrine in Africa," 57–67.
5. Solodovnikov, "The Soviet Union and Africa," 8–10; and Kanet, "African Youth," 161–75.
6. Blakely, *Russia and the Negro,* 132–33.
7. PRO, CO 1017/400.
8. Rosen, *The Development of Peoples' Friendship University in Moscow,* 1–17; Rosen, *Soviet Training Programs for Africa,* 1–2, 10; and *Afrika 1956–61,* 253.
9. Prokofiev, Chilikin, and Tulpanov, *Higher Education in the USSR,* 6–8; Shimkin and MacLeod, "Medical Education in the USSR," 795–801; and Hobson, "Medical Education in Europe," 815–33.
10. Cooper, "Education for the Health Professions in the Soviet Union," 412–18.
11. Shariff, interviewed in Freetown; and Saccoh, interviewed in Freetown. These doctors were trained in Yugoslavia and Bulgaria respectively. See Tadic, "The Development of Medical Education in Yugoslavia," 868–86; and Rowin, "Medical Training in Poland," 1052–58.
12. Larson, *The Rise of Professionalism,* xii, 253.
13. Hinman and Pease, "International Assistance in Medical Education," 1042–51.
14. Olu-Williams, interviewed in Freetown; and *Report of the Commission Appointed to Advise on the Possibility of Establishing a Medical Faculty at Fourah Bay College,* 1–22.
15. PRO, DO 35/9346.
16. Moigula, interviewed in Freetown; and Johnson-Taylor, interviewed in Freetown.
17. Blakely, *Russia and the Negro,* 74, 125, 128.
18. Roberts, interviewed in Freetown.
19. Lee, "*Visible Man: Black among the Reds,*" B1, B4.
20. Blakely, *Russia and the Negro,* 135.
21. Raymond Awooner-Renner, interviewed in Freetown; *Laws of Sierra Leone 1960;* and *Legislation of Sierra Leone 1965.*
22. "Bills," a supplement to the *Sierra Leone Gazette.*
23. Roberts, interviewed in Freetown.
24. Ibid.
25. Evans-Anfom, interviewed in Accra, Ghana. See also NAG, *Ghana, Medical and Dental Council Report.* On surgeons and order of certification for the FRCS, Samuel Manuwa, Nigeria, was the first in Anglophone West Africa; Charles Odamten Easmon, Ghana, was the second (1948); followed by Evans-Anfom, Ghana (1955); and Olu-Williams, Sierra Leone (1956).
26. Wellesley Cole, *An Innocent in Britain,* 331.

27. Olu-Williams, *Report on Activities of the Department of Clinical Studies;* Cobban, "General Practice Training in West Africa," 279–85; and Pobee, "Postgraduate Medical Education for Physicians in West Africa," 242–44.
28. "Editorial," *Ghana Medical Journal,* 173; and Andrew and Iris Thomas, "Medical Impressions of Ghana," 694–708.
29. Raymond Easmon, "Rethinking the Health Services," 8–9.
30. Muchi interviewed at Johns Hopkins Medical School.
31. Adade, "USSR: Training African Professionals," 304–5.

Bibliography

Archival Sources

AUTHOR'S COLLECTION

Beasley, Edward W. Affidavit of financial sponsorship if necessary on behalf of aliens desiring to proceed to the United States. Cook County, Illinois, May 18, 1943.

Belovsky, Sidney A. American consul, Windsor, Ontario, Canada. Letter to Dr. David Ekundayo Boye-Johnson, May 26, 1943.

"Bills." Supplement to the *Sierra Leone Gazette,* vol. 104, no. 5. February 1, 1973.

Boye-Johnson, David Ekundayo. Curriculum vitae. Freetown, Sierra Leone, July 26, 1983.

———. Declaration of identification. Chicago, Cook County, Illinois, April 7, 1941.

———. Personal correspondence to the chief of the visa division, Department of State, Washington, D.C., June 29, 1943.

Broderick, S. M. Personal correspondence with the author. Freetown, Sierra Leone, December 30, 1980.

Commissioner of Police, Chicago Police Department. Letter, May 20, 1943.

Easmon, Raymond Sarif. Letter to Charles Tettey, librarian, Ghana Medical School, March 16, 1984.

Feierman, Steven. Personal correspondence, June 25, 1989, and July 5, 1991.

Gambia Gazette. Vol. 103, no. 14. Banjul. April 14, 1986. List of Gambian doctors.

Kaiser, Thomas. Personal correspondence. May 6, 1992.

The Laws of the Colony and Protectorate of Sierra Leone 1946. Vol. 2. Ord. F/1949/Ord 28/1952. London: Crown Agents for the Colonies, 1946.

Laws of Sierra Leone 1960. Freetown: Sierra Leone Government Printing Office, 1960.

Legislation of Sierra Leone 1965. Freetown: Sierra Leone Government Printing Office, 1965.

The Nigerian Medical Directory 1970–1971. Lagos: CSS Press, 1970. List of Nigerian doctors.

Olu-Williams, A. E. *Report on Activities of the Department of Clinical Studies 1974–1980.* Freetown: Ministry of Health, 1974–80.

Proposal for a College of Medicine and Allied Health Services. Freetown: University of Sierra Leone, 1988.

Report of the Commission Appointed to Advise on the Possibility of Establishing a Medical Faculty at Fourah Bay College in Conjunction with the Building of a National Hospital 1962. Freetown: FBC, University of Sierra Leone Library, 1962, 1–22.

Sinnette, Calvin H. Personal correspondence. Summer 1980 and Summer 1984.

Wilburn, Homer V. Visa division, Department of State, Washington, D.C., April 7, 1943.

BODLEIAN LIBRARY, RHODES HOUSE, OXFORD (BLO)

MSS. British Empire R. 4. 3 vols. Peter Alphonsus Clearkin. "Ramblings and Recollections of a Colonial Doctor, 1913–1958."

MSS. British Empire S22, vo. G248. Reprint from *Lancet,* September 4, 1912.

MSS. British Empire S22, vol. G248. M. C. F. Easmon to Rev. J. H. Harris, organizing secretary, September 18, 1912.

MSS. British Empire S22, vol. G248. Michael Lewis Jarrett Report on African medical doctors in the service to Rev. J. T. Robert, secretary ASAPS, Sierra Leone, February 8, 1913.

MSS. British Empire S22, vol. G248. R. H. Griffin to Dr. M. C. F. Easmon. Correspondence on employment in WAMS, October 10, 1912.

MSS. British Empire S22, vol. G248. West African medical men: 1912, Dr. Easmon's case. Aborigines' Rights Protection Society Papers.

MSS. British Empire S22, vol. G248. "African Medical Practitioners." *Nigerian Chronicle,* February 23, 1912.

NATIONAL ARCHIVES, ACCRA, GHANA (NAG)

Adm. 5/1/217. Annual Report of the Medical Services of Ghana, 1967.

Adm. 5/4/268. Confidential correspondence relating to the training of medical students and medical assistants in British West Africa, 1927.

Adm. 11/1107. Awuna native affairs 1878–1901. Case no. M.P. 1154/01, Gold Coast, 1901.

Adm. 11/1577. Gold Coast colony, government scholarships to African students for the purpose of studying medicine in the United Kingdom, 1943.

Adm. 11/1577. Minute Office of the director of medical services by the selection board for the award of medical scholarships, 1943–44.

Adm. 12/5/143. Employment of native medical men, March 29, 1919.

Adm. 12/15. Secretary of State. Confidential dispatch, October 1897.

Adm. 14/2/10. Gold Coast colony, Legislative Council debates, session 1924–25, March 6, 1924.

Adm. 14/2/11. Gold Coast colony, Legislative Council debates, sessions, 1925–26.

Ghana Gazette. List of Ghana doctors trained in the Soviet bloc. No. 48, Friday, November 23, 1984.

Ghana Gazette. List of medical practitioners and dentists registered in Ghana as on January 1, 1958. No. 99, January 18, 1958.

Ghana, Medical and Dental Council Report for the Period July 1974–December 1975. Accra: Ministry of Health, 1975.

Ghana Medical Association: Regulations of a Company Limited by Guarantee. Accra: Ghana Medical Association, 1963.

Gold Coast Civil Service List. Government Printing Office, 1925.

NATIONAL ARCHIVES, IBADAN, NIGERIA (NAI)

CSO 26 File no. 16631, 2:246. "Medical Students: Maintenance of (Yaba at King's College, England)." W. B. Johnson, Director of Medical and Sanitary Service (Nigeria) to the Honourable Chief Secretary of the Government, February 5, 1931.

CSO 26 File no. 43212/S.19. "The Award of Scholarships, 1947/48, from Medical Departments." W. E. S. Merrett, Dean, University College Ibadan, to Director of Medical Services, February 5, 1949.

E112. Approved medical schools in USA, 1950–52. Robert Ross, American consul, to the Medical Department, Lagos, Nigeria, February 20, 1952.

4797 10.2.42. Correspondence. Classified staff list from chairman to DMS, no. 2/1, January 1, 1943.

4797 10.2.46. Memorandum no. 1136. October 30, 1942, and rules and regulations.

4797 7.12.49. Formation of British Medical Association: West Africa, July 12, 1949.

PUBLIC RECORDS OFFICE, KEW GARDENS, ENGLAND
(PRO); COLONIAL OFFICE (CO), (DO), WAR OFFICE (WO)

CO 92/224. Record of service of Dr. J. F. Easmon, assistant colonial surgeon, Gold Coast Colony, submitted 1892.

CO 92/296. Gold Coast medical officers, November 27, 1897.

CO 96/164. Appointment of Dr. Easmon for special leave privileges and permanent retention at Accra. Governor Young to Lord Derby (Colonial Office), February 9, 1885.

CO 96/164. Dr. J. D. McCarthy on Easmon to Governor Easmon. Application for leave, January 31, 1884, and enclosure: Dr. Easmon's letter to CMO, January 9, 1885.

CO 96/224. Dr. J. F. Easmon applies for appointment as colonial surgeon of Sierra Leone. But the recommendation is refused, as he is invaluable to the colony, June 25, 1892.

CO 96/224. Record of service of Dr. J. F. Easmon, assistant colonial surgeon, Gold Coast Colony, June 25, 1892.

CO 96/244. Dr. W. A. Murray, recommends promotion of March 2, 1894.

CO 96/247. Petition of Dr. B. W. Quartey-Papafio, August 24, 1894.

CO 96/266. Africa trade section of the Incorporated Chamber of Commerce of Liverpool, April 5, 1895.

CO 96/269. *Gold Coast Chronicle,* June 23, 1894, vol. 5, no. 161.

CO 96/269. Secretary to the Chamber of Commerce, April 15, 1895.

CO 96/286. Maxwell, "Affairs of the Gold Coast Colony, Address." September 4, 1896.

CO 96/296. *Gold Coast Independent,* August 3, 1895.

CO 96/296. Acting colonial secretary to Dr. Easmon, Accra, June 12, 1897.

CO 96/296. Confidential dispatch, 1897. Documents contain report of commission of inquiry against Dr. J. F. Easmon.

CO 96/296. Dr. Easmon to the colonial secretary, Medical Department, Victoriaborg, June 2, 1893.

CO 96/296. Government Gazette [Extraordinary], Accra, Gold Coast, Friday, April 23, 1897.

CO 96/296. Medical Service request information on British and native doctors, April 5, 1895.

CO 96/296. Report of Commission of Enquiry, May 22, 1897.

CO 96/297. Dr. J. F. Easmon explains his reasons for being dissatisfied with administration of the Medical Department, July 24, 1897.

CO 96/297. Governor Maxwell to J. Chamberlain, secretary of colonies, July 24, 1897. Unfavorable opinions toward Dr. Easmon.

CO 96/299. Colonial surgeon, November 25, 1897.

CO 96/299. "A" dissenting against Minutes to J. Chamberlain, December 31, 1897.

CO 96/299. Dr. J. F. Easmon to the acting Chief Medical Officer, November 19, 1897.

CO 96/299. Governor Maxwell to J. Chamberlain, Easmon resignation, November 25, 1897.

CO 96/307. Dr. Easmon's appeal to the secretary of state through the governor, June 17, 1897.

CO 96/307. Dr. Easmon's application for sick leave, June 14, 1897.

CO 96/307. Dr. J. F. Easmon. Charges against him, July 31, 1897.

CO 96/307. Dr. J. F. Easmon from Adelphi Hotel, Liverpool, to the undersecretary of state, Colonial Office, Downing Street, London, July 23, 1897.

CO 96/307. Dr. J. F. Easmon submits appeal to charges against him to the secretary of state for the colonies, August 5, 1897.

CO 96/307. Letter from Mr. W. Waters to Dr. Easmon, dated at Weymouth, August 5, 1897.

CO 96/402. West African medical students protesting against exclusions of West Africans from the staff, March 19, 1902.

CO 96/403. Johnson cites Minutes of April 29, 1902, by Chamberlain.

CO 98/19. Gold Coast Minutes of the Legislative Council, 1912–16.

CO 267/40. Governor C. MacCarthy to colonial establishment, Dr. William Fergusson for employment, July 22, 1815.

CO 267/44. William Fergusson to colonial establishment, November 30, 1816.

CO 267/57. William Fergusson to colonial establishment, October 18, 1822.

CO 267/59. William Fergusson from Chatham to Thomas Harrison, Esq., African Institution, Whitehall, London, May 29, 1823.

CO 267/159. Governor R. Doherty, Government House, Sierra Leone, to colonial establishment, William Fergusson appointment, August 30, 1840.

CO 267/164. John Carr, Esq. or to the officer administering the government of Sierra Leone, July 12, 1841.

CO 267/166. Lieutenant Governor Fergusson to directive of appointment, dispatch July 12, 1841. "God Save the Queen." September 3, 1841.

CO 267/184. N. W. MacDonald proclamation, appointment of William Fergusson as lieutenant governor, May 1, 1844.

CO 267/187. Proclamation, Williamm Fergusson appointment as governor in chief over colony of Sierra Leone, July 15, 1845.

CO 267/189. Fergusson's observations on three reports from Dr. Butts, November 26, 1845.

CO 267/196. William Fergusson, Jr., letter on behalf of mother, Mrs. Charlotte Fergusson, with memorial for pension. Piccadilly, March 20, 1846.

CO 267/196. William Fergusson, Jr., on board the barque *Funchal,* Cork Harbor, February 5, 1846.

CO 267/549. Dr. John F. H. Broadbent, to Colonial Office, August 8, 1912.

CO 267/549. Governor Edward Mereweather to Colonial Office (L. V. Harcourt, M.P.) on employment of Dr. M. C. F. Easmon, May 28, 1913.

CO 267/549. Native medical officer, appointment of Dr. M. C. F. Easmon, May 18, 1913.

CO 267/550. Native medical officers: Dr. Easmon appears to be better qualified, June 10, 1913.

CO 267/604. From the medical officer, Bo, to the DMSS. Freetown, May 21, 1924.

CO 267/604. From the principal medical officer to Dr. M. C .F. Easmon, Kabalia, May 3, 1921.

CO 267/604. Governor A. R. Slater to J. H. Thomas, M.P., on Dr. Easmon's promotion, June 10, 1924.

CO 267/646. African medical officers. Petition for revision of conditions of service, 1934.

CO 267/646. Arnold Hudson (Government House, Sierra Leone) to Fiddian, Colonial Office, May 8, 1934.

CO 267/646. From the African medical officers, Sierra Leone, to the secretary of state for the colonies, January 26, 1934. Dr. Easmon and colleagues compiled this list to support their claims against the government.

CO 267/646. From the director of Medical and Sanitary Services to the colonial secretary, May 15, 1934.

CO 279/112. Petitioners Philip C. Randolph, president, and D. Scakey QuarcooPome, honorary secretary, Gold Coast auxiliary of the Anti-Slavery and Aborigines' Protection Society, Accra, January 23, 1913.

CO 537/7172. Award by King Farouk of Egypt of 30 annual scholarships at El Azhar University, Cairo, to Nigerian Muslims. Banned by Nigerian government, 1951.

CO 554/11. List of native medical practitioners registered at Freetown, Sierra Leone, April 21, 1913.

CO 554/11. Native Medical Officers, Memo by Dr. Langley, secretary of state's dispatch no. 1033, November 18, 1912.

CO 554/11. Native medical officers, May 13, 1913.

CO 554/58. The National Congress of British West Africa: Resolutions, March 13, 1923.

CO 554/78/4067. Report of the committee appointed by the secretary of state for the colonies to formulate a scheme for the establishment in British West Africa of a college for the training of medical practitioners and the creation and training of an auxiliary service of medical assistants. (Accra 1928), enclosure in Gold Coast confidential, T. S. Thomas (acting governor) to L. S. Amery, July 7, 1928.

CO 554/82/4179/4212. Admission of West Africans to the WAMS, March 12, 1929.

CO 544/82/4179/4214. Summary of the WAMS policy of discrimination, "Colour Bar," 1901–29.

CO 554/638. A school for medical assistants at Kano in northern Nigeria, February 2, 1952.

CO 554/1000. Policy of recruitment of Africans to government senior service post in the Gold Coast—Africanization 1954–56.

CO 554/1186. Minutes of meetings of West African directors of medical services, 1954–56.

CO 554/1186. West African directors of medical services conferences, 1954–1956. Minutes, March 22, 1956.

CO 554/2097. R. B. Hunter. Report on the Future of Kano Medical School, January 17, 1958.

CO 583/74. War bonus for native medical officers, April 25, 1919.

CO 859/63/4. Draft memorandum on the proposal for the establishment of a School of Tropical Medicine at McGill University, December 3, December 14, 1943.

CO 859/63/4. Memorandum on proposed diploma course in tropical medicine at McGill University, December 1943.

CO 859/1270. Registration as medical practitioners in the Colonies, 1957–59.

CO 859/1271. British colonial medical students in North America by the adviser for colonial scholars, 1957.

CO 859/1271. Dr. H. P. S. Gillette, OBE, medical adviser to the federal government of the West Indies. S/O letter, 1957–59.

CO 859/1271. Legislation and categories. B. Mellor, adviser for colonial scholars in North America, October 1957. British Embassy, Washington, D.C.

CO 859/1271. Note on British colonial medical students in North America, 1957.

CO 859/15614. Dr. R. B. Wellesley Cole, 1940s.

CO 872/72. Report of the Committee to Discuss a Scheme for the Amalgamation of the Medical Services in the West African Colonies and Protectorates, January 1902.

CO 876/248. Students in the United States: evaluation and recognition of U.S. degrees, April 1950.

CO 877/9/2. Appendix 13. Memorandum by the registrar on the subject of reciprocity with the British dominions and with foreign countries, October 1930.

CO 877/9/2. Canadian medical qualifications. Medical reciprocity as between this country and Canada, 1932.

CO 877/9/2. Correspondence from Mayor J. M. Macdonnell, Toronto, to Major R. D. Furse, DSO, Colonial Office, Whitehall, London, England, October–December 1931.

CO 877/32/4. Minutes: Mr. J. M. Martin, Mr. Cohen, Sir Charles Jeffries from J. B. W., May 22, 1950.

CO 877/322/4. Medical Practitioners and Dentists Registration (Amendment) Ordinance 1950.

CO 879/31. Report of committee on "Blackwater Fever," March 28, 1889.

CO 879/99. British Medical Association to the Colonial Office, correspondence relative to the WAMS, December 6, 1901.

CO 879/99. Confidential correspondence December 1901–December 1908 relative to WAMS, West Africa no. 918.

CO 879/99. Enclosure no. 1, preliminary report of the West African Medical Service Committee, December 6, 1901.

CO 879/99. No. 31, Memorandum as to the employment of native medical officers in West Africa, 1901–8.

CO 879/116. Nigeria. The governor-general to the secretary of state, confidential. F. D. Lugard, governor-general, 1915.

CO 1017/369. Confidential. HMOCS: possible developments for references to Cold War, 1954.

CO 1017/369. Confidential. 1954–56. Future of the Colonial Service, draft statement.

CO 1017/369. (Secret) to the secretary of state for the colonies, Overseas Civil Service, May 12, 1954.

CO 1017/399. HMOCS. Central pool: staffing problems in colonies achieving independence, 1956.

CO 1017/400. HMOCS: reactions of White Paper CMD 9768. Dispatch Circular 771/56.

CO 1017/404. HMOCS: reaction in Sierra Leone, 1954–56.

CO 1017/403. HMOCS: reaction in the Gold Coast, 1954–56.

DO 35/9306. Resistance to Soviet penetration in Ghana (top secret), 1958–60.

DO 35/9346. Ghana's relations with Soviet bloc, 1957–60.

DO 35/9451. Interchange of doctors and nurses between National Health Services and Overseas Medical Services, 1957–60.

DO 35/10479. Soviet representative in Nigeria (top secret), 1959–60.

WO 43/869. "Training of African Natives as Army Surgeons," 1853–55.

SIERRA LEONE PUBLIC ARCHIVES, FREETOWN (SLPA)

Annual Confidential Report. 1901, secretary of state confidential dispatches, colony of Sierra Leone.

Annual Medical and Sanitary Report, 1912. No. 1592 (July 16, 1913).

Governor's confidential dispatches 1910, January–June.

Governor's confidential dispatches 1916, January–December.

Governor's confidential dispatches to the secretary of state 1882–88, January 13, 1882–November 12, 1882.

Governor's confidential dispatches to the secretary of state, 1882–88, November 8, 1886. Sierra Leone Confidential no. 22.

Governor's Council Minutes, March 29, 1841.

Governor's Council Minutes, May 1841.

Governor's Council Minutes, September 3, 1841.

Governor's Council Minutes, September 17, 1841.

Governor's Council Minutes, December 20, 1845.

Governor's Council Minutes Book, 1840–46, July 27, 1840–May 16, 1846.

Governor's dispatches to secretary of state, 1844–45. November 4, 1844–December 26, 1845 (contains Governor William Fergusson: Report on the Annual Blue Book of Sierra Leone for the year 1844, enclosed in no. 35, May 18, 1845).

Letters to the Gold Coast 1874–87, September 4, 1874–July 1, 1887 (with index).

Liberated African Department, 15, Letter Book, February 11, 1827–August 19, 1828.

Liberated African Department, 15, Letter Book, 1828–30.

Minute Paper, 1132/1909. The Medical Practitioners Ordinance 1908: Inquiry by Rev. J. R. Frederick as to qualifications of a Dr. E. M. Boyle of USA (Howard University College of Medicine) under the order.

Minute Paper 985/1907. Alleged disadvantage of the West African Medical Service.

Minute Paper 4100/1909. Foreign and colonial degrees and diplomas recognized by the General Medical Council for registration purposes.

Minute Paper 4250/1903. Application from Dr. Renner to be placed on the same footing as regards salary with WAMS officer.

Minute Paper Confidential 10/1902. Amalgamation of medical services in the 6 West African colonies and protectorates.

Minute Paper Confidential 56/1906. Application from Dr. Renner for appointment of PMO.

Minute Paper Confidential 73/1902. West African Medical Staff: Establishment of doctors in Sierra Leone, approved.

Minute Paper Confidential 85/1904. As to salary to be given in future appointments to native medical officers.

Minute Paper Confidential 141/1904. Native medical officers, approval of salary, Sierra Leone.

Minute Paper Confidential 150/1906. Dr. Renner's application for senior medical officer, and to act when the SMO of WAMS is acting PMO.

Minute Paper CS 236/1918. Report on the Epidemic of Influenza in Freetown. September 14, 1919.

Minute Paper M46/1917. Application of Dr. M. C. F. Easmon to sit for the Mende language examination, March 29, 1917.

Minute Paper M46/1917. From PMO, June 22, 1917. Recognition of Dr. Easmon's services in the Cameroons.

Minute Paper M83/17. From the medical officer in Moyamba to the PMO, "Application for Increment," July 2, 1917.

Minute Paper M88/1918. Report on outbreak of influenza at Sherbro. November 25, 1918.

Minute Paper M90/1919. Annual Report 1918. July 14, 1919.

Minute Paper M93/1917. Recognition of Dr. Easmon's services in the Cameroons, June 22, 1917.

Minute Paper M101/1917. From the PMO to the colonial secretary. Minute Paper July 1917. Application from Dr. M. C. F. Easmon for a duty or personal allowance.

Minute Paper M131/1918. Influenza outbreak: insufficiency of the medical officers to cope with the present situation. September 17, 1918.

Minute Paper M151/1917 (October). Subject: Dr. Wood-Mason's thesis on the relationships of blackwater fever to malaria.

Minute Paper M174/1918. Influenza epidemic report by Dr. Easmon. October 30, 1918.

Minute Paper M179/1918. Dr. Easmon's complaint of unusual, uncivil reception accorded him by the OFC.WAFF, Makene.

Minute Paper M179/1918. PMO to the colonial secretary. December 9, 1918. Travel and amenities.

Minute Paper, Rf. 1048. 756/10. Medical Department, July 27, 1910.

Requisitions of medicines, materials, and instruments for the use of the Liberated Africans in Sierra Leone for 12 months. Liberated African Department, 1826–June 30, 1834.

St. George Cathedral, Freetown, Sierra Leone. Notes, February 20, 1985.

Sierra Leone Gazette. September 23, 1985, 858–60.

Sierra Leone Ministry of Health. List of Sierra Leone doctors trained in USSR and Eastern bloc countries. Freetown, Sierra Leone, 1984–85.

Sierra Leone Royal Gazette, vol. 88, no. 20. Thursday, March 21, 1957. Government Notice 246 MP 12862/1.

No. 887, from PMO, April 25, 1913. Retirement of Dr. W. Awooner-Renner, medical.

CSOM 56/36. Junior medical officers. Sierra Leone, appointment of 1936.

UNIVERSITY OF BIRMINGHAM MAIN LIBRARY,
BIRMINGHAM, ENGLAND

CAI/05–6. William Fergusson to CMS, September 1843.

CAI/017. William Fergusson and correspondence to CMS with medical certificates, 1820–44.

CAI/0117/1–23. James Africanus B. Horton. Army staff assistance: Educated by CMS: Anamabue and Cape Coast Castle (Gold Coast) 1859–63. Letters between J. A. B. Horton and CMS, governor of the Gold Coast, Educational Committee (War Office) . . . training of African doctors.

CAI/0117/7. Charles Callaghan, staff and army surgeon, principal medical officer, to the director general, army medical officer, December 13, 1861.

CAI/0117/7. Governor Rich Pine, Government House, Cape Coast, to J. A. B. Horton, MD, Anamabue, October 29, 1863.

CAI/0117/7. James Africanus B. Horton, MD, staff and surgeon, to the earl de Grey and Ripon, Educational Committee, War Office, November 13, 1863.

CAI/0144/1, 2, 9. File contains the other letters mentioned.

INTERVIEWS

Akabi-Davis, Nathaniel Ebenezer. February 13, 1985, Freetown, Sierra Leone.

Awooner-Renner, Ada, age 85 (1900–92). March 10, 1985, Freetown, Sierra Leone.

Awooner-Renner, Raymond. February 12, 1985, Freetown (commentary and notes).

Awooner-Renner, Walter. December 8, 1984, Freetown, Sierra Leone (tape 3, sides A and B), and at other times in Sierra Leone and the United States.

Barnor, M. A. January 7, 1985, Accra, Ghana.

Boyle, Sidney. August 28, 1984, Birmingham, England.

Davies, Marcella. March 14, 1985, Freetown, Sierra Leone.

During, Ola Elsie Palmira. March 6, 1985, Freetown, Sierra Leone.

Easmon, Charles Odamten. January 9, 1985, Accra, Ghana (tapes A and B).

Easmon, Raymond Sarif. August 4, 1983, Freetown, Sierra Leone (tapes A and B).

Evans-Anfom, E. January 14, 1985, Accra, Ghana.

Horton, Edna Elliot. July 24, 1983, Freetown, Sierra Leone.

Johnson-Taylor, Ivan. April 10, 1985, Freetown, Sierra Leone. USSR-trained doctor.

Moigula, Frederick B. February 15, 1985, Freetown, Sierra Leone. Eastern bloc–trained doctor.

Muchi, J. A. July 25, 1986, Johns Hopkins Medical School Complex. USSR-trained doctor (MD, Tanzania). Baltimore (tape side A).

Nicol, Davidson S. H. W. February 6, 1985, Freetown, Sierra Leone, and at other times abroad.

Olu-Williams, A. E. February 25, 1985, Freetown, Sierra Leone (tapes A and B).

Roberts, W. B. O. March 6, 1985, Freetown, Sierra Leone. USSR-trained doctor.

Saccoh, S. M. February 19, 1985, Freetown, Sierra Leone. Eastern bloc–trained doctor (Bulgaria).

Shariff, W. E. February 19, 1985, Freetown, Sierra Leone. Eastern bloc–trained doctor (Yugoslavia).
Thompson, Leone Boyle Easmon. August 31, 1980, Rockville, Maryland (tape no. 1).
Waddy, B. B. July 23, 1980, Winchester, England.

Secondary Sources

Abbott, Andrew. *The System of Professions: An Essay on the Division of Expert Labor.* Chicago: University of Chicago Press, 1991.
Adade, Charles Quist. "USSR: Training African Professionals—Change of Course." *West Africa* 3783 (February 26–March 4, 1990): 304–5.
Adeloye, Adelola. *African Pioneers of Modern Medicine: Nigerian Doctors of the Nineteenth Century.* Ibadan: Ibadan University Press, 1985.
———. *Dr. E. Latunde Odeku: An African Neurosurgeon.* Ibadan: Ibadan University Press, 1975.
———. "Nigerian Pioneer Doctors and Early West African Politics." *Nigerian Magazine,* no. 121 (1976): 1–18.
———. *Nigerian Pioneers of Modern Medicine.* Ibadan: Ibadan University Press, 1977.
———. "Some Early Nigerian Doctors and their Contribution to Modern Medicine in West Africa." *Medical History* 18, no. 3 (July 1974): 275–93.
Afrika 1956–61. Moscow: Institute Afriki, 1961.
Agbabiaka, Tunde. "Doctors' Associations Banned." *West Africa,* no. 3523 (March 4, 1985): 437.
Agboideka, Francis. "Sir Gordon Guggisberg's Contribution to the Development of the Gold Coast, 1919–27." *Transactions of the Historical Society of Ghana* 13, no. 1 (June 1972): 52–64.
Africanus, Leo. *The History and Description of Africa.* Translated by John Pory. New York: Burt Franklin, 1896.
Alteras, Isaac. "The Roles of Spanish Jewish Physicians During the Thirteenth and Fourteenth Centuries." *Illinois Quarterly* 44, no. 1 (Fall 1981): 43–51.
Asmis, W. "Law and Policy Relating to the Natives of the Gold Coast and Nigeria." *Journal of the African Society* 12 (October 1912, January 1913): 17–51, 136–64.
"The Association and Medical Practice in the Colonies." *British Medical Journal,* supp. 2 (July 1931): 2–5.
Ayandele, E. A. *African Historical Studies.* London: Frank Cass, 1979.
Ballhatchet, Kenneth. *Race, Sex, and Class under the Raj: Imperial Attitudes and Policies and Their Critics, 1793–1905.* London: Weidenfeld and Nicolson, 1980.

Bark, Dennis L., ed. *The Red Orchestra: The Case of Africa,* vol. 2. Stanford: Hoover Institution Press, 1988.

Barnor, M. A. "A History of Medical Societies in Ghana." *Ghana Medical Journal* 1, no. 1 (September 1962): 4–7.

Beck, Ann. "The British Medical Council and British Medical Education in the Nineteenth Century." *Bulletin of the History of Medicine* 30, no. 2 (March–April 1956): 150–52.

Berridge, Virginia. "Health and Medicine." In *The Cambridge Social History of Britain, 1750–1950: Social Agencies and Institutions,* ed. F. M. L. Thompson, vol. 3. Cambridge: Cambridge University Press, 1990.

Bissell, Richard E. "The Brezhnev Doctrine in Africa." In *The Red Orchestra: The Case of Africa,* ed. Dennis L. Bark, vol. 2. Stanford: Hoover Institution Press, 1988.

Blakely, Allison. *Russia and the Negro: Blacks in Russian History and Thought.* Washington, D.C.: Howard University Press, 1986.

Boahen, Adu. "Politics of Ghana, 1800–1874." In *The History of West Africa,* ed. J. F. A. Ajayi and Michael Crowder, vol. 2. London: Longman, 1974.

Bolt, Christina. *The Anti-Slavery Movement and Reconstruction: A Study in Anglo-American Cooperation 1883–77.* London: Oxford University Press, 1969.

———. *Victorian Attitudes Toward Race.* London: Routledge and Kegan Paul, 1971.

Boye-Johnson, David Edkundayo. "Concerning the Promotion of Public Health in the Colony and Protectorate of Sierra Leone." Ph.D. diss., London School of Hygiene and Tropical Medicine, n.d.

Brown, Spencer H. "British Army Surgeons Commissioned 1840–1909 with West Indian/West African Service: A Prosopographical Evaluation." *Medical History* 37, no. 4 (1993): 411–31.

Bullough, Vern and Bonnie. "The Causes of the Scottish Medical Renaissance of the Eighteenth Century." *Bulletin of the History of Medicine* 45, no. 1 (January 1971): 13–28.

Callaway, Helen. *Gender, Culture and Empire: European Women in Colonial Nigeria.* Urbana: University of Illinois Press, 1987.

———. "Purity and Exotica in Legitimating the Empire: Cultural Constructions of Gender, Sexuality, and Race." Unpublished paper, 1992.

Casely-Hayford, Adelaide and Gladys. *Memoirs and Poems.* Freetown: University of Sierra Leone Press, 1983.

Cell, John. "Anglo-Indian Medical Theory and the Origins of Segregation in West Africa." *American Historical Review* 91, no. 2 (1986): 307–35.

Chaudhuri, Nupur, and Margaret Strobel, eds. *Western Women and Imperialism: Complicity and Resistance.* Bloomington: Indiana University Press, 1992.

Cheverton, R. L. "The District Medical Office." In *Health in Tropical Africa During the Colonial Period*, ed. E. E. Sabben-Clare, D. J. Bradley, and K. Kirwood. Oxford: Clarendon, 1980.

Chitnis, A. C. "Medical Education in Edinburgh, 1790–1826, and Some Victorian Social Consequences." *Medical History* 17, no. 2 (April 1973): 173–85.

Cissoko, Sekene-Mody. "Famines et Epidémies à Timboutou et dans la Boucle du Niger du XVIe au XVIIIe Siècle" (Famines and Epidemics in Timbuktu and the Niger Bend from the 16th to the 18th Century). *Bulletin de l'I.F.A.N.* 3, no. 3 (1968): 806–21.

Civil Service List. Sierra Leone Government. Freetown: Government Printing Office, 1926.

Cobban, K. "General Practice Training in West Africa." *Journal of the College of General Practitioners* 6, no. 4 (May 1963): 279–85.

Cole, Abayomi. "Obituary of Dr. MaCormack Charles Farrell Easmon." *Medical Practitioners Union Annual Magazine* (Sierra Leone), no. 8 (December 1972): 19–27.

Cole, Robert Wellesley. *An Innocent in Britain: Document Autobiography.* London: Campbell Matthews, 1988.

"Colonial Medical Services: Work and Problems." Special Colonial Supplement to *British Medical Journal* 2 (July 4, 1931): 1–20.

Cooper, John A. D. "Education for the Health Professions in the Soviet Union." *Journal of Medical Education* 46, no. 5 (May 1971): 412–18.

Coppens, Yves. "East Side Story: The Origin of Humankind." *Scientific America* 270 (May 1994): 88–95.

Craemer, Willy De, and Rene C. Fox. *The Emerging Physician: A Sociological Approach to the Development of a Congolese Medical Profession.* Stanford: Hoover Institution Press, 1968.

Cromwell, Adelaide M. *An African Victorian Feminist: The Life and Times of Adelaide Smith Casely-Hayford 1868–1960.* London: Frank Cass, 1986.

Curtin, Philip D. *The Image of Africa.* Madison: University of Wisconsin Press, 1964.

———. "Medical Knowledge and Urban Planning in Tropical Africa." *American Historical Review* 90, no. 3 (June 1985): 594–613.

———. "The White Man's Grave: Image and Reality, 1780–1850." *Journal of British Studies* 1, no. 1 (November 1961): 94–110.

Curtin, Philip D., Steven Feierman, Leonard Thompson, and Jan Vansina. *African History.* Boston: Little, Brown, 1978.

Darnton, John. "In Poor, Decolonized Africa: Bankers Are New Overlords." *New York Times,* June 20, 1994, 1, 8–9.

———. " 'Lost Decade' Drains Africa's Vitality: Survival Test. Can Africa Rebound?" *New York Times,* June 19, 1994, 1, 10.

"The Declaration of Alma-Ata Primary Health Care Is the Key to Health for All Alma-Ata (1978)." Report of the International Conference on Primary Health Care. Alma-Ata, USSR September 6–12, 1978. Jointly sponsored by WHO and the UNC fund.

Denzer, LaRay. "Abolition and Reform in West Africa." In *The History of West Africa*, ed. J. F. A. Ajayi and Michael Crowder, vol. 2. London: Longman, 1974.

Dibner, Bern. *Wilhelm Conrad Rötgen and the Discovery of X-Rays.* New York: Franklin Watts, 1968.

Dols, Michael W., trans. *Medieval Islamic Medicine: Ibn Ridwän's Treatise "On the Prevention of Bodily Ills in Egypt."* Arabic text ed. Adil S. Gamal. Berkeley: University of California Press, 1984.

Dumett, Raymond E. "The Campaign Against Malaria and the Expansion of Scientific Medical and Sanitary Services in British West Africa 1898–1910." *African Historical Studies* 1, no. 2 (1968): 153–97.

———. "Disease and Mortality among Gold Miners of Ghana: Government and Mining Company Attitudes and Policies, 1900–1938." *Social Science and Medicine* 37 (1993): 213–32.

———. "John Sarbah the Elder and African Mercantile Entrepreneurship in the Gold Coast in the Late Nineteenth Century." *Journal of African History* 14, no. 4 (1973): 653–79.

Easmon, John Farrell. "Notes of a Case of Blackwater Fever, with Remarks." *Medical Times* (August 29, 1885): 277–80.

Easmon, M. C. F. "Conditions of Medical Work in a West African Bush Station." *Journal of Tropical Medicine and Hygiene* 28 (March 1925): 128–31.

———. "Helminthiasis in the Sierra Leone Protectorate." *Journal of Tropical Medicine and Hygiene* (November 15, 1924): 305–7.

———. "A Nova Scotian Family." In *Eminent Sierra Leoneans (in the Nineteenth Century)*, ed. M. C. F. Easmon and Davidson Nicol. Freetown: Government Printing Office, 1961.

———. "Sierra Leone Doctors." *Sierra Leone Studies*, n.s., no. 6 (1956): 81–96.

———. "Sierra Leone Doctors of the Nineteenth Century." In *Eminent Sierra Leoneans (in the Nineteenth Century)*, ed. M. C. F. Easmon and Davidson Nicol. Freetown: Government Printing Office, 1961.

Easmon, Raymond Sarif. "Rethinking the Health Service." *Sierra Leone Medical and Dental Association* 1, no. 2 (January 1974): 6–19.

E.C.D. "Native v. European Doctors." *African Mail*, January 7, 1910.

"Editorial." *Ghana Medical Journal* 8, no. 3 (September 1969): 173.

"Editorial." *West African Medical Journal* 8, no. 4, n.s. (August 1959): 1.

"Editorial: Final M.B., B.S. (London) in Special Relationship." *West Africa Medical Journal* 10, no. 1 (February 1961): 2.

Ephson, Ben. "Herbs in Pharmacy." *West Africa* 3439 (July 11, 1983): 1605–7.

Estes, J. Worth. *The Medical Skills of Ancient Egypt.* Canton, Mass.: Watson Publishing International, 1989.

Feierman, Steven. "Popular Control over the Institutions of Health: A Historical Study." In *The Professionalisation of African Medicine,* ed. Murray Last and G. L. Chavunduka.

———. "Struggles for Control: The Social Roots of Health and Health in Modern Africa." *African Studies Review* 28, nos. 2–3 (June–September 1985): 73–148.

Fendall, N. R. E. "A History of the Yaba School of Medicine, Nigeria." *West African Medical Journal and Nigerian Practitioner* 16, no. 4 (August 1967): 118–23.

Finch, Charles S. "The African Background of Medical Science." *Journal of African Civilization* 4, no. 1 (April 1982): 8–24.

Fulton Daily Sun-Gazette, March 5, 1946.

Fyfe, Christopher. *Africanus Horton 1835–1883: West African Scientist and Patriot.* New York: Oxford University Press, 1972.

———. *A History of Sierra Leone.* London: Oxford University Press, 1962.

Gailey, Harry A. *A History of the Gambia.* New York: Praeger, 1965.

Galdston, Iago. "Trade Routes and Medicine." *Bulletin of the New York Academy of Medicine* 35, no. 5 (May 1961): 342–58.

Gale, George W. "Medical Schools in Africa: A Short Historical and Contemporary Survey." *Journal of Medical Education* 34, no. 8 (August 1959): 712–19.

Gale, T. S. "The Disbarment of African Medical Officers by the West African Medical Staff: A Study in Prejudice." *Journal of the Historical Society of Sierra Leone* 4, nos. 1, 2 (December 1980): 33–44.

———. "Official Medical Policy in British West Africa 1870–1930." Ph.D. dissertation, University of London, 1972.

———. "Segregation in British West Africa." *Cahiers d'Etude Africaines* 20 (1980): 495–507.

———. "Sir Gordon Guggisberg and His African Critics." *Transactions of the Historical Society of Ghana* 14, no. 2 (December 1973): 271–75.

Gann, L. H. "The Soviet Union and Sub-Sahara Africa: 1917–1974." In *The Red Orchestra: The Case of Africa,* ed. Dennis L. Bark, vol. 2. Stanford: Hoover Institution Press, 1988.

Gann, L. H., and Peter Duignan. *The Rulers of German Africa 1884–1914.* Stanford: Stanford University Press, 1977.

Gold Coast Civil Service List. London: Waterlow and Sons, 1925.

Harris, John Hobbis. *Dawn in Darkest Africa.* New York: Dutton, 1912.

Hartwig, Gerald W., and K. David Patterson, eds. *Disease in African History: An Introductory Survey and Case Studies.* Durham, N.C.: Duke University Press, 1978.

Heilbroner, Robert L. *The Future as History.* New York: Grove, 1959.

Henige. *Colonial Governors from the Fifteenth Century to the Present.* Madison: University of Wisconsin Press, 1970.

Hinman, E. Harold, and Clifford A. Pease. "International Assistance in Medical Education." *Journal of Medical Education* 36, no. 9 (September 1961): 1042–51.

Hirschberg, H. Z. (J. W.) "The Problem of the Judaized Berbers." *Journal of African History* 4, no. 3 (1963): 313–39.

Hobson, W. "Medical Education in Europe." *Journal of Medical Education* 37, no. 9 (September 1962): 815–33.

Horton, James Africanus. *West African Countries and Peoples.* Edinburgh: Edinburgh University Press (1868), 1969.

Hunter, Yema Lucilda. *Road to Freedom.* Ibadan: African Universities Press, 1982.

Inan, Muhammad Abdalla. "Al-Jami al-Azhar wa Rihlat al-Alf Gana" (The Azhar Mosque: a thousand years of history). *Al-Arabi* 287 (October 1982): 56–57.

Jackson, James Grey. *An Account of Timbuktu and Housa by El Hage Abd Salam Shabeeny.* London: Frank Cass (1820), 1969.

Jenkins, Ray. "Gold Coasters Overseas, 1880–1919; With Specific References to Their Activities in Britain." *Immigrants and Minorities* 4, no. 3 (November 1985): 5–52.

———. "In Pursuit of the African Past: John Mensah Sarbah (1864–1903), Historian of Ghana." In *Under the Imperial Carpet: Essays in Black History 1780–1950,* ed. Rainer Lotz and Ian Pegg. Crawley, England: Rabbit, 1986.

Johnson, Terence J. "Imperialism and the Professions: Notes on the Development of Professional Occupations in Britain's Colonies and the New States." In *The American Sociological Review,* ed. Paul Halmos. Monograph 20. Keele, England: Keele University Press, 1973.

———. *Professions and Power.* London: Macmillan, 1972.

Jones-Quartey, K. A. B. "Sierra Leone's Role in the Development of Ghana, 1820–1930." *Sierra Leone Studies* 18 (1958): 73–84.

Joyce, R. B. *Sir William MacGregor.* London: Oxford University Press, 1971.

July, Robert W. *The Origins of Modern African Thought: Its Development in West Africa During the Nineteenth and Twentieth Centuries.* New York: Praeger, 1967.

Junaidu. *The Relevance of the University to Our Society.*

Kanet, Roget E. "African Youth: The Target of Soviet African Policy." *Russian Review* 27, no. 2 (April 1968): 161–75.

Khaldun, Ibn. *Histoire des Berbers: Et des Dynasties Musulmanes de l'Afrique Septentrionale* (History of the Berbers: Muslim Dynasties of North Africa). Trans. Le Baron de Slane. Paris: Librairie Orientaliste, Paul Genther, 1927.

Kilson, Martin. *Political Change in a West African State: A Study of the Modernization Process in Sierra Leone.* Cambridge, Mass.: Harvard University Press, 1966.

Kimble, David. *A Political History of Ghana: The Rise of Gold Coast Nationalism 1850–1928*. Oxford: Clarendon, 1963.

Kirk-Greene, Anthony H. M. *A Biographical Dictionary of the British Colonial Governor*, vol. 1. Stanford: Hoover Institution Press, 1980.

Larson, Magali Sarfatti. *The Rise of Professionalism*. Berkeley: University of California Press, 1977.

Last, Murray. "The Professionalisation of African Medicine: Ambiguities and Definitions." In *The Professionalisation of African Medicine*, ed. Murray Last and G. L. Chavunduka.

Last, Murray, and G. L. Chavunduka, eds. *The Professionalisation of African Medicine*. Manchester: Manchester University Press, IAI, 1986.

Lee, Gary. "*Visible Man: Black among the Reds:* A View from the Back of the Soviet Bus. My Four Years on the Racial Firing Line." *Washington Post,* editorial, April 21, 1991, B1, B4.

Legum, Colin. *Congo Disaster*. Baltimore: Penguin Books, 1961.

Leiser, Gary. "Medical Education in Islamic Lands from the Seventh to the Fourteenth Century." *Journal of the History of Medicine and Allied Sciences* 38, no. 1 (January 1983): 52.

The London School of Tropical Medicine, Sessions 1899–1900, Seamen's Hospital Society. London: E. G. Berryman and Sons, Steam Works, 1899.

Lumpkin, Beatrice, and Siham Zitzler. "Cairo-Science Academy of the Middle Ages." *Journal of African Civilization* 4, no. 1 (April 1982): 25–38.

Lynch, Hollis R. *Edward Wilmot Blyden: Pan-Negro Patriot*. New York: Oxford University Press, 1967.

Mabayoje, Olu. "The Nigerian Medical Association: A Short Historical View, 1951–1971." *Journal of the Nigerian Medical Association* 1, no. 1 (January 1971): 14–19.

McCall, Daniel F. *Africa in Time Perspective*. New York: Oxford University Press, 1969.

Mann, Kristin. *Marrying Well: Marriage, Status, and Social Change among the Educated Elite in Colonial Lagos*. Cambridge: Cambridge University Press, 1985.

Manson-Bahr, Sir Philip. *History of the School of Tropical Medicine in London (1899–1949)*. London: H. K. Lewis, 1956.

Marcus, Harold G. *A History of Ethiopia*. Los Angeles: University of California Press, 1994.

Mbaeyi, Paul Mmegha. *British Military and Naval Forces in West African History 1807–1874*. New York: Nok Publishers, 1978.

"M. C. F. Easmon, O.B.E., M.D." Obituary. *The Times*, May 9, 1972.

"M. C. F. Easmon, O.B.E., M.D." Obituary. *British Medical Journal* (July 29, 1972).

The Medical Directory, 144th edition, part 1. London: Lewis's of Gower Street, 1988.

"The Medical Practitioners Union, 1968–69." *Medical Practitioners Union Annual Magazine* (Sierra Leone) 3 (December 1970).

Mejia, Alfonso, Helena Pizurki, and Erica Royston. *Physicians and Nurse Migration: Analysis and Policy Implications.* Geneva: World Health Organization, 1979.

Melson, Robert, and Howard Wolpe. "Modernization and the Politics of Communalism: A Theoretical Perspective." *American Political Science Review* 64, no. 4 (December 1970): 1112–30.

Newsome, Fredrick. "Black Contributions to the Early History of Western Medicine." *Journal of the National Medical Association* 71, no. 2 (1979): 27–39.

Nicol, Davidson. *Black Nationalism in Africa 1867: Africanus Horton.* New York: Africana Publishing, 1969.

———. "Brazil, Canada, Nova Scotia, and the Guinea Coast: A Literary and Historical Overview of the African Diaspora." *Presence Africaine.* Paris, 1984.

———. "The Formation of a West African Intellectual Community." *The West African Intellectual Community: The Congress for Cultural Freedom, Freetown, Sierra Leone.* Ibadan: Ibadan University Press, 1962: 10–47.

Nketia, J. H. "Program in Gold Coast Education." *Gold Coast and Togoland Historical Society* 1, no. 3 (1953): 1–9.

Nkwam, Florence Ejogha. "British Medical and Health Policies in West Africa c. 1920–60." Ph.D. dissertation, School of Oriental and African Studies, University of London, 1988.

Oliver, Caroline. *Western Women in Colonial Africa.* Westport, Conn.: Greenwood, 1982.

Oliver, Roland. *The Missionary Factor in East Africa.* London: Longman, 1969.

Osler, Sir William. *The Evolution of Modern Medicine.* New Haven, Conn.: Yale University Press, 1921.

Patai. *The Vanished Worlds of Jewry.* New York: Macmillan, 1980.

Patterson, K. David. "Disease and Medicine in African History: A Bibliographical Essay." *History in Africa* 1, no. 1 (1974):141–48.

———. *Health in Colonial Ghana: Disease, Medicine, and Social-Economic Change, 1900–1955.* Waltham, Mass.: Crossroads, 1981.

———. "Health in Urban Ghana: The Case of Accra, 1900–1940." *Social Science and Medicine* 13b (1979): 251–68.

———. "The Influenza Epidemic of 1918–19 in the Gold Coast." *Journal of African History* 24, no. 4 (1983): 485–502.

———. "River Blindness in Northern Ghana, 1900–1950." In *Disease in African History: An Introductory Survey and Case Studies,* ed. Gerald W. Hartwig and K. David Patterson.

Patterson, K. David, and Gerald F. Pyle. "The Diffusion of Influenza in Sub-Saharan Africa During the 1918–1919 Pandemic." *Social Science and Medicine* 17, no. 17 (1982): 1299–1307.

————. "The Geography and Mortality of the 1918 Influenza Pandemic." *Bulletin of the History of Medicine* 65, no. 1 (1991): 4–22.

Patton, Adell, Jr. "Dr. John Farrell Easmon: Medical Professionalism and Colonial Racism in the Gold Coast, 1856–1900." *International Journal of African Historical Studies* 22, no. 4 (1989): 601–36.

————. "E. Mayfield Boyle: 1902 Howard University Medical School Graduate's Challenge to British Medical Policy in West Africa." *Journal of Negro History* 67, no. 1 (Spring 1982): 52–61.

————. "Howard University and Meharry Medical Schools in the Training of African Physicians, 1868–1978." In *Global Dimensions of the African Diaspora,* ed. Joseph Harris. Washington, D.C.: Howard University Press, 1993.

Peterkin, A., William Johnston, and Robert Drew, eds. *Commissioned Officers in the Medical Services of the British Army 1660–1960.* London: Wellcome Historical Medical Library, 1968.

Peterson, M. Jeane. *The Medical Profession in Mid-Victorian London.* Berkeley: University of California Press, 1978.

Pickering, Sir George. "Medicine and Education." In *Medicine and Culture,* ed. F. N. L. Poynter. London: Wellcome Institute of the History of Medicine, 1969.

Pobee, J. O. M. "Postgraduate Medical Education for Physicians in West Africa." *Journal of the Royal College of Physicians of London* 16, no. 4 (October 1982): 242–44.

Prokofiev, M. A., M. G. Chilikin, and S. I. Tulpanov. *Higher Education in the USSR,* no. 30. UNESCO, 1961.

"Qualifying Degrees and Diplomas." *British Medical Journal* (September 1949): 537–42.

Rawlinson, George. *The History of Herodotus,* vol. 2. New York: D. Appleton, 1889.

Reader, W. J. *Professional Men.* New York: Basic Books, 1966.

Rosen, Seymour M. *The Development of People's Friendship University in Moscow.* Washington, D.C.: U.S. Department of Health, Education, and Welfare, 1973.

————. *Soviet Training Programs for Africa, Bulletin 1963, No. 9.* Washington, D.C.: U.S. Department of Health, Education, and Welfare, 1973.

Rowin, Ksawery. "Medical Training in Poland." *Journal of Medical Education* 36, no. 9 (September 1961): 1052–58.

Rudin, Harry R. *Germans in the Cameroons 1884–1914: A Case Study in Modern Imperialism.* New Haven, Conn.: Yale University Press, 1968.

Saad, Elias N. *Social History of Timbuktu: The Role of Muslim Scholars and Notables 1400–1900.* London: Cambridge University Press, 1983.

Schram, Ralph. *A History of the Nigerian Health Services.* Ibadan: Ibadan University Press, 1971.

Seamon's Hospital Society. The London School of Tropical Medicine. Report for the Years 1899–1911: Number of Students Attending Each Course since Foundation, 1899–1911. Photographs of graduates. London: London School of Tropical Medicine, 1913.

Selwyn-Clarke, Sir Selwyn. "The Bight of Benin and Beyond: Some Experiences in the Colonial Medical Services." *Lancet* 1 (January–June 1953): 843–45.

Shepherd, John A. *A History of the Liverpool Medical Institute.* Liverpool: Liverpool Medical Institution, 1979.

Shimkin, Michael B., and Colin M. MacLeod. "Medical Education in the USSR." *Journal of Medical Education* 34, no. 8 (August 1959): 795–801.

Sigerist, Henry E. *The Great Doctors: A Biographical History of Medicine.* New York: Dover Publications, 1971.

———. *A History of Medicine,* vol. 1. New York: Oxford University Press, 1951.

Slade, Ruth. *The Belgian Congo: Some Recent Changes.* London: Oxford University Press, 1960.

Solodovnikov, V. G. "The Soviet Union and Africa [Friendship Societies/ Origin]." *New Times* 21 (28 May 1969): 8–10.

Spitzer, Leo. *The Creoles of Sierra Leone: Responses to Colonialism 1870–1945.* Madison: University of Wisconsin Press, 1974.

Stepan, Nancy. *The Idea of Race in Science: Great Britain 1800–1960.* Hamden, Conn.: Archon Books, 1982.

Stevens, Siaka. *What Life Has Taught Me.* London: Kensal, 1984.

Stone, Lawrence. "Prosopography." *Daedalus* 100, no. 1 (Winter 1971): 46–79.

Suret-Canale, Jean. *Afrique Noire l'Ere Coloniale 1900–1945* (Black Africa in the Colonial Era). Paris: Editions Sociales, 1964.

Sutton, J. E. G. "The Aquatic Civilization of Middle Africa." *Journal of African History* 15, no. 4 (1974): 527–46.

Tadic, R. M. "The Development of Medical Education in Yugoslavia." *Journal of Medical Education* 37, no. 9 (September 1962): 868–86.

Tettey, Charles. "Medical Practitioners of African Descent in Colonial Ghana." *International Journal of African Historical Studies* 18, no. 1 (1985): 139–44.

Thomas, Andrew L. and Iris D. "Medical Impressions of Ghana, West Africa." *Journal of Medical Education* 36, no. 6 (June 1961): 694–708.

Thomas, Deanna. "Sir Milton Margai: A Study of the Man and His Regime." M.A. thesis, Fourah Bay College-University of Sierra Leone, Freetown, 1972.

Toungara, Jeanne Maddox. "The Apotheosis of Côte d'Ivoire's Nana Houphouët-Boigny." *Journal of Modern African Studies* 28, no. 1 (1990): 23–54.

Vaucel, M. A. "Le Service de Santé de Troupe de Marine et la Médecine Tropicale Française" (The Military Health Service and French Tropical

Medicine). *Transactions of the Royal Society of Tropical Medicine and Hygiene* 59, no. 2 (January 1965): 226–33.

Waddy, B. B. "Arabian Literature and Sleeping Sickness in Northern Nigeria." *Transactions of the Royal Society of Tropical Medicine and Hygiene* 58, no. 3 (1964): 283.

———. "A District Medical Office in North-West Ghana." In *Health in Tropical Africa During the Colonial Period,* ed. E. E. Sabben-Clare, D. J. Bradley, and K. Kirkwood. Oxford: Clarendon, 1980.

———. "The Present State of Public Health in the African Soudan." *Transactions of the Royal Society of Tropical Medicine and Hygiene* 56, no. 2 (1962): 92–115.

"The West African Medical Staff." *Sierra Leone Weekly News,* November 6, 1909, 1–8.

Wilkinson, Frederick D., ed. *Directory of Graduates, Howard University 1870–1963.* Washington, D.C.: Howard University Press, 1965.

Winterbottom, Thomas. *An Account of the Native Africans in the Neighborhood of Sierra Leone.* London: Frank Cass (1803), 1967.

Wrath, R. E. *Guggisberg.* London: Oxford University Press, 1967.

Wyse, Akintola J. G. *H. C. Bankole-Bright and Politics in Colonial Sierra Leone 1919–1958.* Cambridge: Cambridge University Press, 1990.

———. "Searchlight on the Krio of Sierra Leone: An Ethnographical Study of a West African People." Institute of African Studies. Fourah Bay College, Occasional Paper no. 3 (1980): 1–42.

Yakobson, Yakobson. "Russia and Africa." In *Russian Foreign Policy,* ed. Ivo J. Lederer. New Haven: Yale University Press, 1962.

Index

Edinburgh University—*continued*
status of, 63–64; students' protest at,
131–32; training at, 64, 77, 78
education: and Creolization, 197;
development of, 90; and diaspora,
199; and race, 207. *See also* universities
Egypt: history of, 45–48, 86; medical
practices in, 46–47, 50; schools in,
35, 51
Elder Dempster Shipping Line, 162
Elections Before Independence Movement (EBIM) party, 235
Elizabeth II (queen of England), 216
Elliott, Selina, 85
environment, and disease, 43–44, 63.
See also climate
epidemics: effects of, 53–54, 78; timing
of, 43; types of, 43–44, 175. *See also*
disease; influenza pandemic
Episcopal Cathedral of St. George, 210
Epson College, 163
ether, 68
Ethiopia: delegations from, 263, 268;
history of, 48, 50; Soviet cooperation
with, 226; study on, 253
ethnicity: bias based on, 110–13; and
social structure, 152; transformation
of, 195, 210
Europe: certification in, 26–28; medical
centers in, *27;* partition of, 223–24;
transformations in, 127–28. *See also*
Europeans; Eastern Europe; France;
Great Britain
European physicians: attitudes of, 140;
compared to African physicians,
188; and decolonization, 213; exodus of, 215–16, *217,* 250; language
difficulties of, 166; salaries of, *130,*
172–73
Europeans: claims of, 21; and
epidemics, 78; medical leave for,
68–69, 82–83; mortality of, 62–63,
74, 127; physicians for, 107, 205; and
treatment for malaria, 95, 114. *See
also* European physicians

Evans-Anfom, Emmanuel, *241,* 241–42,
299n. 25
eye diseases, 69–70. *See also* river blindness

Faderin, Kubolaje, 173
famines, effects of, 53–54
Fanti Confederation (1868), 124
Fanti people, 79, 124
Farmer, Solomon, 98
Feierman, Steven, 122, 182, 216
FéKuw (Fanti National Political Society), 164
Fergusson, Charlotte, 74
Fergusson, William: background of, 55;
career of, 64–65, 67–69, 106; death
of, 73–76; as governor, 69–73; influence by, 83; on ward system, 198
Fergusson, William, II, 73
fevers, 84, 101–2, 144. *See also* malaria;
yellow fever
FIDES (Fonds pour l'Investissement
pour le Développement
Economique et Social), 25
Finch, Charles, 47
Forde, Robert Michael, 139–40
Forna, Mohammed Sorie, 39
Fourah Bay College: and certification,
27; establishment of, 60; expansion
of, 83; students of, 88, 97, 110
fracture boxes, 68
France: and African training, 25,
155–56; and control of Africa, 95,
123; physicians from, 60; policies of,
23–26; schools in, 23
Franklin, S. O., 213
Frederick, Rev. J. R., 148
Freetown (Sierra Leone): description of,
59–60; disease in, 66, 175; governance of, 29, 141; hospitals in, 38,
87, 168–69; as intellectual community, 60, 145; landowners in, 160;
newspapers in, 125; schools in, 72,
76, 98, 110, 146, 199; social structure
in, 152
French Colonial Corps, 23

Richards, Judge E. H., 116
Ridwän's, Ali ibn, 52
Ripon, marquis of, 108, 110
river blindness (onchocerciasis), 2, 17, 44
Robbin-Coker, Daniel Josephus Ol-
ubami, 39
Roberts, Rev. J. T., 165
Roberts, William, 239–40
Robinson, George Frederick (marquis
of Ripon), 108, 110
Rochefort (France), school in, 23
Rockefeller Foundation, 231
Röntgen, Wilhelm Conrad, 153
Ross, Donald, 104
Ross, Palmer, 135
Ross, Robert, 220
Rotifunk (Sierra Leone): missionaries
in, 199; physicians in, 36
Rotifunk Village Primary School, 199
Royal African Colonial Corps, 65, 70
Royal Asiatic Society, 113
Royal College of Nursing, 38
Royal College of Physicians: accredita-
tion by, 34; certification by, 26, 139;
as clearinghouse, 102; staff for, 163
Royal College of Surgeons: accredita-
tion by, 34; certification by, 26, 33,
64, 78, 139; president of, 99; social
class in, 14; staff for, 163
Royal Military Asylum (England), 75
Royal University (Ireland), 139
Royal Victoria and Albert Docks, 126

Saad, Elias, 51
Sadi, Muhammad, 51
Sagoe, K., 187
St. Andrew's College, 29, 78
St. George's Hosptial (London), 99
St. John's Maroon Town Church, 191
St. Mary's Hospital Medical School,
163, 168, 194
St. Paul's school, 163
St. Vincent Island, governance of, 70
salaries: of African physicians, 132–34,
136–37, 157, 180–81; of Awooner-
Renner, 168; in Colonial Medical

Service, 106, 127; and Depression
years, 189–90; of European physicians, *130,* 172–73; and language
proficiency, 174; of nurses, 188; and
reorganization of medical service,
132–33
Salisbury University of Rhodesia, 35
Samaru-Zaria (Nigeria), 34
Sanders, Edith, 86
Sankarani, 43
sanitation: and conditions, 103; districts
for, 185; improvement of, 2; inspectors of, 184; methods of, 155
Sapara, Oguntola Odunbaku: beliefs
of, 129, 145; career of, 89, 133, 143;
petition by, 173
Sarbah, J. Mensah, 164
Savage, Agnes Yewande, 28, 192
Savage, Richard Akiwande, 28,
143–44
Schram, Ralph, 34–35, *35*
science: and gender stratification, 192;
intellectual centers for, 89–91; lack
of teaching in, 83; and scientific
public, 252–53
Scotland: benefits of, 89–92; medical
culture in, 89–92; schools in, 102;
training in, 61, 78. *See also* Edinburgh University
segregation: and education goals,
71–72; and health concerns, 21
self-teaching, 49
Senegal: Communist delegations to,
261; delegations from, 265–66,
268–70; schools in, 24, 32–34, 156;
Soviet support for, 226
Sessional Paper 22 (1928), 33
Sey, J. W., 164
Shabeeny, Al-Hajj Abd Salaam, 54
Sherbro people, 178, 195
Sierra Leone: administrative areas of,
170; associations in, 159, 191, 212,
221, 233, 238; certification in,
237–38; delegations from, 265;
Europeans in, *100;* exodus from,
217; foreign policy of, 237; governance of, 55, 69–73, 94, 236–37;